MASTERING MENOPAUSE -

A Doctor's Candid Guide

to

Estrogen Hormone Therapy

MASTERING MENOPAUSE -

A Doctor's Candid Guide

to

Estrogen Hormone Therapy

Emine Cay Masters, MD, FACOG

The material presented in this book is designed to provide information on the topics addressed in the publication. It is based upon research and the clinical and professional experience of the author. The information contained herein is not meant to diagnose, treat, cure or prevent any diseases. The reader is advised to consult their physician to obtain medical advice regarding their individual health needs.

Any reference to specific medications or particular supplements is for informational purposes only. The author acknowledges the copyrighted and trademarked status, and trademarked owners, of various products referenced in the book, which have been used without the permission of the owners. The owners did not authorize the author's publication and use of these trademarks. The author receives no compensation or benefits from endorsing any medicines or products in this book.

The author and publisher specifically disclaim all responsibility for any liability, loss or risk, personal or otherwise, that may be incurred as a consequence, directly or indirectly, of the use and application of the contents in this book.

ISBN 978-0-9967029-0-4 (pbk)
ISBN 978-0-9967029-1-1 (ebk)
ISBN 978-0-9967029-2-8 (ebk)

Library of Congress Control Number: 2015949180

Consultant: E. Seref Cay, MD
Editor: Cheryl A. Kelley
Cover Design: Najla Qamber Designs

Medical Specialty Publishing
Ormond Beach, FL

www.MasteringMenopause.com

For my husband,
Richard A.P. Masters,

My son,
Noble Sky Masters,

And Dedicated to All Women

Contents

Over 75% of menopausal Ob-Gyn physicians take estrogen replacement therapy, yet only 5% of their menopausal patients leverage estrogen's power for symptom relief, health maintenance, and disease prevention. What insight into hormone therapy do these doctors have that other menopausal women may not be aware of? If hormones are truly as dangerous as some claim, why are so many women doctors using estrogen when they go through menopause?

As a gynecologist, I have had the privilege of taking care of thousands of menopausal women for over thirty years. By integrating updated scientific information with thoughtful clinical judgment, I have been able to help patients throughout their menopausal journey and beyond. Since a woman will spend over 30 years of her life in the postmenopausal state, effective therapeutic intervention should alleviate bothersome menopausal symptoms, prevent degenerative diseases, and promote healthy living.

Menopause represents more than simply making it through several years of annoying hot flashes and sleep deprivation, only to decline and trail down a gloomy shade of gray and somber infirmity. Surviving beyond her body's capacity to reproduce naturally, a menopausal woman exists beyond her ovaries' ability to generate health-sustaining hormones. Female hormones matter and appropriate estrogen replacement therapy allows a woman to sail through menopause and enjoy her golden years. Not only does estrogen safely treat menopause symptoms, curb weight gain, and lift libido, women on estrogen feel better, look better and age better than their estrogen-deprived counterparts.

Menopause marks a pivotal crossroad in every woman's life. How well a woman travels through her menopausal years, and which hormonal path she follows, determine her health and happiness, long after menopause has come and gone. Menopause provides a window of opportunity for establishing the foundation of wholesome aging and preserving a woman's quality of life. Decades of clinical research and analysis involving millions of women worldwide have finally clarified controversial issues regarding a woman's health connection to her ovarian hormones. Now that the dust has settled on the risks versus benefits of estrogen replacement, it's time to have that candid discussion about appropriate hormone therapy for menopausal women.

The scope and dominion of menopause hormone therapy cannot be covered during a 15-minute visit with your doctor, so this book provides thorough explanations on everything about estrogen. The impact of hormones is best understood in the context of what goes on during a woman's reproductive years, as well as what occurs before, during and after her final menstrual period. From head-to-toe, a woman's body needs estrogen to function optimally, so menopause is a complex issue with far-reaching consequences.

For easy reference and targeted reading, each chapter in the book can stand alone on its topic. Due to the versatile nature of multitasking hormones, some descriptive elements necessitated repeating. When tied all together, these passages weave an illuminating tapestry of estrogen's influence on a menopausal woman's physical, mental, sexual, and spiritual well-being.

Mastering menopause through well-orchestrated estrogen replacement therapy is the key to sustained vitality and dignified longevity for menopausal women of all ages.

INTRODUCTION

Modern humans have been walking the earth for over 200,000 years, yet it has only been within the past 100 years that large populations of women are living for decades beyond their menopausal years. Despite all the glories and expansions of the Roman Empire, the average citizen only lived to be 25. It was not until the Industrial Revolution of the 1800s that the standard of living for the general population began to improve. As recent as the early 1900s, average life expectancy for a woman was still just 49 years, and she spent half her life either pregnant or lactating.

Before the advent of "unnatural" improvements such as proper sanitation, antibiotics, and modern medical care, few women survived long enough to reach menopause. Living as Nature intended, without vaccines, without utilities, without clean surgery, etc., meant that most women died before they developed ovarian failure. Women outliving their ovaries was not part of Nature's plan. Nowadays, a woman who reaches her 50th birthday can expect to live well into her 80s. Whether or not she survives beyond menopause is no longer extraordinary or exceptional. What matters now is how well she's going to live the last 30 years of her life. Will she be vital and relevant or feeble and inconsequential? Hormones, menopause, and meaningful longevity did not become significant issues until the mid-20th century.

Every woman who has ever experienced a menstrual period will go through menopause. When her ovaries run out of follicles/oocytes (eggs) for reproduction, a woman is no longer fertile, and her ovaries stop producing female hormones. For most women, menopause occurs naturally between ages 46 to 56. Despite women living longer, the average age for menopause is still 51 years old. Surgical removal of the ovaries instantly precipitates menopause, and permanent ovarian insufficiency can result from radiation, chemotherapy, and various diseases. Regardless of the cause of menopause, every woman who outlives her ovaries exists in a compromised hormone deficient state.

Since menopause is a natural process women journey through, it may not be viewed as a medical condition warranting treatment. Although menopause comes with dozens of symptoms, and lack of estrogen results in severe health problems, ovarian failure in a middle-aged woman is not considered a pressing clinical issue. There are no menopause emergencies, and there is no immediate risk of dying upon reaching menopause. Yet, every day thousands of women die from the harmful effects of estrogen deprivation brought on by menopause.

When a woman's ovaries no longer produce a healthy balance of estrogen, progesterone and testosterone hormones, she develops menopausal symptoms. Hot flashes, insomnia, mood swings, vaginal dryness, irritable bladder, decreased libido, crushing fatigue, weight gain, memory problems and heart palpitations signal ovarian failure. Some women suffer from many menopausal symptoms, others experience a hot flash here and there, and a few don't even notice menopause.

Every organ system in a woman's body uses ovarian hormones to keep metabolic, physical and mental functions operating optimally. Whether a woman is burdened by menopausal symptoms or sailing through menopause symptom-free, her system sustains damage from the lack of estrogen. It takes 10 to15 years of estrogen deprivation for diseases and degenerative conditions exacerbated by estrogen deficiency to manifest themselves. By slowing down tissue degradation and organ malfunction brought on by hormone deficiency, estrogen replacement therapy allows a woman's mind and body to perform optimally during the aging process. Properly managed hormone therapy is a menopausal woman's most effective and holistic strategy for maintaining vitality and aging with dignity.

1 out of 3 postmenopausal women develops dementia. 70% of women over the age of 70 have urinary incontinence. 1 out of 2 postmenopausal women suffers an osteoporosis-related fracture, and hip fractures carry a worse prognosis than breast cancer. Over 85% of women diagnosed with breast cancer will be long-term survivors; whereas, 20% percent of women die within a year of breaking their hip, and 50% of the remaining survivors are terminally sequestered in a nursing home. Hip fractures, Alzheimer's dementia, and urinary incontinence are the most common disabilities confining older women to nursing homes. These miserable infirmities could have been avoided if ovarian hormone deficiency had been treated appropriately.

Furthermore, the incidence of cardiovascular disease, diabetes, depression, and colon cancer is reduced with appropriate menopause hormone therapy. Far more women will die from these preventable conditions than will ever be diagnosed with breast cancer. Breast cancer survivors are the largest constituent of all cancer survivors. Over 45% of women die from cardiovascular disease compared to 3% of women who succumb to breast cancer.

Although women are 10 times more likely to die from heart disease than breast cancer, a woman dreads breast cancer over any other diagnosis. Unfortunately, overwhelming fear of breast cancer prevents many women from treating their ovarian hormone deficiency properly. They mistakenly assume that they are helping themselves avoid breast cancer by shunning menopausal estrogen therapy, when in fact, women taking estrogen replacement decrease their risk of breast cancer by 23%. A woman does not prevent breast cancer by denying herself the myriad health benefits of menopause hormone therapy.

Estrogen replacement therapy does not cause breast cancer. If estrogen triggered the creation of cancer cells, there would be an epidemic of breast cancer in young women. Reproductive-aged women maintain much higher levels of estrogen than postmenopausal women. A woman would have to consume a century's worth of her menopause hormone pills to equal the staggering output of female hormones produced during the last three months of pregnancy. Breast cancer is a disease of aging, not estrogen replacement.

MEN'S TESTOSTERONE vs. WOMEN'S ESTROGEN

As a result of trauma, surgery or aging, men develop a condition similar to women's menopause, called male hypogonadism. Colloquially this is referred to as "low T" or "andropause." Male hypogonadism means that a man's testicles (gonads) are no longer producing enough testosterone hormones to keep him healthy and happy. When the underlying cause of his symptoms is determined to be testicular hormone deficiency, a man is offered testosterone replacement, no matter how old he is. Replacing his testosterone restores libido, boosts energy, blunts depression, improves concentration, maintains bone density and strengthens muscles. A man's overall quality of life improves with appropriate testosterone replacement therapy. If a man's testicles are not producing enough testosterone, and he has low testosterone levels, then his sex hormone deficiency is treated with long-term testosterone replacement therapy, regardless of his age.

Although they experience a similar type of life-diminishing glandular problem, women with estrogen deficiency or "low E" are treated very differently. When a menopausal woman's gonads, her ovaries, stop producing hormones, she now suffers from female hypogonadism or ovarian hormone deficiency. A menopausal woman with low estrogen levels due to female hypogonadism is not regarded the same as a man with low testosterone levels due to male hypogonadism. Since a menopausal woman can no longer reproduce, it has become acceptable for her to endure the hardships of estrogen deficiency. She is encouraged to get by without hormones and exist without the health benefits of appropriate estrogen replacement therapy. Instead, she is persuaded to meditate, meander or muscle her way across this hormonal divide and just make it through menopause.

Deprived of hormones, menopausal women explore alternative therapies to relieve distressing symptoms caused by estrogen deficiency (low E) due to female hypogonadism, also known as, ovarian failure. They seek out herbs and dietary supplements, purchase magnets, try acupuncture, and practice yoga. Prescriptions are written for antidepressants to reduce menopausal hot flashes, sleeping pills to battle insomnia, and non-estrogen drugs to fortify bones and dampen vaginal dryness. Regrettably, none of these approaches treats the root cause of menopausal symptoms, nor do they prevent the damaging consequences of estrogen deficiency.

There is no mystery to menopause. It is simply a condition of hormone deficiency in a woman; wherein her aging ovaries fail to produce adequate amounts of female hormones. There are no health benefits to denying a woman her estrogen. In fact, by avoiding appropriately timed and properly managed hormone replacement therapy, a menopausal woman is unwittingly compromising her quality of life, both during her "freshly menopausal" years, as well in her older, "geripausal" years.

LET the SUNSHINE IN

The key to any type of hormone replacement therapy is managing the hormone deficiency properly. A 50-year-old woman navigating through menopause is very different from a 79-year-old survivor of estrogen deficiency. Blanketing all postmenopausal women spanning a 30-year age gap with the same dose of a single type of hormone preparation is bound to be problematic. Once menopause has become a distant memory, it may be too late to initiate estrogen therapy. At this late juncture, estrogen cannot reconstitute tissue loss or reverse organ damage already sustained by years of hormone deprivation. Replacing hormones of any type, whether it is thyroid, insulin, adrenal or ovarian hormones, requires a far more individualized approach.

Estrogen replacement therapy is not an antidote for poor lifestyle habits, and hormones will not eliminate diseases a woman is genetically programmed to develop. Although well-managed menopause hormone therapy is a many-splendored thing, it is neither a miracle drug nor an elixir of youth for an aging menopausal woman. By maintaining cellular components, tissue architecture, and organ integrity, estrogen does, however, slow down decline exacerbated by estrogen deficiency.

Hormone replacement therapy should be based on a menopausal woman's clinical presentation, her medical and family history, along with laboratory tests and diagnostic evaluations. Recommendations are then made in accordance with her particular needs for alleviating menopausal symptoms, as well as her personal desire to prevent debilitating diseases. Consistent with standard medical practice for managing all other hormone deficiencies, estrogen replacement dosing and therapeutic adjustments are fine-tuned further with hormone testing and clinical assessments.

For menopausal women in the 21st century, sustained vitality, enhanced sexuality, and dignified longevity involve treating ovarian hormone deficiency appropriately. Establishing hormone harmony through properly timed and well-orchestrated estrogen replacement therapy allows women of all ages to journey safely and naturally to the sunny side of menopause.

The ERA of WHI

In the summer of 2002 the principal results of the Women's Health Initiative (WHI) landmark study on the use of estrogen-plus-progestin hormone therapy in healthy postmenopausal women were released with dramatic and widespread media fanfare. Then, in the spring of 2004, WHI released the results of the estrogen-only arm of the hormone study. This aspect of the WHI study evaluated postmenopausal women who had undergone a hysterectomy in the past, and then embarked on estrogen therapy using only conjugated equine estrogen (Premarin).

WHI's well-publicized findings on the risks vs. benefits of menopause hormone therapy were inconsistent with established medical wisdom and clinical practice. Physicians and patients were also alarmed that, due to safety concerns, both the estrogen-plus-progestin and the estrogen-alone arms of the study had been terminated early. Bewildered and dismayed by the repeated proclamations of the WHI study, women's use of hormone therapy plummeted from nearly half of all menopausal women enjoying the benefits of hormone therapy, down to just 5% using estrogen replacement.

For decades, estrogen had been the mainstay treatment for hot flashes, vaginal dryness, bone density maintenance, and heart disease protection in menopausal women. Then, based on generalized conclusions promulgated by WHI's hormone studies, menopause hormone therapy became "hormona non grata." Estrogen replacement therapy was reduced to the medication of last resort for treating symptoms linked to estrogen deficiency, or for use in any disease process exacerbated by estrogen deficiency. For example, even though the WHI studies confirmed that menopause hormone therapy significantly decreased the incidence of osteoporosis-related fractures, estrogen was kicked to the curb in favor of other bone-sparing medications, despite cumbersome logistics and serious side effects caused by these other prescription drugs.

In January 2003, within 6 months of the publication of the WHI results, the FDA slapped a Black Box Warning label against the use of estrogen and estrogen-plus-progestin "to reflect the increased risk of heart disease, stroke and breast cancer in postmenopausal women using these products as confirmed by results of the WHI published in July 2002." If nothing else worked, then a woman may consider trying "risky" menopause hormone therapy, at the lowest possible dose and for the shortest time possible.

Because the lumped and clumped conclusions of the WHI hormone trial were prevalent in any discussion involving menopausal issues, it took a while for the clouds looming over estrogen replacement therapy to pass. As raw data from the WHI studies was stratified according to women's ages and follow-up results assessed, the age-specific risks and benefits of different types of menopause hormone therapy became clearer.

WHI STUDY DESIGN

In 1991, the first woman to head the National Institutes of Health (NIH), cardiologist, Dr. Bernadine Healy, established the Women's Health Initiative (WHI) to address the most common causes of death and disability in postmenopausal women, which are cardiovascular disease (heart attacks and strokes), cancer and osteoporosis.

In its entirety, the WHI study included more than 160,000 postmenopausal women who were aged 50 to 79 at the time they enrolled. They were to participate in randomized clinical trials (RCTs) and observational studies involving menopause hormone therapy, calcium and vitamin D supplementation, as well as dietary modifications. 40 study clinics across the nation would recruit women, and funding was obtained directly from Congress in the form of a discrete line item, with a budget of $625 million over the life of the 15-year study. The WHI study is one of the largest U.S. prevention studies of its kind.

To determine if estrogen therapy decreases the risk of cardiovascular disease and osteoporosis-related fractures, the hormone therapy component of the WHI involved asymptomatic postmenopausal women between the ages of 50 to 79 participating in two randomized placebo-controlled trials (RCTs). Since coronary heart disease is the number one cause of death in postmenopausal women, it became the primary clinical outcome of interest. Additional outcomes monitored included strokes, blood clots, endometrial uterine cancer, colon cancer, hip fractures, and death from other causes. Due to concerns over the relationship between hormones and breast cancer risk, breast cancer was selected as the primary adverse outcome.

The WHI hormone trial was officially launched in 1993, and each arm of the randomized controlled trial (RCT) using menopause hormones was to last 9 years, and then there would be a follow-up phase, which would last until 2010.

There were two arms to the WHI hormone therapy trials:

1) The WHI Estrogen-plus-Progestin Study involved 16,600 women with a uterus, who were randomly assigned to receive either a hormone pill containing estrogen-plus-progestin (Prempro) or a placebo (sugar pill). Prempro is a combination of 0.625mg conjugated equine estrogen (Premarin) with 2.5mg medroxyprogesterone (Provera); hence the trade name Prempro. To prevent the possibility of estrogen-induced endometrial uterine tissue overgrowth or uterine cancer, menopausal women who have not had a hysterectomy need to have progesterone added to their estrogen replacement therapy.

2) The WHI Estrogen-Alone Study involved 10,700 women without a uterus, who were randomly assigned to receive either an estrogen containing hormone pill (Premarin) or a placebo (sugar pill). The

conjugated equine estrogen (Premarin) pill's dose in the study was 0.625mg. Women who have had a hysterectomy do not need to worry about endometrial uterine cancer.

The WOMEN of WHI

The average age of the postmenopausal women participating in these WHI trials was 63, with 70% over the age of 60. Most of these ladies were at least a decade past their menopausal years. Only 3.5% of the participants were between the ages of 50 to 54. Women suffering from significant menopausal symptoms were excluded from participating in the WHI trials, due to concerns that those receiving the placebo (sugar pill) would drop out of the studies prematurely, to seek relief for their bothersome hot flashes and vaginal dryness.

Essentially, the WHI study evaluated women who were well beyond menopause and did not suffer from menopausal symptoms. 70% of the participating women were either overweight or obese, and nearly half of the women were already being treated for high blood pressure. 40% had been smokers in the past, and 10% were still smoking at the time they enrolled in these trials. Although these women were considered "average," upon focused analysis, few were freshly menopausal and most were not all that healthy when they initiated hormone therapy.

EARLY TERMINATIONS

Interim monitoring of the combined estrogen-plus-progestin (Prempro) treatment group showed an increased risk for breast cancer, with some increase in the risk for heart attacks. These risks outweighed the health benefits of menopause hormone therapy, so the Data Safety and Monitoring Board (DSMB) recommended that the WHI Estrogen-plus-Progestin Study be terminated early. After 5.2 years of data collection, the study was stopped in 2002.

In 2004, NIH also terminated the WHI Estrogen-Alone Study early, after 6.8 years of data collection, despite the DSMB's determination that none of the predefined stopping boundaries had been crossed. NIH indicated that estrogen-alone (Premarin) did not appear to affect the risk of coronary heart disease, but it had increased the risk of strokes. They felt that the results were unlikely to change if the study was continued until 2005, as originally planned, so the estrogen-alone arm of the trial was stopped in 2004.

WHI RESULTS

Although 70% of the study's participants were over age 60, when the principal conclusions of the WHI hormone therapy trials were released, all women spanning the ages of 50 to 79 were blended into one homogenous group. Painting all women between the ages of 50 to 79 with the same broad hormonal brush stroke is biologically inaccurate. There are considerable metabolic and physiological differences between a 50-something freshly menopausal woman and a 79-year old woman who is decades beyond her final menstrual period. A lot of changes occur over the course of 30 years of aging, and menopause hormone therapy does not neutralize age differences.

Principal results from the WHI Estrogen-plus-Progestin Study published in 2002 showed that, when compared to women taking a placebo, women taking the combined estrogen-plus-progestin hormone therapy (Prempro) experienced fewer osteoporosis-related fractures, decreased risk of colon cancer, and decreased risk for developing diabetes. On the other hand, women taking the oral estrogen-plus-progestin combination had an increased risk for breast cancer, coronary heart disease, stroke, blood clots and gallbladder problems.

Since women suffering from bothersome menopausal symptoms, such as hot flashes, depressive symptoms and sexual satisfaction issues, were excluded from WHI trials, it is not surprising that after taking estrogen-plus-progestin for one year, hormone therapy did not have a meaningful effect on improving quality of life in women who were not suffering from menopausal symptoms.

Principal results from the WHI Estrogen-Alone Study published in 2004 showed that, when compared to placebo, women taking estrogen-alone hormone therapy experienced fewer osteoporosis-related fractures, decreased risk for developing diabetes, and surprisingly, estrogen therapy decreased a woman's risk of breast cancer. Estrogen-alone therapy slightly decreased the risk of coronary heart disease, and it had no effect on the risk of colon cancer. Women taking the oral conjugated equine estrogen (Premarin) had an increased risk for stroke, blood clots and gallbladder problems.

Increased risks for adverse effects common to both regimens of oral menopause hormone therapy, such as stroke, blood clots, and gallbladder problems, as well as the increased risks for breast cancer and coronary heart disease linked to the estrogen-plus-progestin arm of the WHI, were in the order of 30% increased relative risk.

What does this 30% increased relative risk really mean? Well, let's say that just by being alive, 3 out of 100 women who were not taking any hormones develop one of these medical problems. If all 100 women were on menopause hormone therapy, then 4 of them might develop one of these medical issues. The 30% increased relative risk translates into an increased risk of the event occurring in 1 person out of a hundred, which is an increased absolute risk of 1%. The individual's risk of the problem affecting a particular woman is still very low.

As a consequence of these sensationalized WHI results, what was once considered a beacon of menopausal health and vitality burned down in flames. Because the risks of estrogen replacement seemed to exceed its benefits, women and physicians simply abandoned menopause hormone therapy. Since over 85% of menopausal women experience bothersome symptoms that stem from estrogen deficiency, women without hormones suffered considerably.

Deprived of estrogen replacement to treat estrogen hormone deficiency, women were left scrambling for alternative therapies. They sought herbs and other substances to alleviate bothersome menopausal symptoms. The pharmaceutical industry stepped up marketing of alternative drugs and chemicals for treating osteoporosis. Low-dose antidepressants for hot flashes, different statins to lower cholesterol and more "gotta go, gotta go" bladder pills came into vogue. A wide variety of vaginal moisturizers and lubricants popped up in drugstores. Estrogen-deficient, but physically active menopausal women muscled their way through hot flashes, while others took up yoga, and some calmed their menopausal mayhem with paced breathing. Most women, however, muddled their way through an unpleasant and disconcerting menopausal odyssey, only to end up on the dark side of aging.

No matter how an estrogen-deprived woman navigates the turbulence or tranquility of her menopausal journey, she still has to cope with the long-term consequences of estrogen deficiency. Prolonged estrogen deprivation exacerbates the degenerative processes of aging, such as cardiovascular disease (heart disease and strokes), osteoporosis, mental decline, lagging libido, vaginal dryness and urinary incontinence. Without estrogen replacement therapy to treat her estrogen loss, a woman's quality of life is compromised, both during her early menopausal years and into her elderly years. Women age better and experience more meaningful longevity when they use menopause hormone therapy.

It has been over a decade since the principal results of the WHI hormone therapy trials saw the dawn of the 21st century. Since then, focused analysis of data, subsequent follow-up evaluations, and additional clinical studies have clarified and supplemented WHI's initial findings. Fortunately, these landmark studies helped refine our understanding of the myriad beneficial effects of appropriately timed and properly managed menopause hormone replacement therapy.

SHADES of MENOPAUSE

It's inevitable, it's unavoidable, and it's universal. Every woman will go through menopause. Why menopause exists or why women go through menopause when they do is unknown. 50 million American women are between the ages of 40 and 60, and every day 6,000 women are marching into menopause.

Menopause occurs when a non-pregnant or non-lactating woman has not had a menstrual period for 12 consecutive months. On average, this happens around age 51. The age range for normal menopause extends for 5 years on either side of 51, so 90% of women experience their final menstrual period between the ages of 46 to 56. Often the age of menopause is genetically determined, so a woman's age at menopause tends to correlate with her mother's timeline. 10% of women experience "early menopause," that is, their final menstrual period occurs between the ages of 40 to 45. 1% of women are less than 40 years old when they lose ovarian function, so they face "premature menopause," also known as premature ovarian failure.

Menopause marks the end of a woman's fertility and the beginning of ovarian hormone deficiency. Each woman is born with a finite number of oocytes/follicles (eggs) housed in her ovaries. These are all the oocytes/follicles (eggs) she will ever have. Once her last oocyte/follicle (egg) ovulates and she has her final menstrual period, a woman can no longer get pregnant naturally. Her reproductive years are over. At the same time, ovarian production of female hormones plummets.

The overwhelming majority of mammals die very soon after their reproductive capabilities end. Not so for humans and a few others. Female gorillas, chimpanzees, rhesus monkeys, elephants and lions live beyond their reproductive years. The older females help take care of the younger members of their clan. The "grandmother hypothesis" holds that an older woman who can no longer bear babies of her own is now available to help take care of her grandchildren. Weakened by age and depleted by prior pregnancies, an older woman can achieve more reproductive genetic success by caring for her grandchildren than by bearing more children of her own. By spending more time foraging than younger mothers, Stone Age grandmothers improved their grandbabies' chance for survival. This built-in ovarian obsolescence may have helped perpetuate the menopausal gene for future generations.

Starting around age 35, the quantity and quality of a woman's ovarian follicles/oocytes (eggs) rapidly deteriorate. Not only is it harder for her to get pregnant, but because of her older eggs, there is also a higher risk that the baby will suffer from a genetic abnormality. Aging ovaries lead to erratic estrogen production, either too much or too little, and declining egg quality results in decreased progesterone production. When estrogen production is too low, then hot flashes, vaginal dryness, and migraines can occur. When estrogen levels are too high, relative to poor progesterone levels generated by older eggs, the woman experiences more problems with "estrogen dominance." This amplifies fibrocystic breast changes, increases uterine fibroid growth, and causes irregular heavy periods and menstrual dribbling.

Natural menopause happens gradually for most women. Ovaries don't stop functioning abruptly; they slow down, producing less and less female hormones. Eventually, menstrual periods disappear. The path of declining ovarian function leading up to menopause is known as perimenopause. Perimenopause may either extend for years, over a long and winding road, or be just a quick hop and a skip into menopause. Although there are common symptoms that women share during the menopausal transition, each woman experiences her vacillating hormonal fluctuations differently. For most women, the perimenopausal journey is a bumpy ride of hormonal ups and downs, lasting 2 to 8 years, preceding her ovaries' final menopausal destination.

With the onset of menopause, the ovarian follicles/oocytes (eggs) are depleted, so there are no follicles left to produce estrogen, and there are no eggs left to ovulate and produce progesterone. A menopausal woman's estrogen levels plummet by 90%, and since she cannot get pregnant, progesterone is nowhere to be found. Although aging ovaries still produce a trickle of testosterone, and the adrenal glands continue to produce androgens, a menopausal woman's testosterone levels decrease by 50%. These hormonal shifts upset her estrogen to testosterone ratio, tipping the balance in favor of masculinizing androgens. This generates unwanted facial hair, elevated cholesterol, scalp hair loss and increased abdominal (visceral) fat.

The dramatic loss of female hormones triggers bothersome symptoms in over 85% of menopausal women. Loss of ovarian function has a huge impact on a woman's physical, mental, sexual and spiritual well-being. Colored by a kaleidoscope of symptoms, every woman perceives menopause differently. Some women waltz through menopause without being tainted by uncomfortable shades of estrogen deficiency, while others agonize through menopause meltdown. Although menopausal women can live without estrogen, their quality of life is compromised, and for so many, their extended longevity is tarnished by disease and disability exacerbated by prolonged estrogen deprivation. Very few women are genetically blessed to fend off degenerative diseases compounded by estrogen loss.

Everything that occurs during the menopausal years may not only be due to estrogen deficiency. Irregular menstrual periods can occur because of ovarian cysts, abnormal growths in the uterus, thyroid problems, hepatitis C or celiac disease (sprue). Vaginal dryness may be due to Sjogren's syndrome. Night sweats could be a sign of tuberculosis, heart valve infection, hyperthyroidism, lymphoma, Parkinson's, HIV/AIDS, or other diseases. Antidepressants and corticosteroid medications can cause night sweats. Other medical or gynecological conditions should not be overlooked or go untreated, just because they share symptoms with menopause.

Menopause is a natural event, but for most women it is not a serene organic passage into senior citizenship. Just like any other biological situation associated with a hormone deficiency, such as diabetes, thyroid problems, adrenal issues, etc., estrogen loss leads to organ damage, disease, and disability. From head-to-toe, estrogen receptors are found throughout a woman's body, so estrogen is vital to helping her stay happy and healthy. Without estrogen, cellular connections are disrupted; collagen structures collapse, and tissues dry out. Menopause is a physiologically distressing ride down the falls of hormone withdrawal into the rapids of accelerated aging and relentless deterioration.

Degenerative loss of tissue architecture with organ dysfunction accelerates the aging process. Estrogen acts as a hormonal lubricant, keeping a woman's cellular tissues supple, flexible, and resilient. Although still aging, a menopausal woman's organs function more smoothly with hormone replacement, so she looks younger and stays healthier longer. Metaphorically speaking, with estrogen maintaining parts and services, a woman's sexy sedan does not deteriorate into a postmenopausal jalopy quite as quickly. Sadly, as time goes by, an estrogen-deprived elderly chassis could end up housebound or garaged in a nursing home – immobilized, melancholy and leaking fluids.

Menopause Symptoms include:

- Thermostat turmoil - hot flashes/hot flushes, night sweats, and cold chills
- Sleep disturbances - trouble falling asleep, trouble staying asleep, increased snoring, increased sleep apnea, increased restless legs, sleep disrupted from frequent trips to the bathroom due to a twitchy bladder
- Sexual dysfunction - decreased libido, decreased sexual arousal and orgasms, painful sex, dry sex, no sex
- Anxiety, irritability, mood swings, depression
- Feeling overwhelmed and apprehensive, panic attacks
- Memory problems, difficulty concentrating, decreased word retrieval

- Dizziness and lightheadedness, vertigo
- Crushing fatigue
- Increased migraines and headaches
- Vaginal woes - vaginal dryness, decreased tissue turgor and elasticity, painful intercourse (dyspareunia), vaginal irritation and tissue tears, changes in vaginal odor, vulvar dystrophies
- Bladder blunders - urinary urgency, frequency, incontinence, prolapse, recurrent urinary tract infections
- Slower metabolism
- Weight gain with body shape-shifting, from an hourglass to a pear and then to an apple, with increased abdominal (visceral) fat deposition, increased cellulite
- Decreased muscle tone and decreased muscle mass
- Decreased breast firmness, droopy breasts
- Acne
- Premature wrinkling
- Dry, itchy, thinning skin
- Creepy, crawly, tingling sensations
- Changes in body odor
- Softer fingernails, thicker toenails
- Increased facial hair, thinning scalp hair
- Dry eyes, fading vision
- Decreased hearing, tinnitus
- Dry mouth, burning tongue, gingivitis, and halitosis
- Heart palpitations, irregular heartbeat
- Cholesterol and blood pressure increase
- Diabetes risk increases
- Allergies and asthma problems increase
- Gastroesophageal reflux (GERD) and indigestion increase
- Bloating, gas and constipation increase
- Joint pain, muscle and tendon aches increase
- Rheumatoid arthritis, osteoarthritis and gout increase
- Decreased bone density
- Exacerbations and worsening of other preexisting medical conditions

Prolonged Estrogen Deprivation Leads to More:

- Heart disease
- Strokes
- Dementia, Alzheimer's disease, Parkinson's disease
- Osteoporosis
- Joint replacements
- Urinary incontinence
- Vaginal atrophy and shrinkage
- Stool incontinence
- Loss of vision
- Loss of hearing
- Loss of teeth
- Loss of balance
- Dependent living
- Decreased quality of life
- Increased mortality

Some menopausal maladies are temporary, e.g.- hot flashes and sleep disturbances, while others, e.g.- vaginal dryness, leaky bladder, brittle bones and memory loss, get progressively worse. Everyone ages, but that doesn't mean a woman needs to succumb to the misery of menopause or the wretched hardships of prolonged estrogen deficiency. Menopause hormone therapy is not an elixir of youth, nor can it compensate for years of poor lifestyle choices, but it does slow down tissue degradation and organ dysfunction exacerbated by estrogen loss.

Women are far more than the just the sum of their breasts, uterus, and vaginal tissue turgor. Estrogen affects over 400 functions in a woman's body. Because everything in a menopausal woman's life goes better with the right estrogen, at the right dose, at the right time, women simply age better and are healthier with appropriate estrogen replacement. Well-orchestrated hormone therapy provides meaningful longevity with dignified aging to menopausal women of all ages.

MENOPAUSE – TYPES and TIMING

The climacteric, from the Greek word for "ladder, climax" is an older, less frequently used term applied to a woman's transition through menopause. It indicates the interval of time in a woman's life during which she climbs down the ladder of reproduction, and steps into menopause. Her reproductive distance from menopause identifies where a woman is during this transition. These stages are further identified as premenopause, perimenopause, menopause, postmenopause, and geripause (the elderly years). Let's describe these menopausal stages further.

PREMENOPAUSE... *Before Menopause*
Premenopause refers to the time from a woman's first menstrual period (menarche), usually occurring around age 12, to her last regular monthly menstrual period. This is considered the most fertile time of a woman's reproductive years. Every month either the right or the left ovary releases an oocyte/egg (ovulation) for potential fertilization.

The length of menstrual cycles is every 28 days, plus or minus 7 days on either side of 28, so normal menstrual bleeding can occur every 21 to 35 days. Cycle length varies from woman to woman, and can vary from month to month, within that every 21 to 35 days' range, in the same woman. Menstrual cyclical bleeding that occurs every 3 to 5 weeks is acceptable. After age 35, the quality and quantity of a woman's follicles/oocytes (eggs) decrease rapidly, fertility declines and older eggs generate more chromosome abnormalities in the offspring.

PERIMENOPAUSE… *Around Menopause*

The literal translation of perimenopause is "around menopause." It refers to the stage of declining ovarian function that lasts for 2 to 8 years prior to a woman's final menstrual period. The woman is transitioning between her reproductive years to her infertile menopausal years. Typically, women experience perimenopausal symptoms in their 40s. Since the follicles/oocytes (eggs) are now older, not only is it harder for a woman to get pregnant, these older eggs do not produce hormones efficiently.

Erratic perimenopausal hormone fluctuations can bring on uncomfortable menopausal symptoms, irregular uterine bleeding and gynecological conditions requiring medical/surgical interventions. A woman may experience problematic premenstrual syndrome (PMS) and fibrocystic breast changes. The nature and length of her menstrual cycles may vary; the menstrual flow may increase, decrease or sputter. She may experience either more menstrual cramping or less pelvic discomfort with her periods.

Gynecological conditions such as uterine fibroids, endometriosis, adenomyosis, polyps, vaginal infections, dysfunctional uterine bleeding and ovarian cysts are exacerbated with perimenopausal hormone fluctuations and require medical or surgical intervention. As she gets closer and closer to her final menstrual period, a woman may experience more problems with vaginal dryness, urinary incontinence, hot flashes, sleeping disturbances, decreased libido, moodiness, and other unpleasant symptoms of full-blown menopause. Only 10% of women cease menstruating abruptly with no perimenopausal irregularity.

MENOPAUSE…

From Greek *meno-* meaning "month," and *pause,* meaning "cease or stop;" by definition, a woman is menopausal when she experiences 12 consecutive months without a menstrual period. At this point, she cannot get pregnant naturally, and her ovaries fail to produce adequate female hormones to keep her healthy and happy. With the onset of menopause, her estrogen levels drop by 90%, her testosterone levels drops by 50%, and since she is no longer ovulating, progesterone is totally absent.

In response to low estrogen levels, the pituitary gland in the brain secretes more follicle-stimulating hormone (FSH), trying to encourage disappearing ovarian follicles to secrete more estrogen. Because there are no follicles/oocytes (eggs) left to ovulate, the ovaries no longer produce progesterone. In response to low levels of progesterone, the pituitary gland secretes more luteinizing hormone (LH), trying to stimulate the empty ovaries to release an egg (ovulate) and luteinize and produce progesterone. Sustained elevations of blood serum FSH and serum LH levels, coupled to low estrogen levels, are diagnostic of menopause. Since women who have had a hysterectomy cannot rely on uterine bleeding to diagnose menopause, blood hormone levels establish their menopausal status.

A cardinal feature of menopause is the inability to regulate body temperature properly. Over 85% of menopausal women experience hot flashes, night sweats, and in some cases, cold flashes. Vaginal dryness with painful sex is the other menopausal irritation for which women frequently seek gynecological care. Estrogen withdrawal also precipitates imbalances in brain chemicals called neurotransmitters. Neurotransmitters relay signals between brain cells and other nerve cells throughout the body. Deficiencies involving serotonin, norepinephrine, and dopamine neurotransmitters are connected to depression, anxiety, irritability, palpitations, tingling extremities, and insomnia. There are dozens of other distressing menopausal symptoms, as well. 7 to 10 years after a woman's final menstrual period, some bothersome menopausal symptoms resolve or the woman has simply adapted to them. Unfortunately, due to lack of estrogen, silent tissue damage and organ degradation continue their merciless decline into disease and disability.

INDUCED MENOPAUSE occurs when menopause is brought on by damage to ovaries or by surgical removal of ovaries. Damage may be due to chemotherapy, radiation, toxins, infectious diseases or autoimmune conditions. Menstrual cycles may also stop if a woman's body fat dips below a critical amount. This can occur in female athletes and women suffering from anorexia nervosa and other eating disorders. Stress can also disrupt the brain-to-ovary hormone feedback loop, causing menstrual cycles to stop. Since nicotine compromises blood flow to the ovaries, smokers go through menopause 2 to 3 years earlier than non-smokers. Women who have had a hysterectomy without removal of their ovaries may go through menopause several years earlier than otherwise expected. Removing the uterus compromises some of the blood flowing to the ovaries, and this may cause menopause to arrive sooner.

EARLY MENOPAUSE – 10% of women go through menopause before age 45.

PREMATURE MENOPAUSE – 1% of women go through menopause before age 40, and 0.1% of women experience premature ovarian failure by age 30. Other than being an induced menopause, early or premature menopause may be due to genetic issues. Most of the time the cause for menopause coming sooner than expected is unknown.

POSTMENOPAUSE… *After Menopause*

A woman is postmenopausal the day after the 12th consecutive month of not having any menstrual bleeding. After this point, any postmenopausal vaginal bleeding is considered abnormal and should be thoroughly evaluated by a gynecologist. One year after her final menstrual period, a woman is now living with ovarian failure, and she will be postmenopausal for the rest of her life. Fortunately, if appropriately managed hormone replacement therapy is initiated within 10 years of menopause, not only will her bothersome menopausal symptoms be treated naturally and holistically, disease and disability exacerbated by estrogen deprivation will be minimized.

GERIPAUSE… *Long After Menopause*

Once a decade or more has passed since a woman has had her final menstrual period, menopause is a distant memory. Well beyond the turbulence of her freshly menopausal years, a geripausal woman exists in the tundra of prolonged estrogen deprivation. For most women, this occurs when they reach their mid-60s, when the golden years are supposed to be shining.

If a postmenopausal woman has not started estrogen replacement therapy within a decade of menopause, then permanent damage to organs throughout her body is silently already occurring. Arteries supplying oxygenated blood to her heart and brain are now hardened and narrowed by cholesterol plaque build up in a process called atherosclerosis, from the Greek word *athero-*, meaning "gruel or paste," and *sclerosis*, meaning "hardening." Atherosclerotic blood vessels render a postmenopausal woman vulnerable to heart attacks, strokes, and sudden death. Confined by congestive heart failure, her workouts become limited to shuffling trips to the bathroom.

Estrogen-deprived vaginal tissues have lost architectural integrity, elasticity, and responsiveness, so not only is sex painful, sexual responsiveness and orgasms are vague historical memories. Without estrogen, her eye retinas have degenerated even faster, so she cannot read, drive or recognize faces. Estrogen deficiency decreases saliva production and weakens periodontal ligaments. This ailing oral cavity is connected to osteoporotic alveolar jawbones, so an older postmenopausal woman keeps losing teeth. Concentration difficulties and episodic forgetfulness lapse into minimal cognitive impairment (MIC), which withers into Alzheimer's dementia. At one time, a menopausal woman could rely on panty liners for intermittent urinary incontinence, but as the years of estrogen deprivation sabotage bladder function, she depends on diapers. Without estrogen, she has lost bone density, skeletal muscle mass, and agility, so a simple slip and fall can prove deadly. An osteoporosis-related hip fracture could be an older woman's unpleasant one-way ticket to a nursing home.

For maximum protection from the misery and anguish of estrogen deficiency, it is best to start hormone replacement therapy close to menopause and adjust hormone dosing and therapeutic preparations as the years go by. Postmenopausal women younger than 60 years old, who start female hormone replacement therapy soon after menopause, have a 30% lower rate of death from all causes. Without estrogen replacement, an older postmenopausal woman's golden years become riddled with debilitating chronic diseases, which have been exacerbated by estrogen deficiency. For a menopausal woman, improved quality of life and aging with dignity are achievable with well-orchestrated estrogen replacement therapy.

WHAT'S LIFE EXPECTANCY GOT TO DO WITH IT?

Produced by glandular organs, a hormone is a chemical messenger that travels through the bloodstream to reach its target organ. Upon arriving at its destination, the hormone locks onto a receptor site on the recipient tissue, and this triggers the tissue's response to the hormone's directive. Through this signaling system, the body regulates vital functions, controls metabolism, growth and development, and modulates sexual activity, reproduction and mood. Hormones make it all happen, so if any gland is not functioning properly, hormone balance is disrupted, and the whole body suffers.

Hormones are powerful. Just tiny amounts have huge impact on organ functions throughout a woman's body, and they are essential to her health and happiness.

There are two leagues of hormones in the body, the majors and the minors. Adrenaline (epinephrine), cortisol, insulin and thyroid hormone are crucial for life-sustaining functions such as regulating heart rate and metabolism, maintaining blood pressure, providing blood sugar for cellular nourishment, and managing inflammation and swelling for tissue repair and healing. If a woman is missing any of these major hormones, she will get sick quickly and not live very long. These hormones keep a person alive, so if there is loss of any of these hormones, they are replaced immediately.

Estrogen and testosterone, our major sex hormones, operate in the minor leagues. Progesterone is needed only to sustain a pregnancy, and DHEA is a precursor hormone, so low levels may not even be addressed. Although loss of a minor league hormone is not a life-threatening emergency, nor does lack of a sex hormone precipitate a life-compromising coma, withdrawal of any hormone is traumatic to the body.

Women experience declining estrogen levels differently, but very few women sail through menopause unscathed. Estrogen deficiency causes a litany of bothersome symptoms in over 85% of menopausal women. Regardless of whether or not a woman notices menopausal discomforts, without appropriate estrogen replacement she will endure the long-term physical, psychological, sexual and emotional consequences of ovarian hormone deficiency. As years of estrogen deprivation unravel, a postmenopausal woman will not feel well, but she will most likely attribute her decline in health and function to normal aging. She may not realize that loss of ovarian hormones, in particular the lack of estrogen, is contributing to her declining quality of life. She may rationalize that if Nature had wanted her to have sex hormones after turning 50, her ovaries would still be producing estrogen well into her elderly years.

The truth of the matter is that Nature was not really planning for most women to live past the age of 50, so there was no need for postmortem hormone production. Indeed, prior to "unnatural" improvements in modern sanitation, milk pasteurization and contemporary obstetrical and surgical practices, very few women made it past their 49th birthday. Until the early 1900's, a woman considered herself immensely fortunate to have survived the delivery of her children. The most common cause of death for women during the Victorian era was not tuberculosis, nor smallpox, nor old age. Astonishingly, childbirth was the number one killer, with 1 out of 25 women dying during the birth of a baby, regardless of their social or economic status. Back then, poverty and malnutrition played little part in determining the rate of maternal mortality

Unlike death from other conditions involving sick people dying from contagious diseases or other afflictions, death during childbirth involved healthy women who had been well enough to get pregnant in the first place. Infant survival was also bleak, with only 50% of babies born making it to their first birthday. It was not until the 1930's that nurses and surgeons routinely washed their hands and gloved for procedures, and attendants delivering babies finally started wearing facial masks to prevent coughs and sneezes from contaminating the delivery room. And then in 1940, there was an abrupt and steep reduction in women dying during childbirth, which could not be explained by natural factors, but coincided with the antibiotic revolution in medicine. Use of the antibiotic sulfonamide started in 1937, followed by the utilization of penicillin in the early 1940's. Survival rates from pregnancy improved dramatically by simply overcoming maternal infection with the infusion of antibiotics. Then in the 1950's, ergotamine use stemmed the tide of post-partum hemorrhage.

For thousands of years, healthy young women had needlessly succumbed to childbirth. Then, within the span of a few decades, maternal mortality rates decreased from a dismal 1 in 100 women dying from childbirth in 1940 down to 1 in 10,000 women dying from pregnancy-related complications today. Over the course of human history, post-partum infections, hemorrhage, toxemia of pregnancy and illegal abortions tragically ended healthy young women's lives and crippled families. By reigning in these pregnancy-related four horsemen of death, the risk of dying from pregnancy was nearly eliminated during the 20th century.

Fortunately, most women are now living for decades past their final menstrual period. Women who reach 51 years of age can expect to live to 86 years old. Instead of merely surviving her golden years, a menopausal woman can thrive naturally and holistically by simply bringing her hormones into the 21st century. Diseases that rarely occur in a well-estrogenized woman routinely afflict her estrogen-deficient postmenopausal counterpart. It does take at least a decade of estrogen deficiency for these serious diseases to surface, so many women and health care providers do not make the connection between menopause and the onset of chronic diseases. Heart ailments, strokes, dementia, diaper-clad urinary incontinence, and osteoporosis do not occur immediately after menopause. It takes years of estrogen deprivation for tissues to sustain enough damage to manifest obvious organ malfunction. After 10 to15 years of estrogen deficiency, arteries have hardened and narrowed with cholesterol plaques, brain cells have tangled, bones have thinned, joints have rusted, and vaginal tissues have collapsed.

These crippling infirmities plague postmenopausal women and lead to life-restricting disability.

Everyone ages, but that doesn't mean a woman needs to succumb to the drudgery and hardships that come with ovarian failure. Everyone agrees that a healthy lifestyle is crucial to maintaining a healthy life, but menopausal problems are precipitated by ovarian hormone deficiency, and subsequent degenerative processes are exacerbated by the lack of estrogen. As a woman goes through menopause and shuffles her way from one doctor to another doctor, medication after medication is added to her pillbox to help her cope with one organ after another estrogen-deprived organ breaking down. She ends up on the medical merry-go-round of pill after pill, injection after injection, procedure after procedure, side effect after side effect, all relentlessly corroding her aging system.

Instead of squandering away her postmenopausal years in a downward spiral of ailing misery, a woman can help sustain her health and happiness by simply having her ovarian hormones replaced appropriately. User-friendly with proven reliability, estrogen replacement therapy not only alleviates bothersome menopausal symptoms, it naturally prevents damage exacerbated by estrogen deficiency. Elegantly simple in design and fundamental to meaningful longevity with dignified aging, no other therapy takes care of a hormone-deficient menopausal woman like estrogen replacement.

LIFESTYLE - LIVE LONG and AGE WELL

Menopausal women will feel better and enjoy healthier living with estrogen replacement therapy, but hormones alone cannot overcome harmful lifestyle choices. Over 75% of health care spending is for chronic diseases that can be prevented or cured with healthier lifestyle habits. Over 75% of all cardiovascular-related deaths can be prevented simply with adequate changes in lifestyle.

Heart disease is the #1 killer of women, and heart disease kills more women than all forms of cancers combined. Each year, 1 in 3 women dies from heart disease, while 1 in 36 (just 3%) dies from breast cancer. Women fear breast cancer above any other medical diagnosis, yet more than 10 times more women die from heart disease than will ever succumb to breast cancer. Heart problems are rare in women prior to menopause, but adverse and lethal cardiac events markedly increase after the age of 50. When a woman loses her estrogen, she loses her biological edge over heart disease. Menopause increases a woman's risk for cardiovascular diseases, such as heart attacks, strokes, and sudden death. Estrogen deficiency contributes to harmful alterations in cholesterol ratios, increased blood pressure, increased insulin resistance and diabetes, and increased weight gain, with shape shifting towards more unhealthy abdominal (visceral) fat deposition.

Estrogen works best with healthy lifestyle choices. Paving the way for vitality and relevance into her golden years, beneficial lifestyle considerations for a menopausal woman include:

✓ **A healthy weight**. Body mass index (BMI) should be between 18.5 and 25, and a woman's waist size should be no more than 35 inches. Devised in the early 1800's by a Belgian mathematician, the BMI is a method of assessing how much an individual's body weight departs from what is healthy for their height. BMI is calculated by taking a person's weight (kilograms) and dividing it by the square of their height (meters)^2 or by taking a person's weight (pounds) and dividing it by the square of their height (inches)^2 and then multiplying this number by 703.

A healthy BMI ranges between 18.5 to 25.

A woman over the age of 50 can usually consume about 1,500 kcal/day without gaining weight. The more physically active a woman is, the more she can eat.

In addition to the afflictions of diabetes, heart disease, stroke and joint replacements, overweight (BMI 25 to 29.9) and obese (BMI > 30) women are at much higher risk of developing breast cancer, uterine and ovarian cancer, blood clots, and colon cancer. 1 out of 3 cancer deaths is linked to excess body weight.

✓ **Proper nutrition**. The Mediterranean diet, along with a small amount of wine (5 ounces serving two to three times a week), is the healthiest diet on the planet. 7 fruits and vegetables a day helps keep disease away.

✓ **To soy or not to soy...** Soybeans, like any other bean, are rich in cholesterol-free protein, fiber, nutrients, and antioxidants. In Asia, thoroughly cooked and properly prepared intact soy protein has been a dietary staple for thousands of years. The traditional fermentation process broadens soy's nutritional value by increasing its digestibility and the bioavailability of its nutrients. Soy contains isoflavones, plant-derived compounds with weak estrogenic influence, and this nutritional bonus helps explain why women in Asia experience less discomfort from hot flashes and night sweats. Naturally cultivated and traditionally prepared soy can be good food.

✓ A **multivitamin** specifically designed for menopausal women taken several times a week can help make up for dietary micronutrient shortcomings. A menopausal woman no longer has menstrual uterine bleeding, so she does not need iron supplementation. Iron levels that are desirable earlier in life during growth and reproduction are not beneficial in a woman's postmenopausal years. Excess iron may contribute to heart attacks, strokes and diabetes in older individuals.

✓ **After the age of 65, a chewable baby aspirin (81mg)** several times a week helps decrease clot-related strokes, heart attacks, breast cancer and colon cancer in older women.

✓ **Sleeping 8 hours a night** is critical to healthy longevity. Adults are created to spend a third of their lives sleeping to reboot their brain and rest their body.

✓ Adequate **calcium and vitamin D** intake are needed not only for bones but for the rest of the body, as well. Daily oral intake, meaning how much is consumed through diet plus supplements per day, of calcium and vitamin D should follow the rule of "1000 & 1000" – 1000mg of calcium per day and 1000 IU of vitamin D per day. Since most women usually get 500mg of calcium in their diet every day, a 500mg calcium supplement with one meal per day will round out their calcium needs.

Unless low vitamin D blood levels indicate a need for increased dosing, an over the counter supplement of vitamin D3 1000 IU every day takes care of a woman's "sunshine hormone" needs. It's okay if the vitamin D supplement is in addition to the 400 IU of vitamin D found in a multivitamin.

✓ **Locomotion.** Taking a 30-minute walk on most days of the week boosts metabolism and increases longevity. Walking at a steady pace is just as effective as jogging or running for heart health and bone health. A woman does not grind down her knees or traumatize her hips by walking. I've yet to see a jolly jogger happily running along.

Most women only take 5,000 steps a day. Walking 10,000 steps a day keeps disease and cancers away.

✓ **Tobacco-free** existence. People are not human chimneys, so avoid smoking and stay away from secondhand (environmental) smoke. Cigarettes kill. Lung cancer is the leading cause of cancer death, killing more people than breast, colon and prostate cancers combined. Every year twice as many women die from lung cancer than breast cancer. Although 1 out of 8 women who live into their 80s develops breast cancer, the chance that breast cancer will kill a woman is only 1 in 36 (3%). Meanwhile, 1 out of 16 women will develop lung cancer, and 50% of them will die within a year of their diagnosis. The chances of surviving lung cancer are dismal – the 5-year survival rate is only 15%, compared to breast cancer's impressive 5-year survival rate of 90%. Women smokers are also at increased risk for gynecological cancers, such as cervical, vaginal, vulvar and ovarian cancers.

In addition to lung cancer, smokers are at much higher risk for a daunting list of other cancers: mouth, throat, larynx (voice box), esophagus, stomach, pancreas, colon, bladder, kidney and leukemia. Women who smoke triple their risk of having a heart attack or a stroke compared to women who are not around cigarettes. Smoking not only damages internal organs, but looks also go up in smoke, as well. Smoking accelerates facial wrinkles, breasts drooping and butts sagging. Vexing cellulite increases with smoking. Smoking discolors nails, stains teeth and promotes tooth loss. The winning smile is lost, but the bad breath stays. When a woman quits smoking, she pulls the plug on deteriorating looks and diseases linked to noxious tobacco smoke.

✓ Practice **safe sex**. Outside of a mutually monogamous relationship, a sexually active woman is at risk of sexually transmitted diseases (STDs). She can acquire syphilis, genital herpes, gonorrhea, genital warts and other STD's at any age. HIV is found in body fluids such as blood, semen, and vaginal secretions, and the virus can enter the body through any opening or scratch in the skin or mucosal surfaces. The incidence of HIV transmission after isolated sexual contact with an HIV-positive person is unknown, but it is estimated to be approximately 1 to 2 per 1,000 cases after vaginal penetration, and 1 to 2 per 100 cases after anal penetration. Postmenopausal women are at special risk because their thin, fragile vaginal tissues are more susceptible to tearing. To help decrease the transmission of HIV, a person who seeks medical care within 72 hours after exposure to an individual known to have HIV, may receive a 28-day course of antiretroviral therapy to help decrease their chance of acquiring HIV.

✓ Evaluate **thyroid** function. 1 in 8 women develops thyroid disease, and it is 8 times more common in women than men. Thyroid problems increase as women age, so thyroid hormone levels should be checked every 1 to 2 years.

✓ Get **vaccinated**. As people age, their immune system fades, so they are more vulnerable to all types of infections. Tetanus, for example, is not just limited to stepping on a rusty nail. Tetanus spores remain infectious for decades and are found in the soil and even in house dust. From the flu vaccine to the shingles vaccine, vaccines help an aging immune system fend off infections.

✓ Make use of **health screening services**, such as a cervical Pap smear every 3 years, a screening mammogram every 1 to 2 years, and screening for glaucoma and colon cancer. Bone density scans detect and help direct treatment for osteopenia and osteoporosis.

✓ **Minimize stress**. Stress causes the adrenal glands to release the steroid hormone, cortisol. Although generally considered a "bad stress hormone," cortisol is involved with important functions critical to survival. It aids in the metabolism of fats, protein, and carbohydrates. Cortisol stimulates the normal breakdown of stored fats and starch into glucose for the body's energy needs. Cortisol helps maintain blood pressure and cardiac function. It also decreases inflammation and modulates the immune system. Just like anything else, too much of a good thing is bad.

When chronic stress exposes the body to a relentless stream of cortisol, cells become desensitized to all this cortisol floating around. Unchecked inflammation goes wild, and cells of the immune system are unable to respond properly. A stressed person is more vulnerable to acquiring infections, and their wounds are slower to heal. Stress also interferes with the immune system's cancer surveillance capabilities. Chronic inflammation damages blood vessels and brain cells, leads to insulin-resistance and diabetes, and promotes painful joint diseases. Stress messes with circadian rhythms, so sleep cycles are disrupted; meanwhile, the body thinks it needs more reserves to handle stress, so weight gain occurs. Reduce stress peacefully by choosing one thought over another and letting go of what you can't change. Exercise diffuses stress and improves coping mechanisms.

✓ Although a diamond is just a chunk of charcoal that did well under pressure, human carbon life forms live better when they find a stress-free, rewarding, healthy **passion**. So, somehow, someway, somewhere, there's a place for participation.

COMPLEMENTARY and ALTERNATIVE THERAPIES

Menopausal issues stem from estrogen deficiency. To avoid replacing needed female hormones, complementary and alternative therapies have evolved to try to cope with bothersome menopausal symptoms. These include black cohosh, paced breathing, ginseng, kava, acupuncture, yoga, Dong quai, Evening primrose oil, St. John's wort, chanting, self-compassion and magnetic therapy.

In addition, chemicals found in certain plants, such as isoflavones from soybeans and red clover, as well as lignans from flaxseed, are categorized as phytoestrogens ("phyto" meaning plant), because they possess weak estrogenic activity. The predominant isoflavone found in soybeans, genistein, may help some women with their hot flashes, but it can take several months to a year for isoflavones to reach their maximal effectiveness in reducing hot flashes by just 25%. Evidence suggests that for soy or flaxseed phytoestrogens to reduce a woman's risk of breast cancer, consumption of these foods during childhood and adolescence is required. Whether adult soy food intake reduces breast cancer risk is unclear. Because of possible weak estrogenic behaviors associated with isoflavones and lignans, questions remain about the safety of women with breast cancer consuming products containing phytoestrogens. Derived from the roots of wild yams, some over the counter progesterone skin creams contain the phytoestrogen, diosgenin. Diosgenin is not converted into progesterone within the human body, so it does not provide sufficient amounts of absorbable progesterone for uterine safety. Consensus reviews of studies involving phytoestrogens reveal no conclusive evidence that these dietary supplements significantly reduce a woman's risk for heart disease, improve her bone density or reduce her cancer risk.

Just because a product is labeled "natural" does not automatically mean that it is essentially safe and free from potentially damaging chemicals. Black cohosh and kava, for example, can cause severe liver damage. Since food or nutritional supplements are considered dietary products, they are not subject to the same rigors of establishing efficacy and potency as pharmaceutical products. In contrast, prescriptions drugs and over the counter medications are required to provide "full product information," along with warnings and possible side effects, listed on the package labeling.

Similar to drug-drug interactions, there are herb-drug interactions that can interfere with therapeutic goals. Dong quai and some species of red clover contain chemicals called coumarins. Coumarins are weak blood thinners, so if these dietary supplements are consumed while a woman is on anticoagulants, such as warfarin (Coumadin), clopidogrel (Plavix) or aspirin, her risk of bleeding increases.

Tamoxifen (Nolvadex) is a selective estrogen receptor modulator (SERM) oral medication used to treat and prevent breast cancer. The liver's CYP2D6 enzyme converts tamoxifen to its breast-protecting metabolically active form, endoxifen. Endoxifen is the metabolite that actually binds to estrogen receptors in breast cells and prevents the occurrence or recurrence of breast cancer. St. John's wort and black cohosh interfere with the CYP2D6 enzyme, decreasing tamoxifen's effectiveness in protecting breast tissue. Relizen, also known as Femal or Serelys, is a non-hormonal herbal supplement made from pollen extract harvested in southern Sweden. Relizen reduces menopausal hot flashes without interfering with the CYP2D6 enzyme action needed for effective tamoxifen therapy.

In general, clinical trials have not shown that complementary or alternative treatments are clearly superior to a placebo in relieving hot flashes or menopausal symptoms. A "placebo effect" occurs when a person perceives that they have a good response to an inert substance or intervention when there is no true objective effect. Alternatively, a "nocebo effect" occurs when a harmless substance that is taken by a person is associated with harmful effects due to the person's negative expectations. Since these alternative modalities are non-prescription therapies, many women consider these strategies a more natural approach to coping with the physical, sexual and psychological disruptions brought on by estrogen deficiency. Because of the inherently high 50% placebo rate involved with any intervention for menopausal hot flashes, women may register relief with a variety of approaches.

None of these complementary and alternative therapies address the root cause of menopause, nor do they prevent the damages associated with estrogen deficiency. As long as these coping strategies entail minimal risk with no toxicity and do not interfere with other therapeutic agents, they may help some women through their menopausal journey. Regular exercise, notably brisk walking and yoga, are particularly helpful in improving overall physical and spiritual health. Whether a woman marinates in herbs, meditates with candles, muscles to Zumba or just muddles her way through menopause, she still faces the grim reality of tissue degradation and organ dysfunction exacerbated by ovarian hormone deficiency. Although a menopausal woman can survive without estrogen, she lives healthier and happier with her estrogen on board.

HORMONE HISTORY

It was not until the mid-1900s that women consistently survived long enough to experience the hardships of menopause and the detrimental effects of estrogen deficiency. Over the past 70 years, we have learned quite a bit about menopause, and how estrogen loss adversely impacts a woman's health. Through clinical research and focused analysis of data, we have refined our understanding of the importance of replacing a menopausal woman's estrogen in a timely manner, using appropriate types and dosing of hormones, and adjusting hormone therapy as the woman ages. This informed and individualized approach allows a woman to navigate comfortably through her menopausal years and safely journey into her golden years. Estrogen replacement therapy is not designed to keep a woman nubile and young forever, but it will help keep her healthier and happier as she ages with dignity.

HORMONE THERAPY is BORN

In 1878, while describing aspects of a woman's "change of life" in his immensely popular book entitled, The Physical Life of Woman: Advice to the Maiden, Wife and Mother, Philadelphia gynecologist, George H. Napheys, M.D. writes, "After a certain number of years, a woman lays aside those functions with which she has been endowed for the perpetuation of the species, and resumes once more that exclusively individual life which had been hers when a child. The evening of her days approaches, and if she has observed the precepts of wisdom, she may look forward to a long and placid period of rest, blessed with health, honored and loved with a purer flame than any which she inspired in the bloom of youth and beauty."

Wow. A woman can almost visualize herself sitting in a beautiful garden, sipping iced tea while the sun is shining, and birds are singing. In his book, Dr. Napheys does go on to describe bothersome menopausal symptoms and reminds women that, "All intelligent physicians know that there are in very many cases a most unpleasant train of symptoms that characterize this epoch in the physical life of a woman. They are alarming, painful, often entailing sad consequences, though rarely fatal." He goes on to point out that, among physicians, "… there are too many who are inclined to ridicule such complaints, to impute them to fancy, and to think that they have done their full duty when they tell the sufferer that such sensations are merely indicative of her age, and that in a year or two they will all pass away. Such medical attendants do not appreciate the gravity of the sufferings they have been called to relieve."

Under "Precautions and Remedies," Dr. Napheys states that, "some simple remedies will suffice to allay the disagreeable [menopausal] symptoms, and the knowledge that most of them are temporary, common to her sex, and not significant of any peculiar malady, will aid her in opposing their attacks on her peace of mind." He suggests some dietary and lifestyle modifications, such as, "liquor, wines, strong tea, coffee and chocolate should be avoided… cool bathing regularly observed… and care taken to avoid excitement, severe mental or bodily effort, and exhaustion…" If simple remedies fail to be of service, then "opium plaster" applied over the stomach is recommended.

As more and more women lived long enough to "turn the half-century mark," they sought relief for menopausal ailments from their doctors. At the beginning of the 20th century, cannabis, opium, amyl nitrite and belladonna were used to help women make it through menopause. Lydia E. Pinkham's vegetable compound for women contained black cohosh and 40% proof to alleviate hot flashes. During this time, Ovariin, a flavored powder made by desiccating and pulverizing cow ovaries, was used to treat "ovarian problems."

Estrogen's existence was not established until the 1920s. Estradiol, also known as 17beta-estradiol, is the estrogen produced by a woman's ovaries, so it is the primary type of estrogen circulating during her reproductive years. Any estrogen preparation whose chemical structure is identical to the chemical structure of the estradiol produced in a woman's body is considered "body"-identical or bioidentical. Initially, oral estradiol did not lend itself to being used as estrogen replacement therapy for alleviating menopausal symptoms, because it was deactivated in the gastrointestinal tract. Since natural substances cannot be patented, alternative oral estrogen replacement hormones were sought for the burgeoning menopausal market.

Collaboration between a Canadian pharmaceutical company and McGill University endocrine researcher, J. Montreal led to the discovery of Emmenin, the first orally active (water-soluble) estrogen in 1930. Before this conjugated estrogen product, the only estrogen therapy available were human steroids from female cadavers, and these estrogens had to be administered by injection. Emmenin was made by extracting the conjugated estrogens obtained from the urine of pregnant Canadian women and became commercially available in 1933. Emmenin could not be made fast enough to keep up with market demand, so it soon became clear that there was a need for a more potent, better smelling, estrogen preparation with a lower production cost. Consequently, attention was turned to other potential mammalian sources.

Researchers in Germany studied the urine of all mammals in the Berlin zoo and reported that the urine of pregnant equines (zebras and horses) included significant quantities of potent, water-soluble, conjugated estrogens. This discovery led to the production of conjugated equine estrogen, and Premarin was born. Its name is a clever shortened version of *pre*gnant *ma*re u*rin*e (Premarin). When the FDA approved the use of Premarin in 1942, it was meant to treat menopausal symptoms associated with the reduced production of estrogen by the ovaries. If a woman had her ovaries removed during a complete hysterectomy, then Premarin was given to her postoperatively.

By the mid-20th century, for the first time in human history, large populations of women were living decades beyond their childbearing years, so the incidence of cardiovascular disease and osteoporosis in postmenopausal women was increasing substantially. With the intent of preventing osteoporosis-related fractures and cardiovascular events following menopause, while also simultaneously alleviating bothersome menopausal symptoms, hormone replacement use increased throughout the 1950s.

In 1966, in his book Feminine Forever, Brooklyn gynecologist, Robert A. Wilson, MD, proselytized that estrogen replacement therapy could accomplish more than menopausal symptom relief for women. It could reverse the bodily changes typical of middle age, and it would restore a woman's sexual function. An estrogen-rich woman's "breasts and genital organs will not shrivel. She will be much more pleasant to live with and will not become dull and unattractive."

Micronized estradiol (Estrace), where soy-derived bioidentical estradiol is made into tiny crystals for better oral absorption, did not become available until the early 1980s; meanwhile, conjugated equine estrogen (Premarin) was galloping along as the premier estrogen replacement therapy for menopausal women. Premarin was widely marketed as a "completely natural estrogen complex," showing women in a highly glamorized light, surrounded by handsome men, happy families, and having fun. As part of "upscale" menopause therapy, estrogen replacement was considered a panacea for aging skin, thinning hair, and declining libido.

In the mid-1970s, after studies found that giving women estrogen-only increased their risk of uterine cancer, progestin was added to their estrogen replacement therapy. The same problem of inadequate intestinal absorption linked to bioidentical oral estradiol was found with bioidentical oral progesterone, as well. A synthetic progesterone substitute, an oral progestin, was coupled to Premarin estrogen therapy, usually medroxyprogesterone (Provera). Effective bioidentical oral micronized progesterone, (Prometrium), which is made from peanut oil, did not become available until 1998.

The Womens Health Initiative (WHI) hormone trial, which used the combination conjugated equine estrogen (Premarin) with the synthetic progestin, medroxyprogesterone (Provera), known as Prempro, was launched back in 1991. It was well on its way long before the advent of FDA-approved, pharmaceutical grade, bioidentical progesterone.

By the 1990s, menopause hormone therapy using either the estrogen-plus-progestin combination found in Prempro, or in the case of a woman who has had a hysterectomy, Premarin only, became the principal medical therapy for bothersome menopausal symptoms. Furthermore, based on data from epidemiologic observational studies, menopause hormone therapy was being prescribed to older postmenopausal women as treatment for established heart disease and osteoporosis. From the 1960s through the mid-1990s, research and clinical trials on menopausal women revealed that, overall, menopause hormone therapy decreased a woman's risk for heart disease by 50%, and also reduced her risk of osteoporosis-related fractures by 50%. These were truly impressive reductions in debilitating and deadly diseases.

OBSERVATION vs. RANDOMIZATION

When it comes to evaluating menopause hormone therapy, observational studies involve collecting and analyzing populations of women who choose to use or choose not use hormones. By observing and recording data over many years, observational studies reveal an association between activities, but they do not establish a direct cause-and-effect.

To establish the effectiveness of a medication, eliminate potential biases, and provide information about side effects, a randomized control trial (RCT) is considered the gold standard of clinical studies. People are allocated at random (by chance) to either receive a trial medication or a placebo (sugar pill). What happens to the people receiving the medication is then compared to the control group (the people receiving the placebo). Data is collated, statistically analyzed, and a conclusion is drawn as to whether there is a possibility of a direct cause-and-effect relationship between the medication and treatment goals.

Over the past 15 years more randomized controlled trials (RCTs) have come along to establish a direct cause-and-effect, whether good, bad or indifferent, between menopause hormone therapy and its impact on major causes of morbidity and mortality in postmenopausal women. Because trial participants in clinical research trials may not represent the patient population as a whole, some results from randomized control trials (RCTs) cannot be applied and generally spread across all individuals. For example, in the landmark Women's Health Initiative (WHI) menopause hormone therapy trials, women suffering from bothersome hot flashes and night sweats were excluded from participating in the study. Since 85% of menopausal women suffer from hot flashes, the women selected for participation in the WHI study may not have been representative of the general population, at large.

In 2002 and 2004, the WHI's principal results of traditional menopause hormone therapy in healthy postmenopausal women were published. Considerable media publicity and fanfare surrounded the investigators' stunning conclusions regarding estrogen replacement therapy in menopausal women. Although all women between the ages of 50 to 79 were collectively painted with the same broad hormonal brush, WHI's sensationalized results effectively cast doubt on the purpose and safety of menopause hormone therapy.

WHI revealed that when a large group of asymptomatic menopausal women between the ages of 50 to 79 were all given the exact same dose and preparation of hormones, specifically conjugated equine estrogen (Premarin) with or without the synthetic progestin, medroxyprogesterone (Provera), there were some benefits to hormone therapy, but there were some adverse outcomes, as well. In particular, strokes, blood clots, and increased dementia occurred more often in older women, who were at least a decade beyond menopause when they embarked on hormone therapy. Younger, freshly menopausal women did not sustain these risks. Surprisingly, estrogen-only did not increase a postmenopausal woman's risk of breast cancer; however, coupling estrogen replacement with a synthetic progestin increased her risk of breast cancer slightly. Subsequent well-designed clinical trials showed that other types of progesterone do not carry this same slight increased risk.

The WHI trial's overall negative assessment regarding hormone therapy rocked the world of menopausal women and their health care providers. Estrogen replacement therapy was dramatically, and mistakenly, abandoned on an unprecedented scale. Subsequently, further analysis took a closer look at WHI's participant profile, their conclusions were stratified according to the postmenopausal women's ages, and relevance to type and timing of hormone replacement were considered. Eventually, and in particular amongst those specialists with a clinical focus on menopausal women's health care, estrogen replacement therapy rose up from its ashes to its proper place as the safest and most effective health maintenance strategy for menopausal women. Nothing takes care of a menopausal woman like estrogen.

The most biologically accurate method for addressing any hormone deficiency is by replacing the deficient hormone appropriately. This is the universal standard of care with respect to any glandular problem, whether it is thyroid hormone deficiency, adrenal hormone deficiency, insulin deficiency in diabetics, or growth hormone deficiency. And, for all forms of hormone therapy, the type and dose of the hormone that is replaced is individualized and well-orchestrated for each patient. We now know this holds true for menopausal hormone therapy, as well. Appropriately timed and properly managed menopause replacement therapy is pivotal to preserving a woman's naturally safe and holistically healthy connection to estrogen.

ESTROGEN RECEPTORS – HERE, THERE and EVERYWHERE

Estrogen is here, there and everywhere in a woman's body. Not only is estrogen responsible for a woman's feminine characteristics, sexuality and reproductive capabilities, estrogen has a positive impact on her cardiovascular health, bone formation, brain function, bladder integrity, skin aging, and many other organ systems. Although estrogen was discovered in the 1920s, it would be decades before estrogen receptors were identified. Estrogen receptor-alpha (ER-alpha) was recognized in the late 1950s, and estrogen receptor-beta (ER-beta) in the 1990s. Deciphering the lock and key mechanism of hormone action opened the door to improving our appreciation of how estrogen influences over 400 functions in a woman's body.

Ovarian follicles/oocytes (eggs) produce estrogen, which is secreted directly into the bloodstream. Hitching a ride on its sex hormone binding globulin (SHBG), estrogen travels through the bloodstream to reach its target organ. Upon reaching its destination, estrogen disembarks from its SHBG and hooks up with an estrogen receptor in the cell. When estrogen binds to its receptor, this union influences cellular mechanisms, regulates tissue activity and coordinates organ function.

Estrogen receptors are widely distributed throughout a woman's body and are found in tissues well beyond the reach of her breasts or reproductive system. ER-alpha receptors are more prevalent in her reproductive organs and liver, and ER-beta receptors are more commonly found in her heart, blood vessels, kidneys, bladder, lungs, skin, bone and gastrointestinal tract. The brain, breasts, and ovaries contain both ER-alpha's and ER-beta's. From head-to-toe, a woman needs estrogen for her physical, mental, sexual and spiritual health and happiness.

A woman reaching her 50s today can expect to live into her 80s and beyond. Extended longevity opens up a lot of doors to age-related changes and diseases that were not experienced when a woman's average life expectancy was only 49 years. Nature had not planned for a woman to survive beyond her reproductive years, so although life expectancy has increased dramatically, menopause and ovarian failure still occur around age 51. Women are simply outliving their ovaries. Of course, as outliers on the bell curve of life expectancy, there were a few women who made it to their 70s and 80s in the past, but the widespread occurrence of populations of women spending a third of their lives in an estrogen-deprived state is a relatively new phenomenon in human history.

It is no longer a question of how long a woman will survive, but how well she lives out her senior years that's at stake. Will those years truly be golden, as she lives an active and independent lifestyle? Or, will her existence be marred by dementia, incontinence, and debility, as she's languishing in a nursing home somewhere? Just because a woman stops having menstrual cycles, and she isn't reproducing, it does not automatically follow that her body no longer needs estrogen to help her non-reproductive organs. Since a woman is far more than the sum of her breasts and genitals, health-sustaining benefits of estrogen go well beyond sexual reproduction. Estrogen receptors exist in nearly all tissues throughout a woman's body, from her brain to her Achilles' tendons and everywhere in between. Estrogen maintains tissue architecture and organ stability before, during and after menopause.

USE IT or LOSE IT

Estrogen receptors need estrogen to stay alive. Consistent with the "use it, or you lose it" phenomenon, once estrogen is withdrawn, tissues and organs throughout a menopausal body start losing estrogen receptors. If hormone therapy is delayed a decade or more after menopause, there are fewer estrogen receptors left for estrogen to lock onto. Embarking on hormone therapy at this point will not recoup what a woman has already lost. Estrogen-deprived and receptor-depleted, a woman's tissues are now in disrepair, organs are malfunctioning, and diseases have taken root. It takes 10 to 15 years of estrogen deprivation for permanent damage to occur in the heart and brain's blood vessels, so the majority (80%) of heart attacks and strokes in women occur at least a decade after menopause.

The 10 to 15 years' lag between menopause and when debility and death creep in explains one of the disparate findings of the Women's Health Initiative (WHI) study. Amongst the WHI participants, a history of having had surgical removal of both ovaries was not associated with significantly increased risks of fatal heart attacks, heart disease or strokes. Upon closer inspection of the participants and analysis of the raw data, this paradox is understandable.

The women in the WHI analysis were on average 63 years old when they enrolled in the study, and follow-up data collection began decades after most of these women had undergone removal of their ovaries. There was a built-in survival bias to the WHI participants. Women who had already died of estrogen-deprivation did not live long enough to enroll in the WHI study, and half of the women participating in the WHI hormone therapy trial had been on estrogen replacement therapy prior to enrolling in the WHI study. The study's 7.6 years follow-up did not allow enough time to capture adverse events that may not happen until 10 to 15 years of estrogen deprivation have transpired.

Unfortunately, women less than 50 years old who have both of their ovaries surgically removed and are rendered menopausal have a 40% increase in all-cause mortality. Women without estrogen die younger than their well-estrogenized counterparts. Estrogen-deprived women experience more heart disease, strokes, dementia, Parkinsonism, diabetes, osteoporosis, anxiety, and depression, compared to same-aged women who are well-estrogenized. The clinical reality is that for women who are menopausal prior to age 50, life without estrogen is fraught with chronic diseases and accelerated decline.

What about a woman who becomes menopausal after 50 years old? Well, she now exists in the arid and tissue-damaging tundra of estrogen deficiency. Just because she's older when she loses her ovarian hormones does not mean she needs to struggle through the last few decades of her life bearing the brunt of estrogen deficiency. Although she may be a grandmother and no longer producing children of her own, her non-reproductive organs still function better with estrogen.

Without estrogen's head-to-toe protection, a woman's mind and body dry out, break down, and wither away. Her skin wrinkles, her hair thins, her eyes deteriorate, her teeth fall out, her brain cells knot and tangle, arteries supplying her heart and brain harden and narrow from calcified plaques, her bladder leaks, her vagina dries, her joints creak and brittle bones break. Her metabolism slows down, and she packs on unhealthy abdominal (visceral) fat. Sexual desire and pleasantries are distant memories. This sounds dismal.

… And then, along comes menopause hormone therapy…

Relieved of hot flashes, night sweats, and vaginal dryness, a menopausal woman looks and feels better with her female hormones. Although estrogen is not the fountain of youth, it definitely slows down tissue degradation and organ deterioration amplified by estrogen deficiency. Aging is far more pleasant and attractive with custom-tailored menopause hormone replacement therapy.

The "one size fits all" dress is not flattering on anyone, and replacing hormones of any kind should not be a "one dose fits all" prescription, either. In fact, administering the same dose and formula of female hormones to women spanning across a wide range of ages is not a biologically correct method of managing any type of hormone replacement therapy. Thyroid hormone replacement dosing is tailored to each individual. Insulin hormone therapy for diabetics varies from patient to patient. The standard clinical practice of individualization and monitoring applied to the treatment of other types of hormone deficiency should also be extended to the management of female hormone replacement in menopausal women.

Women who experience menopause prior to age 45 usually need higher doses of estrogen to reach adequate physiological replacement levels. Some women also need a touch of testosterone replacement to make up for the 50% drop in testosterone levels precipitated by ovarian failure. Women's bodies produce less than one-tenth the testosterone men manufacture, so just a little bit goes a long way in menopausal women. Once a woman turns 50, adjustments to her hormone replacement therapy can be made for age-appropriate dosing.

Because aging kidneys and the older liver are not as efficient at metabolizing and detoxifying medications, standard clinical practice dictates that lower doses of medicine be prescribed to elderly patients. When a woman reaches her mid-60s, to reduce her risk of strokes and blood clots, step-down reductions and alterations to her hormone dosing, as well adding low-dose aspirin, and depending on her cholesterol levels, a smidge of statin, to her "geripause cocktail," safely maintains hormone harmony throughout her senior years.

Menopause marks the universal crossroads at which point a woman chooses how she wants to live with ovarian failure. Although a woman can exist without estrogen, the real issue is what kind of life will she experience as years of ovarian hormone deficiency unravel. Quality of life is an important consideration, not only during her freshly menopausal years, but throughout her older, geripausal years, as well. Within the historical realm of women's existence, hormone health beyond menopause is a relatively new concept. Fortunately, properly orchestrated hormone replacement therapy weaves a healthy and holistic tapestry of dignified aging for menopausal women of all ages.

GLANDS, GLANDS, GLANDS

Love makes the world go round, and glands make it all happen by powering up hormones. A gland is a group of cells or an organ that produces and secretes chemicals. There are two types of glands, exocrine and endocrine. Exocrine glands release their secretions into ducts or channels that deliver the chemicals to specific areas. Sweat glands release secretions in the skin, salivary glands release their juices inside the mouth, and a woman's breast produces milk delivered to the baby. Endocrine glands, on the other hand, release more than 20 hormones directly into the bloodstream. These hormones are then transported to tissues in other parts of the body. The hypothalamus, pituitary, thyroid, pancreas, adrenal, ovaries and testicles are hormone-producing endocrine glands.

Derived from the Greek word *hormon*, meaning "to set in motion" or "to arouse or excite," hormones are the body's chemical messengers. A hormone is a molecule that travels through the bloodstream to affect other tissues and organs in the body. This petite marvel packs a big punch when it locks onto a receptor site in the target tissue, and then triggers the tissue's response to the hormone's directive. Some of these messengers work on tissue-specific target cells while others work throughout the body. Hormones regulate sexual development, reproduction, childbirth, lactation, digestion, metabolism, and the immune system. Hormones are also involved with temperature regulation, bone integrity, growth and development, sleep/wake patterns, pain relief, fluid and electrolyte regulation and the production of red blood cells. There are many other life-sustaining actions of hormones, so these chemical messengers are essential to one's survival.

The amount of hormones secreted by the glands in the body needs to be maintained at healthy levels. If hormone levels climb too high or fall too low, the person gets sick. How does the body accomplish all this? Well, like so many things connected to human existence, it all starts with our brain.

HYPOTHALAMUS

The endocrine hormone system's central command station is the hypothalamic-pituitary connection located in the basement of the brain. The hypothalamus links the brain and endocrine system to make it all happen-feedings, feelings, and freedom. Located above the brainstem, the almond-sized hypothalamus is the portion of the brain that keeps the body's internal balances in working order. It maintains body temperature, heart rate, and blood pressure, as well as modulates thirst, hunger, sleep, sex drive, moods and circadian rhythms. As the hypothalamus receives signals from the brain and interprets metabolic indicators, it triggers the pituitary to release or withhold stimulating hormones to the rest of the glands in the body.

The thermal neutral zone within the hypothalamus is the body's thermostat. It ensures that the body temperature remains stable regardless of ambient or room temperature. Menopausal-related hot flashes, night sweats, heat waves or cold sweats are due to estrogen withdrawal disrupting the thermostat mechanism in a woman's hypothalamus. This triggers the pituitary to release hormones that cause physiological responses to either cool the body, by increasing blood flow through the skin's capillaries and sweating, or increase body heat, through shivering and reducing blood flow to the skin.

PITUITARY

The pea-sized pituitary gland is a protrusion off the bottom of the hypothalamus, so communications between the "higher power" hypothalamus and the pituitary gland are tightly connected. Located behind the bridge of the nose in the central base of the skull, the pituitary is the only gland housed in its own protective bony enclosure. Because of the bone's resemblance to a Turkish saddle, this enclosure is named the sella turcica. As the "master gland," the pituitary helps maintain the body's overall functioning by secreting hormones that stimulate other endocrine glands to secrete their hormones. Every vertebrate, that is, every creature with a backbone, has a pituitary gland masterminding the endocrine system.

The pituitary delegates tasks by secreting over a dozen hormones and chemicals. It secretes thyroid stimulating hormone (TSH), follicle stimulating hormone (FSH), luteinizing hormone (LH), adrenocorticotrophic hormone (ACTH), growth hormone (GH), antidiuretic hormone (ADH), also known as vasopressin, melanocyte stimulating hormone (MSH), prolactin and oxytocin. The pituitary also produces endorphins, which are chemicals involved with pain relief. Possessing morphine-like effects, endorphins are also involved in natural reward circuits such as drinking, eating, sex and parental behavior.

OXYTOCIN

Oxytocin is a hormone manufactured by the hypothalamus of the brain, and then stored and released by the pituitary gland. Oxytocin stimulates uterine contractions during childbirth, triggers the release of milk during breastfeeding, and promotes bonding between individuals. During the first few weeks of lactation, oxytocin release during breastfeeding causes uterine contractions that help the uterus involute back into its non-pregnant smaller size.

Dubbed the "cuddle hormone," oxytocin is released during hugging, touching and sexual arousal in both sexes. Although both genders produce oxytocin, women produce the hormone in larger quantities than men. It is thought to play a role in monogamous pair bonding, as well as deepening attachment between mother and child. It enhances social relaxation by inducing trust between people.

Oxytocin is destroyed in the intestinal tract, so it must be given intravenously or via nasal spray. Synthetic oxytocin is sold under the trade name Pitocin, and when obstetrically needed, it is used to facilitate childbirth and prevent post-partum hemorrhage. The body degrades oxytocin very quickly, so it administered as a continuous intravenous (IV) drip to stimulate uterine contractions during labor and delivery. When given intravenously, it does not cross the blood-brain barrier, so it cannot enter the brain in any significant quantity.

VASOPRESSIN (ANTIDIURETIC HORMONE)

Vasopressin (antidiuretic hormone) is another hormone manufactured by the hypothalamus, and then stored and released by the pituitary gland. As an antidiuretic hormone, it helps retain water in the body and constricts blood vessels to maintain blood pressure. Very similar in chemical structure to oxytocin, vasopressin is also released directly into the brain after sex. Dubbed the "monogamy molecule," vasopressin is involved in producing long-term attachments in pair bonding. Interestingly, fear of commitment may be due in part from genetic variation in vasopressin receptors located in the reward centers of the brain.

PROLACTIN

As its name implies, the prolactin hormone's purpose is "pro-lactation." It is produced by the pituitary gland to promote milk production during pregnancy and breastfeeding. If a woman does not breastfeed her baby, then her prolactin level drops back down to pre-pregnancy levels.

An abnormal elevation in serum prolactin is known as hyperprolactinemia. Antidepressant medications, antipsychotic drugs, and narcotics reduce dopamine levels in the brain, and this leads to excess prolactin levels circulating in the body. An underactive or slow thyroid gland can cause elevated prolactin levels. Interestingly, chest wall surgery or trauma can increase prolactin, as well. Another cause of elevated prolactin levels is a prolactinoma, a benign tumor of the pituitary gland. 1 in 4 persons will develop a pituitary tumor in their lifetime. This pituitary growth may enlarge significantly, putting pressure on the optic nerve and causing headaches and visual disturbances.

Elevated prolactin hormone levels can cause irregular menstrual cycles, infertility, and galactorrhea. Galactorrhea occurs when a non-pregnant, non-breastfeeding woman experiences unwanted nipple leakage of breast milk.

Elevated prolactin levels can cause symptoms of estrogen deficiency in women and testosterone deficiency in men causing loss of sexual function and decreased libido. Abnormal prolactin elevation can be treated with dopamine-mimicking medications or surgical removal of the pituitary growths.

THYROID

The thyroid is a butterfly-shaped gland located in front of the neck just below the thyroid cartilage or "Adam's apple." Thyroid hormones control how quickly the body metabolizes calories, how the body makes proteins, and how sensitive the body is to other hormones. By influencing all the body processes that use energy, thyroid hormones impact every organ's growth and function. The thyroid gland plays a huge role in breathing, blood circulation, heart rate, body temperature, muscle control, digestion, bowel movements, menstrual cycles, and brain function. The thyroid gland's parafollicular cells produce a hormone called calcitonin, which helps control the levels of calcium in the blood. An imbalance of thyroid hormones can result in problems all over the body.

Thyroid hormone deficiency during embryonic development can lead to severely stunted physical and mental growth in the baby. Iodine is an essential trace element and is required for the synthesis of thyroid hormones. If a pregnant woman does not have enough iodine in her diet, her thyroid gland cannot produce thyroid hormones. Iodine deficiency is one of the most common, and easily preventable, causes of brain damage worldwide. Incidentally, the most common cause of brain damage in babies is alcohol intake by the mother during pregnancy, another totally preventable tragedy.

1 in 8 women will develop thyroid disease, and thyroid disease occurs far more frequently in women than in men. 80% of people with thyroid disease are women. The greater prevalence in women is not attributed directly to the hormonal effects of estrogen, since thyroid conditions can occur before puberty and long after menopause. Many times, however, thyroid malfunction reveals itself at times of major hormonal shifts in women: puberty, post-partum, and during menopause. There may be a genetic link, since a woman is more likely to develop thyroid problems if there is a family history of thyroid disease, and the prevalence of thyroid disease increases

with age. Starting at age 35, thyroid hormone blood tests should be done every 2 years, and when a woman reaches her 60s, her thyroid hormone levels should be checked annually.

Symptoms of menopause transition, such as fatigue, sleep disturbances, mood swings, forgetfulness, heat or cold intolerance, palpitations and altered menstrual cycles, can also reflect thyroid dysfunction, common in midlife women.

Hypothyroidism, a condition involving an underactive thyroid or not having enough thyroid hormone, is 5 times more common than hyperthyroidism, a condition where either an overactive thyroid is secreting too much thyroid hormones or there is too much thyroid hormone in a woman's system. Having excess thyroid hormone turns up the metabolism and body heat, leading to weight loss, heat intolerance, anxiety and nervousness. On the other hand, not enough thyroid hormone turns down metabolism, so one gains weight and feels cold, tired and depressed. Left untreated, either hypothyroidism or hyperthyroidism can be fatal.

HYPOTHYROIDISM

The signs and symptoms of hypothyroidism vary, depending on the severity of thyroid hormone deficiency. Problems tend to develop slowly, often over a number of years. Initially, a woman may attribute her fatigue and weight gain to simply getting older. But as her metabolism continues to slow down, other organ systems show signs of thyroid deficiency.

Increased sensitivity to cold, slowed heart rate, dry skin, thinning hair, puffy face, heavier uterine bleeding or irregular menstrual periods, hoarseness, constipation, muscle aches and weakness, stiffness and swelling in joints, elevated blood cholesterol, depression, slowing down of thought processes, and impaired memory can be symptoms of hypothyroidism. Meanwhile, due to persistent low levels of thyroid hormones, the pituitary gland increases its production and release of thyroid-stimulating hormone (TSH), which may lead to an enlarged thyroid gland (goiter).

Untreated hypothyroidism can progress to myxedema coma, a life-threatening situation that is typically seen in elderly women. Precipitated by an infection, medication, environmental exposure, or other physiological stressors, this foreboding condition requires potentially toxic doses of thyroid hormone replacement, and mortality rates exceed 20%, despite optimum therapy.

SUBCLINICAL HYPOTHYROIDISM

A healthy woman without signs or symptoms of thyroid disease who has an elevated blood serum thyroid-stimulating hormone (TSH) level and normal thyroid hormone concentrations may have subclinical (asymptomatic) hypothyroidism. Before making the diagnosis of subclinical hypothyroidism, repeat thyroid blood work should be done in 3 to 6 months for confirmation.

Subclinical hypothyroidism can be associated with an increased risk of heart disease, heart failure, and mortality. Treating a midlife woman with subclinical hypothyroidism is somewhat controversial, since even without treatment, there is a 50:50 chance her thyroid blood work will spontaneously normalize over the next 5 years. The presence of antithyroid peroxidase antibodies (TPOAb) in blood tests predicts progression of subclinical hypothyroidism to overt or symptomatic hypothyroidism.

If a woman's blood serum TSH is greater than 10 mIU/L, treatment with thyroid hormone is recommended. If her TSH level falls between 4 and 10 mIU/L, and she tests positive for the antithyroperoxidase antibodies (TPOAb+), then she should be considered for treatment, as well. Subclinical hypothyroidism usually does not require high doses of thyroid hormone replacement to achieve normal blood serum TSH levels. Treatment with 25 micrograms to 75 micrograms of thyroxine (T4) usually suffices.

THYROID plus ESTROGEN

If a menopausal woman starts oral estrogen therapy, her thyroid hormone replacement dose may need to be increased. Oral estrogens, but not transdermal estrogens (estrogen patches, topical gels or sprays), increase the liver's production of thyroid-binding globulin (TBG). The thyroid-binding globulin (TBG) ties up thyroid hormones, which reduces the amount of free thyroid hormone in the circulation, so thyroid doses may need to be calibrated accordingly.

Thyroid hormone replacement therapy for hypothyroidism is usually life-long, and doses are adjusted according to regularly monitored blood hormone levels.

HYPERTHYROIDISM

Hyperthyroidism, either due to an overactive thyroid gland, a thyroid cyst or a thyroid hormone producing tumor, or even from ingesting too much thyroid hormone, can also present with a variety of signs and symptoms that may be confused with other medical conditions. These include weight loss, increased appetite, rapid heart rate, palpitations or irregular heartbeat, heat intolerance, sweating, nervousness, anxiety and irritability, tremors, difficulty sleeping, thinning skin, fine, brittle hair, irregular menstrual bleeding, and changes in bowel patterns, especially more frequent bowel movements. All this thyroid hormone overdrive can lead to an enlarged thyroid gland (goiter), fatigue and weakness.

Elderly women with hyperthyroidism are more likely to have either no signs of excess thyroid hormone or manifest subtle symptoms, such as an increased heart rate, heat intolerance, and a tendency to become overly tired during ordinary activities.

GRAVE'S DISEASE

Grave's disease is an immune system disorder that leads to overproduction of thyroid hormones. Although Grave's disease can affect anyone, it is more common in women less than 40 years old. Treatment is usually with radioactive iodine pills or anti-thyroid medication that interferes with the thyroid gland's use of iodine to produce hormones.

Smokers with Grave's disease are at increased risk of developing exophthalmos, a condition where the eyeballs protrude beyond their normal protective orbits. This occurs when there is an abnormal deposition of connective tissue components into the orbit cavity fat and muscles of the eyeball. Since the skull's orbit housing the eyeball is closed off by bone at the back and to the right and left sides of the eye socket, any enlargement of eyeball structures within the orbit will push the eyeball forward. This prevents the eyelids from closing during sleep leading to corneal dryness and damage. Patients may require orbital radiation or decompressing eye surgery to alleviate pressure symptoms and prevent blindness.

HASHIMOTO'S (AUTOIMMUNE) THYROIDITIS

Hashimoto's thyroiditis, also known as chronic lymphocytic thyroiditis, is an autoimmune disease in which the thyroid gland is attacked, and eventually destroyed by the body's own immune system. Hashimoto's thyroiditis is 10 times more common in women than men, usually manifests between ages 40 to 60, and often there is a family history of thyroid issues or other autoimmune diseases.

When inflammatory flare-ups destroy the integrity of thyroid hormone storage within the thyroid gland, excess thyroid hormones may periodically flood a woman's system. As the disease progresses, there may be intermittent bouts of symptomatic hyperthyroidism. The thyroid gland becomes firm and enlarged due to immune cells infiltrating the thyroid gland and scarring from inflammation.

Diagnostic testing involves blood levels for anti-thyroid peroxidase antibodies (TPOAbs), anti-thyroglobulin antibodies, anti-microsomal antibodies, as well as the usual blood work for thyroid function, such as thyroid-stimulating hormone (TSH) and thyroid hormone levels. Eventually, thyroid function is totally compromised, the thyroid gland scars down, and the woman will require lifelong thyroid hormone replacement therapy.

THYROID & OVARY

One percent of all ovarian tumors are an unusual type of dermoid cyst known as struma ovarii. This rare ovarian tumor, usually benign but malignant change can occur in about a third of the cases, is defined by the presence of thyroid tissue compromising more than 50% of the overall mass of the ovary. This ovarian-thyroid tissue tumor can produce excess thyroid hormones, and due to its potential for malignancy, surgical removal of the involved ovary is recommended.

THYROID & BONE

If there is too much of either of the thyroid hormones, triiodothyronine (T3) or thyroxine/tetraiodothyronine (T4), in a woman's system, she is at higher risk for bone-thinning diseases such as osteopenia and osteoporosis. When too much thyroid hormone is around, the bones are subjected to more bone remodeling cycles. After age 30, every bone remodeling cycle is inefficient, so more bone mass is lost than gained with each round. The more bone cycles a woman goes through; the more bone mass is lost.

THYROID & HEART

Women with hyperthyroidism may not be diagnosed with their thyroid condition until they present to the emergency room with heart palpitations, "heart racing" or an irregular heartbeat. Many times, the cardiac arrhythmia known as atrial fibrillation (A Fib) shows up on their electrocardiogram (EKG). As part of every woman's evaluation of a cardiac event, thyroid hormone levels should be checked to make sure her thyroid is functioning normally.

Treatment for hyperthyroidism depends on the cause of excess thyroid hormones. Therapies include radioactive ablation of the abnormal thyroid tissue, medications that interfere with thyroid hormone synthesis, or surgical removal of the thyroid or thyroid hormone generating tumor. Some of these treatment modalities may result in permanent hypothyroidism, so the patient is then placed on lifelong thyroid hormone replacement therapy. Oral levothyroxine, (Synthroid, T4) and liothyronine (Cytomel, T3) are FDA- approved, pharmaceutical-grade bioidentical thyroid replacement hormones, so their chemical structures are identical to the hormones produced naturally by the human thyroid gland.

PANCREAS

Located behind the stomach in the abdomen, the pancreas is an organ that is part of both the digestive system and the endocrine system. As a digestive organ, it secretes pancreatic juice containing digestive enzymes that help breakdown food and help with the absorption of nutrients in the small intestine. It is also an endocrine gland producing the hormones, insulin, and glucagon, which are critical to balancing sugars in the body.

When we eat, carbohydrates are broken down into sugar and enter the bloodstream in the form of glucose. Glucose is the body's source of energy for everything it does, from thinking and working to exercising and sitting. In response to elevated blood sugar, the pancreas responds by secreting insulin. Insulin helps glucose enter cells throughout the body. Any excess blood sugar not taken up by the cells is then stored in the liver in the form of glycogen. Between meals, when blood sugar decreases, the pancreas releases glucagon to stimulate the liver to breakdown its glycogen and release glucose back into the bloodstream for cells to use. This insulin-glucagon hormone duo complements each other and maintains blood sugar levels within a healthy narrow range.

If the pancreas does not produce insulin (type 1 diabetes) or the body has become resistant to insulin's action (type 2 diabetes), glucose stays in the bloodstream, raising blood sugar levels (hyperglycemia). Without insulin to ferry glucose into the body's cells, cells starve and die, despite being bathed by elevated levels of glucose in the bloodstream. A constant stream of glucose is so vital to brain function that the brain is one of the few tissues in the human body that does not require insulin to transport glucose into its cells. Glucose gets a free pass into brain cells.

When blood sugars are either too low or way too high, a person can go into a diabetic coma. Over time, hyperglycemia can permanently damage nerves and blood vessels causing blindness, heart attacks, strokes, kidney failure, infections, numbness, anorgasmia, poor wound healing, and amputations.

ADRENALS

A triangular walnut-sized adrenal gland sits on top of each kidney and produces hormones that affect a variety of bodily functions. The adrenals generate corticosteroid hormones, such as glucocorticoids (cortisol and corticosterone) and mineralocorticoids (aldosterone). These hormones influence the body's immune system, metabolism, and fluid and electrolyte balance. The adrenals also produce the androgen hormones dehydroepiandrosterone (DHEA), androstenedione and testosterone.

PERIPHERAL CONVERSION

DHEA and androstenedione travel to adipose (fatty) tissue, muscles, bone marrow, and the brain, where aromatase enzymes can convert these androgens to testosterone and estrogen. The aromatase enzymes can go on to convert testosterone to even more estrogen. This process, where one hormone is converted to another hormone, beyond the borders of the original gland's anatomical site, is known as "peripheral conversion." All this peripheral conversion of androgens to estrogen by aromatase enzymes housed in adipose (fatty) tissue explains why folks carrying excess body fat are walking around with way too much estrogen, and suboptimal levels of testosterone, in their system.

In times of stress, the adrenals secrete the fight or flight hormones cortisol, adrenalin (epinephrine) and norepinephrine. Cortisol stimulates the release of glucose into the bloodstream. Adrenalin and norepinephrine are released in response to stimulation by sympathetic nerves. They increase heart rate, boost respiratory rate, and airway diameters in the lungs are increased so that more oxygen can be taken in. To allow for fight or flight, blood flow is shunted towards the large skeletal muscles to run and climb, and less blood is sent to internal organs, like the bowel or spleen. All this redirecting is helpful in times of acute or short-term stresses when revved up systems improve focused performance.

Chronic stress, on the other hand, causes sustained elevations in these fight or flight hormones, and this is physiologically problematic. Chronically elevated cortisol levels cause weight gain, diabetes, high blood pressure, infections, fatigue, immune system malfunctions, thinning skin, stretch marks, moodiness and muscle weakness. Without adrenal hormones, a person will die. On the other hand, sustained elevation of any of the adrenal hormones will damage organs.

PINEAL GLAND

Named for its shape resembling a pinecone, the pineal gland is the size of an apple seed, and it is located in the center of the brain. Unlike the rest of the brain, the pineal gland is not isolated from the rest of the body's circulation by the blood-brain barrier. The pineal gland handles the synthesis and secretion of the melatonin hormone.

Melatonin maintains the body's circadian rhythm (sleep-wake cycle), regulates the onset of puberty, and helps protect the body from oxidative cell damage caused by free radicals. In cases where the pineal gland is severely damaged in children, the result is precocious puberty. Melatonin production is stimulated by darkness and inhibited by light, so blind individuals have higher levels of melatonin than sighted individuals. Women who work the "graveyard shift," or cope with night shifts alternating with dayshift work, have lower melatonin levels than their 9 to 5 working counterparts. Lower melatonin levels have been linked to a higher risk of breast cancer in women working these physiologically challenging nightshifts.

Menopausal women have lower melatonin levels, and this may hamper their ability to fall sleep and stay asleep. Calcification of the pineal gland is typical in adults and can be visualized on plain film X-rays. The degree of calcification is significantly higher in patients with Alzheimer's disease compared to other types of dementia.

GONADS – OVARIES & TESTICLES

The hypothalamus of the brain produces GnRH (gonadotropin-releasing hormone), which regulates the pituitary gland's production of FSH (follicle-stimulating hormone) and LH (luteinizing hormone), which regulate the function of ovaries and testicles. Ovaries in females are analogous to testicles in males, in that both function as gonads and endocrine glands. As gonads, they both produce cells for sexual reproduction (gametes). The ovaries maintain follicles/oocytes (eggs) and the testicles produce sperm. When these gametes meet, conception occurs.

As endocrine glands, the ovaries and testicles produce sex hormones that are secreted directly into the bloodstream. The ovary produces estrogen, progesterone, and testosterone, and the testicles produce testosterone and a bit of estrogen. The sex hormones, estrogen, and testosterone, initiate puberty and maintain gender-specific sexual characteristics, such as body shape, muscle mass, facial hair and fertility. Progesterone, the "pro-gestation or pro-pregnancy" hormone prepares and maintains a woman's uterus and breasts for pregnancy.

Low testosterone or "low T" is damaging to men. This condition is also known as "male menopause" or "andropause," and clinically, it is diagnosed as "male hypogonadism" or androgen deficiency. It is considered a medical condition requiring testosterone hormone replacement, regardless of the man's age. Obviously men do not have a final menstrual period marking a clear-cut signpost that their hormone of masculinity has dropped. Androgen or testosterone deficiency in men emerges more gradually. In the normally developing male, testosterone peaks during early adulthood. Once he reaches age 30, testosterone levels naturally decline 1 to 2% a year. 50% of men over the age of 50 have low testosterone levels, a condition marked by blood testosterone levels below 300 ng/dL.

Produced primarily by the testicles, testosterone is a hormone required for male development and reproduction capacity. During puberty, testosterone helps define a man's androgenic qualities, such as increased height, muscle mass, facial and chest hair, and deeper voice. It also influences the male pattern of fat distribution, bone density, and red blood cell production. Testosterone sustains a man's energy level, mental focus, and positive mood. Sperm production, sex drive and performance are fueled by testosterone.

Testicular trauma, surgery, radiation, mumps, or medications used to treat metastatic prostate cancer, precipitate a dramatic drop in testosterone levels. When a man suddenly loses testicular function, he will experience thermostat turmoil, similar to the hot flashes and night sweats that plague menopausal women. Obesity, diabetes, liver or kidney disease, HIV/AIDS, pituitary growths, prescription medications and recreational drugs also cause testosterone levels to drift downwards.

Testosterone is converted to estrogen in fat cells, so overweight and obese men have way too much estrogen flooding their system. All this surplus estrogen drowns out their testosterone. Excess estrogen can cause undesirable breast development in men (gynecomastia). Statins lower cholesterol and cholesterol is the fundamental building block for all male and female sex hormones. Overzealous statin therapy can lower testosterone levels in men, as well as lower estrogen levels in women. Alcohol, anabolic steroids, smoking or marijuana, undermine testosterone levels. Antidepressants, antipsychotic medicines, and narcotics increase the pituitary gland's secretion of prolactin. Prolactin stimulates breast milk production. This can result in unwelcome galactorrhea in a man taking any of these medications. In men, elevated prolactin levels can also suppress testicular function resulting in low testosterone levels, reduced sperm counts, and infertility. In women, elevated prolactin levels suppress ovarian function, as well, resulting in low estrogen levels, vaginal dryness, irregular menstrual periods, and infertility.

Regardless of the cause for male hypogonadism, symptoms of declining or low testosterone levels in men include erectile dysfunction, decreased libido, infertility, decreased beard and body hair, decreased muscle mass with decreased physical strength, increased body fat, difficulty concentrating, decreased motivation, depression, sleep disturbances and thinning bones. Prolonged testosterone deficiency increases a man's risk for heart disease, diabetes, and osteoporosis. Men with lower testosterone levels die sooner than men with normal levels of testosterone. For improved quality of life and overall healthier functioning, long-term testosterone replacement therapy is recommended for men with low testosterone levels.

Similar to how low testosterone is considered damaging to a man and warrants clinical attention with appropriate testosterone replacement therapy, estrogen deficiency due to female hypogonadism or ovarian hormone deficiency is just as detrimental to a menopausal woman and deserves the same clinical focus to appropriate estrogen replacement therapy. Sex hormones do far more than provoke the desire to ride the universal merry go round of meeting and mating. Along the way, they keep the individual healthy, happy, and dancing to the beat of life's passion for love and vitality.

OVARIES – Quality over Quantity

Everything menopausal begins and ends with a woman's ovaries, her gonads. Ovaries are two small organs located in a woman's pelvis, one on either side of the uterus near the open end of the fallopian tubes. In a healthy young woman, each ovary is about the size of a chestnut. As a woman gets older and ovarian function declines, the ovaries decrease in size. Menopausal ovaries are the size of almonds. As the years go by after menopause, ovaries atrophy and shrink down to the size of pine nuts.

Ovaries are the main source of sex hormones that control the development of female body characteristics, such as breasts, body shape and body hair. Estrogen is also responsible for the maturation and maintenance of reproductive organs in their functional state. Progesterone prepares the uterus for pregnancy and the breasts for lactation. Estrogen and progesterone work together to synchronize menstrual cycle changes in the endometrial lining of the uterus. Testosterone enhances estrogen's effects on bone density and sexuality. Ovaries produce 50% of the testosterone found in a woman's body. A woman's level of testosterone is usually one-tenth of a man's.

Astonishingly, a woman's ovaries start aging before she's even born. The greatest number of ovarian follicles/oocytes (eggs) a woman ever possesses occurs while she's still in her mother's womb. A woman is born with all the follicles/oocytes (eggs) she will ever have, and this pool of eggs will never be replenished. At 16-20 weeks of pregnancy, the ovaries of a female fetus contain 6 million eggs. By the time a baby girl is born, her number of eggs has decreased to 2 million. When puberty occurs around age 12, the number of eggs has further decreased to 300,000. By the time a woman enters her thirties, the number of eggs has dropped down to 30,000. Spanning forty years of a woman's reproductive lifetime, only around 450 eggs will mature and be released for potential fertilization. All the other eggs will have degenerated over time as part of a natural process called atresia.

In contrast to a woman's ever-declining egg count, with the onset of puberty, a man's testicles are perpetually producing sperm. Testicles are non-stop sperm-producing factories, generating 100 million sperm per day, week after week, month after month, and year after year. Although quantity and quality of sperm decline with age, until a man dies his aging testicles still produce sperm. Postmortem sperm retrieval of viable and fertile sperm can be harvested up to 36 hours after death.

As women age, they experience a decline in ovarian performance leading to menopause. Dwindling ovarian reserves diminish at a constantly increasing rate, and finally ovarian supplies collapse. When the ovarian follicle bearing the last egg ovulates, there are no more eggs for the ovary to nurture and prepare for potential conception. Menstrual cycles stop, and a woman can no longer get pregnant naturally. For most women, their final menstrual period occurs between ages 46 to 56, on average at age 51.

Once the ovaries are depleted of their eggs, they no longer produce adequate amounts of female hormones, either. The end of a woman's reproductive capability marks the beginning of her ovarian hormone deficiency. Just because her ovaries are programmed for reproductive obsolescence, a woman should not suffer from damages inflicted by ovarian hormone deficiency. A woman's mind, body, and spirit still need estrogen to continue functioning optimally. When menopause arrives, it's time for appropriately managed female hormone replacement therapy. Not only does well-orchestrated estrogen replacement alleviate menopausal symptoms, but it also slows down the aging process by curbing tissue destruction and organ malfunction exacerbated by estrogen deficiency.

DANCING with HORMONES

With the dawn of sexual maturity, a woman's ovaries not only supply oo-cytes/eggs for pregnancy and motherhood, but her ovaries also generate hormones that profoundly affect her mind, body and spirit. During the 40-year span between puberty to menopause, most ovaries produce estrogen, progesterone and testosterone in a well-choreographed ballet of health and fertility. Some women may find the ebb and flow of female hormones troublesome while others rumba to their rhythms.

Eventually, every woman's ovaries swirl, twirl or trudge down the peri-menopausal path to her final menstrual period. Once depleted of ovarian follicles/oocytes (eggs), a menopausal woman cannot get pregnant naturally, and harmony between her trinity of sex hormones ceases. No longer slow dancing or swaying to the music of hormonal harmony, she settles into menopause. Fortunately, well-orchestrated estrogen replacement therapy allows her to continue the waltz and age with dignity.

PUBERTY

The vibrant tempo of sex hormones begins with the glandular rhythm of puberty. Puberty is the physiological process that growing girls (and boys) go through to reach sexual maturity and become capable of reproducing. Most girls go through puberty between the ages of 10 and 14, with their first menstrual period, known as menarche, occurring around age 12 ½.

The "critical fat hypothesis" stipulates that most girls need to reach a certain body mass before puberty begins. Once she reaches 100 pounds, a pubescent girl now has just enough caloric reserves to sustain a pregnancy. Her 25% body fat represents the store of 87,500 calories (25 pounds multiplied by 3,500 calories per pound) needed for pregnancy. It is thought that when a girl reaches this critical body mass, adipose (fatty) tissue releases the hormone leptin, which then travels to her brain's hypothalamus and triggers the pituitary to activate the process of sexual maturity. Melatonin, secreted at night by the brain's pineal gland, affects the onset of puberty, as well. Decreased melatonin production helps launch puberty.

Once a girl's pituitary gland is activated for puberty, it releases hormones that stimulate the ovaries to produce estrogen and testosterone, as well as hormones that encourage the adrenal glands to produce androgen (masculinizing) hormones. Follicle stimulating hormone (FSH) stimulates ovarian follicles/oocytes (eggs) to produce estrogen, luteinizing hormone (LH) stimulates the ovaries to ovulate and produce progesterone. LH also stimulates the ovarian tissue to produce testosterone. The adrenocorticotropic hormone (ACTH) stimulates the adrenal glands to produce androgens and testosterone. Increased levels of estrogen initiate breast development, and increasing androgen levels give rise to pubic hair and axillary hair. The first menstrual period or menarche usually occurs 2 years after breasts develop, and 4 to 6 months after the growth of pubic and axillary hair. It takes 2 to 3 years for the pituitary and ovaries' hormonal syncopated rhythm to mature and generate monthly ovulations with regular menstrual cycles. Irregular uterine bleeding due to sporadic ovulation is common for 2 to 3 years following a girl's first menstrual period (menarche).

MENSTRUAL CYCLE

Derived from the Latin word *menses*, meaning month, menstrual cycles are coordinated by hormones that are secreted by the pituitary gland in the brain and the ovaries in a woman's pelvis. Month after month, year after year, from puberty to menopause, a woman's body prepares for pregnancy.

The hypothalamus secretes gonadotropin-releasing hormone (GnRH) to trigger the pituitary into action. The pituitary secretes follicle-stimulating hormone (FSH), which stimulates ovarian follicles containing oocytes (eggs) to mature and produce increasing estrogen. A woman's testosterone levels increase gradually, as well. Once estrogen levels peak, the pituitary's secretion of luteinizing hormone (LH) surges. This pre-ovulatory LH surge is the basis of the home ovulation kits. While the LH level is peaking, estrogen levels dip back down a little.

With the onset of monthly menstrual cycles, one oocyte (egg) fully matures every month. Then, in response to the LH surge, the mature oocyte/ ovum (egg) is released by its ovarian follicle (ovulation). This emancipated oocyte/ovum (egg) heads toward the fallopian tube in search of a willing and able sperm to hook up with. The human oocyte/ovum (egg) is only viable for 24 hours, but sperm can live up to 5 days inside a woman's reproductive tract. In response to climbing estrogen levels that finally peak just prior to ovulation, the woman's cervical mucus production increases and becomes more watery. Around mid-cycle, a woman notices clear, vaginal discharge that's wetter and stretchable between her fingers. This watery mucus facilitates an easier upstream swim for sperm traveling through the cervical canal, up the uterus, to the fallopian tube.

Certain cells within the ovary, the theca cells, respond to LH stimulation with a surge of testosterone. As part of Nature's plan for ovulated egg to meet earnest sperm, this extra testosterone boosts a woman's interest in sexual activity. Testosterone makes a woman feel more confident, so she becomes more comfortable taking risks. The proverbial, "Mr. Right vs. Mr. He will do for now," scenario comes to mind. In the week following ovulation, testosterone levels decrease, staying at a low, but relatively steady state, until the next ovulation cycle comes around. Residual cells within the ovulated follicle of the ovary form the corpus luteum, which is Latin for "yellow body." After ovulation, the corpus luteum of the ovary produces increasing amounts of progesterone and estrogen in anticipation of potential conception.

Meanwhile, Back at the Uterus...

Prior to ovulation, the estrogen produced by the ovarian follicles has been stimulating the lining of the uterus, known as the "endometrium," to proliferate and thicken, so this pre-ovulatory time of the menstrual cycle is referred to as the "follicular or proliferative" phase.

After ovulation, progesterone produced by the ovary's corpus luteum plumps up the juicy, secretory components of the endometrium, so this post-ovulatory time is referred to as the "luteal or secretory" phase of the menstrual cycle. Estrogen-primed and juiced-up by progesterone, the endometrium is now fully thickened and adequately prepped for a fertilized egg (zygote) to have a soft and spongy landing for implantation and growth in the uterus.

Estrogen is the primary hormone that stimulates breast growth during puberty, but progesterone is required to convert the female breast into a milk-producing organ. As its name implies, progesterone is the "pro-gestation or pro-pregnancy" hormone, so the only time the ovary produces progesterone is after ovulation. Progesterone's only purpose is to prepare and maintain a woman's uterus for pregnancy and prime her breasts for lactation.

The most likely time to get pregnant is during the "fertile window," which lasts around 4 to 5 days every month. A woman's fertile days are a couple of days before ovulation, the day of ovulation, and the day after ovulation. Even when the couple times sex perfectly, the chance that pregnancy will occur that particular joining is about 10%. Trying is half the fun, so by the end of a year of trying, over 90% of fertile couples will be pregnant.

A woman's fertility peaks from ages 20 to 25 and begins to decline after age 30. Women in their 20s tend to be healthy without chronic diseases, so both mom and baby do well. Teenage pregnancy, on the other hand, is complicated by anemia, poor maternal weight gain, placenta problems, pregnancy-induced hypertension and premature labor with delivery of preemie babies. At the opposite end of the fertility curve, a woman's time-honored, biological clock starts to tick-tock loudly in her mid-30s. Due to aging ovaries, her fertility declines rapidly starting at age 37. Fortunately, it's not over until the ovaries are totally depleted. 40% of babies are born to women over age 30, and 15% of babies are born to women over age 35.

Pre-pregnancy health and nutrition are critical to maximizing positive obstetrical outcomes in any age group.

If conception occurs, the ovary continues to produce increasing amounts of estrogen and progesterone. The fertilized egg (zygote) travels down the fallopian tube to implant in the uterus. There, tissues from the embryo, along with the endometrial lining of the uterus at the implantation site, grow together to form the placenta (afterbirth), which nourishes the growing embryo. By the end of the 12th week of pregnancy, the placenta is large enough to take over the production of enough progesterone and estrogen to sustain the pregnancy. If a pregnancy is at risk during these first three months of gestation, bioidentical or "body"-identical progesterone, which is progesterone whose chemical structure is identical to that produced by women's ovaries, is prescribed to support the pregnancy.

If fertilization does not occur, estrogen and progesterone levels drop. No longer supported by elevated estrogen and progesterone levels, the endometrial lining of the uterus sloughs off, taking the unfertilized egg with it, in a process called menstruation. Hormone withdrawal precipitates this menstrual bleeding, and then the cycle starts all over again. During a woman's period of menstrual bleeding, her female hormone levels are at their lowest values in the cycle, and these low levels mirror those of a menopausal woman. Menstrual bleeding generally lasts 3 to 7 days with an average loss of 80cc (1/3 cup) of menstrual fluid per cycle.

The first day of menstrual bleeding is considered the first day of the menstrual cycle. The length of a menstrual cycle is usually 28 days, with 7 days spanning either side of 28, so normal menstrual periods can occur every 21 to 35 days. Cycles longer than 6 weeks are considered unusual. Most variation in cycles arises from the differing lengths of the pre-ovulatory phase. Menses always starts 14 days after ovulation. For example, in a 30-day menstrual cycle, the pre-ovulatory (follicular or proliferative) phase lasts 16 days, ovulation occurs, and the post-ovulatory (luteal or secretory) phase lasts 14 days. In a 22-day menstrual cycle, the pre-ovulatory phase lasts 8 days, ovulation occurs, and the post-ovulatory phase lasts 14 days. With the onset of uterine bleeding, the next menstrual cycle begins.

450 vs. 150

From puberty to menopause, a contemporary woman ovulates 450 times across the span of 40 years, so she spends half her lifetime managing the ebb and flow of 450 menstrual cycles. This is in contrast to eras gone by when a woman experienced only 150 menstrual cycles across her lifespan.

Women are now living into their 80s, but in the early 1900s, average life expectancy for a woman was 49 years. Due to unpredictable and inadequate nutrition back then, most girls did not reach critical fat mass to start menstruating until they were 15 years old, and then women spent most of their reproductive years pregnant or lactating.

Left to Nature, the number of children a mother might expect to have passing through the reproductive ages of 15 to 49, statistically known as the total fertility rate, is 6 children per woman. Calculating 40 weeks' gestation for a full-term pregnancy coupled with one to two years of breastfeeding for each child, a woman spent 14 to 17 years, that is, a third of her short life either pregnant or lactating. Between childhood, childbearing, and child-rearing, there was not much time or energy left for anything else.

With effective family planning, women now have fewer pregnancies and far more menstrual cycles. Despite extended life expectancy, and regardless of the number of pregnancies, the number of menstrual cycles experienced or the use of hormonal contraceptives, the average age for menopause is still 51. Throughout recorded human history, if a woman lived long enough, she usually went through menopause around age 51. An ovary is an ovary is an ovary. Over the millennia, there has been no change in women's ovarian destiny.

OVERT vs. COVERT MENSTRUATION

Overt menstruation occurs when the endometrial lining is shed from the uterus through the vagina to the outside world. This occurs in humans and most primates, although menstrual bleeding in primates is minimal. Humans and primates with overt menstruation are sexually active generally throughout their menstrual cycles. Near the time of ovulation, many female primates' perineal and bottom areas turn bright red and swell up to attract more male attention.

Covert menstruation, on the other hand, means that the endometrial lining of the uterus is not shed to the outside world; it is simply resorbed into the body. Also known as the estrous cycle, this occurs in all other placental mammals, including dogs, cats, horses, elephants, pigs and rats. Dogs have their cycle twice a year, cats once a month, horses every three weeks, and rats go through their cycle every 5 days. Some of these animals, e.g.- dogs, display a bloody discharge from the vagina due to pre-ovulation dips in estrogen levels. This is different from menstruation, because it occurs when the animal is "in heat" at the time of ovulation, and the blood comes from the vaginal walls, not the uterus. Egg-laying animals such as birds, reptiles, amphibians, and fish, do not need a uterus to grow an embryo, so they do not have menstruation of any kind. Female mammals with estrous cycles or covert menstruation are sexually receptive to males only when they're ovulating, so only at those times do they physically and behaviorally display their reproductive availability. Humans, however, can and do have sex at any time during their menstrual cycle, and humans are the only animals that do not advertise their "fertile window." Only the woman knows.

After ovulation, and in preparation for potential implantation of an early embryo, the endometrial lining of the uterus is juiced up with hormones, proteins, fats, and sugars. This thickened endometrium increases the overall metabolic demands of the body. It may seem inefficient for a woman's body to consume energy to build up the endometrial lining of the uterus, only to shed it each month. The menstrual shedding process is more energy efficient than permanently maintaining a fully developed and thickened endometrium indefinitely.

STEADY ESTROGEN & PROGESTERONE

To avoid hormonal fluctuations associated with menstrual cycles, reproductive-aged women can take oral contraceptive pills (OCPs) containing the same low-dose of estrogen and progesterone every day. Most menopausal women requiring both estrogen and progesterone for their hormone replacement therapy use the same dose of estrogen and progesterone hormones daily. After a year of being on these hormone regimens, and as long as she stays on the hormones, a woman will not experience uterine bleeding.

Less jarring than fluctuating hormone levels, a steady state of low levels of female hormones is physiologically therapeutic for many gynecological and medical conditions in women. It is perfectly healthy for these women not to have monthly menstrual bleeding, since they do not have endometrial tissue build up within the lining of their uterus. When delivered on a daily basis, the progesterone component of the hormone preparation neutralizes estrogen's stimulating effect on the endometrial lining of the uterus (endometrium), so the endometrium does not thicken or grow.

The progestin in the Mirena/Liletta intrauterine device (IUD) provides continuous progesterone to the endometrium, as well. After a year of having the progestin-containing IUD in place, 20% of women no longer experience uterine bleeding. Those who still have monthly cycles notice decreased menstrual flow and decreased pelvic cramping.

With regular menstrual cycles, estrogen stimulates the endometrial uterine lining to proliferate and grow and grow. After ovulation, progesterone production stabilizes and ripens the lining's growth. When the endometrial lining is exposed to both estrogen and progesterone on a continuous daily basis, it does not grow. Daily progesterone exposure prevents estrogen from growing the endometrial lining, so the endometrium of the uterus is kept short and smooth, free of polyps and tissue overgrowth. There is no endometrial thickening for the uterus to shed, so no "cleaning out" is necessary.

MENSTRUAL SYNCHRONY

Women who live together may end up cycling together. As a graduate student at Harvard University in 1971, Martha McClintock noticed that the women in her dormitory eventually ended up having their menstrual periods at the same time. She took swabs from the armpits of women at different points in their cycles and then exposed other women to these swabs. The exposed women's menstrual cycles then synchronized to match the cycle from the swab's originator.

Although menstrual synchrony occurs often, it does not occur in every situation. It may depend upon the amount of time the women spend together, or the menstrual phase a woman is in when she contacts others. It is difficult to say what exact effect one woman's menstrual cycle might have on another woman's hormonal milieu, but social interactions can influence ovulatory cycles.

A HIGHER POWER

Women who spend a lot of time together may end up with synchronized menstrual cycles, whereas, women who are under chronic stress or have poor eating habits or exercise too much, may lose their menstrual cycles altogether.

As long as a woman has a uterus and an ovary, the only normal times for her to go without menstrual periods are pregnancy, breastfeeding or menopause. Of course, for women using certain types of hormonal regimens, it's okay for them not to experience uterine bleeding, as well. Otherwise, missing three or more periods in a row is a cause for concern, and is clinically referred to as "amenorrhea," meaning "without monthly flow."

The most common cause for amenorrhea in a reproductive-aged woman is pregnancy. Since 50% of pregnancies are unplanned, many women are surprised when their pregnancy test is positive. If the pregnancy test is negative, then a woman's thyroid and prolactin hormone levels need to be assessed to ensure that these organs are functioning normally and not contributing to her lack of menstrual periods.

Chronic stress in a woman's life can cause menstrual cycles to cease. The stressors may be psychosocial anxieties caused by mental, emotional and situational difficulties, or metabolic distress caused by overwhelming trauma, sustained infections, drugs, malnutrition or a perpetual energy deficit from severe caloric restriction and excess exercise. Regardless of how the difficulties started, all stress-filled pathways lead to the center of her brain, the hypothalamus. As far as the stressed-out woman's hypothalamus is concerned, it is not a good time to ovulate and reproduce. When a woman's menstrual periods cease under these circumstances, it is considered "hypo-thalamic amenorrhea."

As the brain's hypothalamus receives signals from thinking and emotional parts of the brain, interprets stressors, and integrates metabolic indicators, it directs the pituitary to release or withhold hormones that control other glands in the body. The pituitary gland is a protrusion off the bottom of the hypothalamus, so communication between the "higher power" hypothalamus and the pituitary "master" gland is tightly connected. These small structures within the brain (the almond-sized hypothalamus and the pea-sized pituitary) wield remarkable control over the body's protection mechanisms.

When the body is challenged by any stress, it launches into self-preservation mode. The reactive nervous system galvanizes survival mechanisms, and the hypothalamus triggers the pituitary to release hormones to stimulate the adrenal glands. Although adrenal glands generate sex hormones, the adrenals' primary purpose is to help one survive in the face of a threat. Adrenal glands rally all the body's resources into "fight or flight" mode by flooding the system with adrenalin (epinephrine), norepinephrine and cortisol hormones. The adrenalin rush instantaneously increases heart rate, respiratory rate, and blood pressure, shunts blood away from internal digestive organs to skeletal muscles for action, releases energy stores for immediate use, and sharpens the senses. Allowing humans to outrun, outclimb or outwit our predators, these efficient survival tactics are hardwired into our being.

Our bodies were built to handle short-term stress. Rapid reflexes are great for swerving to avoid a car accident or getting out of a burning building. These performance-enhancing mechanisms help us handle challenging physical, professional and social situations, as well. On the other hand, when chronic stress or metabolic distress keeps bombarding the hypothalamus and pituitary, we get into trouble. Chronic stress results in elevated cortisol production by the adrenals. Cortisol is a steroid hormone that normally helps the body modulate inflammation, mobilize energy stores and heal from trauma. Sustained cortisol levels, however, decrease the output of other hormones.

The hypothalamus perceives stress as a threat, and instructs the pituitary accordingly, so they both lock into survival mode and shut down non-essential functions. Since the hypothalamus is not in the mood to wine and dine the pituitary into activating the ovaries or testes, there is no reproductive sex hormone activity going on. Ovulatory menstrual cycles stop, periods become irregular and eventually cease altogether. Most of the time, once the stress is relieved, menstrual cycles resume.

DISORDERED EATING

If a woman is plagued by energy or nutritional deficits caused by disordered eating, severe caloric restriction or excess exercise, she stops menstruating. On the other hand, healthy dieting and exercise, where the goal is to lose weight sensibly to improve health and appearance, does not adversely impact menstrual cycles.

Women struggling with their relationship with food view weight loss as the only way to achieve happiness. Attempting to control life and emotions, they become obsessed with food and appearance. This can occur in women suffering from anorexia nervosa, bulimia nervosa or orthorexia nervosa. These are complex eating disorders driven by psychological issues but can lead to serious physical and medical problems. Anorexics have an intense fear of gaining weight, which is further compounded by a distorted view of body image. They will severely restrict caloric intake because they think they can never be thin enough. Bulimics have frequent episodes of binge eating, followed by frantic efforts to avoid gaining weight through self-induced vomiting, laxative abuse and exercising excessively. Orthorexics are obsessed with eating only certain foods they consider healthy, and not consuming anything else, so they may end up malnourished.

The brain perceives all of these circumstances as starvation, and not a good time for the woman to get pregnant, so the hypothalamus shuts down menstrual cycles until weight and nutritional status improve. Treatment of eating disorders involves a team approach with medical professionals, psychotherapy and nutritional counseling.

FEMALE ATHLETE TRIAD

Exercise and sports are healthy activities for girls and women of all ages; however, when a female athlete focuses too much on being thin, lightweight or featherweight, she eats too little or exercises too much. When she goes to extremes in dieting or exercise, she develops a condition known as the "female athlete triad." This is a combination of three interrelated illnesses: disordered eating, menstrual dysfunction, and premature osteoporosis. When the body perceives too great a gap between limited caloric intake and excess energy expenditure, estrogen levels in the body drop, so menstrual cycles cease. In an overzealous young athlete, the critical fat mass for triggering puberty hormones may not be reached, so she does not even start her menstrual periods. Despite external appearances and all that physical activity, she is unhealthy.

With normal menstrual cycles, ovaries produce estrogen, a hormone that helps keep a woman's bones strong, estrogen strong. Without estrogen, the body loses bone mass, so the young female athlete develops the osteoporosis suffered by postmenopausal estrogen-deprived women. But unlike menopause, where estrogen replacement prevents osteoporosis, merely reconstituting uterine bleeding cycles with estrogen plus progesterone hormone preparations is not as effective in protecting these young athletes' bones from osteoporosis. Only when their body is supplied with adequate calories will bone loss be reversed. Proper counseling, along with meeting the young woman's nutritional needs relative to balanced energy expenditure, will triumph over the female athlete triad.

LEPTIN

Leptin is a satiety hormone produced by adipose (fatty) tissue, and it is an energy signal informing the brain that fat reserves are adequate for survival and reproduction. Loss of critical fat mass drops leptin levels, so the hypothalamus will not receive the signal to launch the reproductive hormone cascade. Without the leptin signal, the hypothalamus will not release gonadotropin-releasing hormone (GnRH) to spark the pituitary gland into activating the ovaries into action. Without GnRH, the pituitary will not release follicle-stimulating hormone (FSH) and luteinizing hormone (LH). Without FSH and LH, the ovarian follicles neither produce estrogen nor ovulate.

About 5% of women develop hypothalamic amenorrhea, and their blood serum hormone levels reflect very low levels of FSH, LH, and estrogen. Neither psychosocial stress nor metabolic distress is a healthy environment conducive to sexual reproduction, so the hypothalamic higher power halts ovulatory menstrual cycles during times of stress.

MITTELSCHMERZ – OVULATION PAIN

The medical term mittelschmerz is derived from German for "middle pain." When ovulation occurs, 20% of women experience pelvic pain and cramping that occurs roughly midway through their menstrual cycle. As a follicle/oocyte (egg) destined for ovulation matures in the ovary, it is surrounded by follicular fluid. During ovulation, the egg, and the fluid, as well as some blood, are released from the ovary. The follicular fluid or blood may irritate the lining of the pelvic cavity, causing pain.

A woman may experience this ovulation indicator either with every cycle or intermittently, and the pelvic pain may be localized enough so that a woman can tell which of her two ovaries provided the egg in a given month. Because ovulation occurs from either ovary, the pain may switch sides from cycle to cycle. If a woman is trying to get pregnant, mittelschmerz discomfort confirms that she is ovulating. The diagnosis of mittelschmerz is made if a woman is mid-cycle, and a pelvic exam and pelvic ultrasound show no gynecological abnormalities. If a woman is not trying to conceive, and ovulation pain is not alleviated with over the counter pain relievers, then suppressing ovulation with either progesterone-only contraceptives or hormonal contraceptive preparations using a combination of estrogen plus progesterone, such as low-dose oral contraceptive pills, patches or a vaginal ring, eliminates mittelschmerz.

PREMENSTRUAL SYNDROME (PMS)

During her reproductive years, a woman experiences the highs and lows of fluctuating levels of female hormones associated with menstrual cycles.

Around the time of ovulation, some women encounter ovulation pain, while some migraine sufferers experience mid-cycle headaches from the slight pre-ovulatory dip in estrogen. Then, when estrogen levels again drop around the time of her menstrual period, she may experience a menstrual migraine. Two migraines a month is two too many. Other bothersome symptoms that can occur a week or so prior to a woman's menstrual period include breast tenderness, acne, bloating and bowel changes, fluid retention and weight gain, fatigue and achiness, food cravings, trouble concentrating, sleep disturbances, along with moodiness and irritability. Known as premenstrual syndrome (PMS), these monthly symptoms go away after a woman's period starts. 85% of women with ovulatory menstrual cycles experience prickly PMS of some sort. Symptoms and symptom severity vary from woman to woman, and symptoms can vary month to month in the same woman.

Seemingly cavalier about calories, premenstrual women zoom in on chocolate treats, comfort carbs, and greasy goodies. There is a biological basis for these predictable food cravings during this phase of the menstrual cycle. When estrogen levels dip before menstruation, serotonin levels decline. Serotonin is a brain chemical that promotes feelings of relaxation, confidence, and security. Serotonin is made from tryptophan, and chocolate contains tryptophan. Tryptophan is an "essential" amino acid because it cannot be made in the body; therefore, it must be obtained from food or supplements. Chocolate's appeal is attributed to its serotonin generating power. Carbohydrates increase insulin secretion. Insulin shifts the pattern of other amino acids in the blood, allowing tryptophan to enter the brain easier, so more serotonin can be manufactured. With the premenstrual decline in estrogen levels, acetylcholine levels also decrease. Acetylcholine is a brain chemical that regulates the rate at which the brain processes information and sensory input. It is the awareness neurotransmitter providing fuel for creativity and memories. Since fat is the building block of acetylcholine, premenstrual women crave fatty foods. PMS is a monthly diet buster.

After ovulation, progesterone competes with aldosterone, an adrenal hormone that stimulates the kidneys to resorb sodium and water back into the bloodstream. When progesterone levels fall just prior to menstrual periods, aldosterone is free to increase absorption of sodium and water, which leads to premenstrual fluid retention, bloating and weight gain. This engorgement can lead to more symptoms with fibrocystic breast changes. These fluid shifts usually dissipate during the woman's menstrual period.

Although testosterone levels remain steady during the premenstrual week, due to drops in estrogen and progesterone levels, testosterone levels are relatively higher compared to lowered female hormones. This slight testosterone dominance may increase libido in some women, but it can also bring on premenstrual irritability, acne, or "sentinel zits," heralding imminent menstrual bleeding.

Moderate to severe PMS affects 20% of reproductive-age women, and severe PMS can adversely affect a woman's life by impairing her work function, her relationships, and social activities. The most severe form of PMS, premenstrual dysphoric disorder (PMDD) is considered a type of depressive disorder affecting 7% of women. PMDD responds to treatment with selective serotonin reuptake inhibitors (SSRI) antidepressants, such as fluoxetine (Prozac, Sarafem), paroxetine (Paxil, Brisdelle) or sertraline (Zoloft). These medications may be taken continuously on a daily basis throughout the month, or intermittently for the 14 days prior to a woman's menstrual period.

The exact cause of PMS is unknown, but there are some risk factors associated with developing troublesome premenstrual difficulties. Women with other health issues are more likely to have PMS, so it is important to evaluate and treat any thyroid disease, or any other medical problem, whose symptoms may be exacerbated during the week prior to a woman's menstrual period. Current mood and anxiety disorders, or a history of depression or mental health issues, are common in women with moderate to severe PMS. Higher levels of perceived stress and higher daily hassles scores have been identified as risk factors for PMS, as well. Also, there is an association between obesity and increased risk for PMS. Gynecological conditions tend to cluster in families, so a woman with PMS may have other female relatives who also suffer from PMS. Despite their considerable placebo effects, evening primrose oil, black cohosh, wild yam root, Dong quai, vitamin B6, and even natural progesterone supplements are not that successful in resolving PMS.

There is no laboratory test or unique physical finding that is diagnostic of PMS. A menstrual diary over the course of several cycles reveals premenstrual clustering of symptoms. Blood serum measurements of sex hormones in women suffering from disruptive PMS are no different than in women without PMS. However, since PMS symptoms consistently occur during the premenstrual phase, when estrogen and progesterone levels descend prior to a woman's period, hormones are obviously involved.

The dominant theory is that women with severe PMS may have an abnormal sensitivity to the normal hormonal fluctuations associated with ovulatory menstrual cycles. Although circulating levels of estrogen, progesterone and testosterone remain within the normal premenstrual range, a PMS-sufferer's system is more sensitive to these normal hormonal changes.

Back in the Victorian era, hormonal fluctuations in women were treated as emotional problems. In fact, the words "hysterical" and "hysterectomy" come from the Greek word for "uterus." By surgically removing the uterus, a hysterectomy would allegedly cut out a woman's hysteria. Fortunately, since then we have come a long way in our understanding and appreciation of female hormones

Many vexing but short-term PMS discomforts associated with monthly premenstrual drops in estrogen and progesterone levels are similar to the years of bothersome menopausal symptoms a woman experiences when her female hormones plummet permanently. PMS can be considered a snapshot view of the future full-length "hormone withdrawal" menopause video.

.

BACK to STEADY HORMONES

Because hormonal fluctuations associated with ovulatory menstrual cycles contribute to the cause of PMS, treatment involves modulating or minimizing the oscillations of estrogen and progesterone, while simultaneously maintaining a woman's healthy female hormone environment. When ovulation is suppressed, there are no more fluctuating levels of hormones, so PMS symptoms resolve. Maintaining smooth and steady levels of sex hormones is safely and easily accomplished by using the hormone preparations found in low-dose oral contraceptive pills (OCPs). OCPs contain a combination of low-dose estrogen plus progesterone that suppresses ovulation, supplants ovarian hormone production and generates a stable hormone environment conducive to many health benefits. In contrast to triphasic OCPs that contain variable doses of hormones from week to week, monophasic OCPs deliver the same dose of estrogen and progesterone in every pill throughout the cycle. Monophasic low-dose OCPs work well for PMS sufferers.

When oral contraceptive pills (OCPs) are used in "extended cycle therapy," that is, a woman takes a hormonally active pill daily for 12 consecutive weeks, then one week of no pills, then a hormonally active pill for the next 12 weeks, then one week of no pills, etc., she will have menstrual bleeding every 3 months. She could safely take a hormonally active OCP pill daily for 365 days a year, but she may then experience unpredictable break through spotting/bleeding. Instead, it's more practical to have predictable menstrual bleeding every 3 months. Mild PMS followed by light menstrual bleeding 4 times a year certainly beats monthly misery.

Using a progesterone-only pill/shot/implant suppresses ovulation and eliminates fluctuating hormones. Progestin-only therapy results in irregular uterine bleeding, bone thinning and does not provide the estrogen needed to maintain a woman's long-term healthy hormonal environment. 15% of progestin-only users develop problems with depression symptoms or weight gain.

Other health benefits of using oral contraceptive pills (OCPs) containing a combination of low-dose estrogen-plus-progesterone include reducing a woman's risk of ovarian cancer, uterine cancer, and colon cancers. These OCPs also reduce fibrocystic breast discomfort, decrease acne, decrease hirsutism, decrease menstrual flow, reduce menstrual cramps, eliminate ovulation pain and increase bone density. OCPs also happen to help protect a woman against ovarian cancer and uterine cancer. Low-dose monophasic OCPs do not increase a woman's risk of breast cancer. With monophasic OCPs, a woman can be PMS-free all the way through menopause.

POLYCYSTIC OVARY SYNDROME (PCOS)

From the time they started menstruating in their early teens, nearly 10% of women encounter lifelong irregular uterine bleeding. Because their ovaries do not ovulate on a regular basis, they do not have monthly menstrual cycles. Instead, they encounter unpredictable uterine bleeding episodes, anywhere from 3 to 8 times a year. Also, if a young woman in her 20s experiences substantial weight gain, her monthly menstrual periods may be lost to irregular, but prolonged, uterine bleeding episodes. Although menopause is still far away, these young women's ovaries rarely ovulate or don't ovulate at all. They have normal thyroid function, normal adrenal glands, and normal prolactin hormone levels. The problem is with their ovaries.

In addition to not ovulating on a regular basis, what these young women share in common are high levels of androgenic or masculinizing hormones, such as testosterone, in their system. This could manifest as acne, hirsutism (male pattern facial hair growth, chest and abdominal hair), increased muscle mass, deeper voice or androgenic alopecia (scalp hair loss). Pelvic ultrasound may reveal polycystic ovaries, that is, both ovaries are enlarged with each containing multiple, small cysts along the ovary's periphery, looking like a "string of pearls." These small cysts are immature egg-bearing follicles whose development has stopped due to disturbed ovarian function. Putting all this together, these women have a condition known as polycystic ovary syndrome (PCOS).

PCOS is a metabolic and glandular disorder that was first described by Dr. Stein and Dr. Leventhal in 1935, so PCOS was commonly known as Stein-Leventhal syndrome. Reflecting multiple potential etiologies and a variable clinical presentation from woman to woman, the exact cause of PCOS is unknown. The ovaries are obviously involved, and like other gynecological conditions, PCOS clusters in families. PCOS is the most common endocrine disorder in women between the ages of 18 to 44 and is best characterized as "hyperandrogenic anovulation."

Most physicians agree that PCOS can be diagnosed clinically in a woman with irregular menstrual cycles, either physical or lab evidence of excess testosterone or androgens in her system, and the ovaries' classic appearance on ultrasound. Only having the classic polycystic ovary appearance on ultrasound is not enough to render a diagnosis of PCOS in a woman who has regular ovulatory menstrual cycles or does not have excess testosterone, since this type of ovarian appearance is seen in 20% of regularly ovulating women.

Over 50% of women suffering from PCOS are obese, and obesity leads to insulin resistance and diabetes. Insulin resistance occurs when the body's ability to use insulin effectively is impaired, so blood sugar levels remain elevated. Excess insulin causes ovaries to produce excess testosterone, which interferes with the ovaries' ability to ovulate. Excess adipose (fatty) tissue in overweight or obese woman with PCOS creates the paradox of having both excess androgens and excess estrogen in her system. Adipose (fatty) tissue contains the enzyme aromatase, which converts androgens to estrogens. Estrogen then stimulates the endometrial lining of the uterus to grow and proliferate. Without ovulation there is no progesterone produced to protect the endometrial lining of the uterus from excess estrogen stimulation, so women with PCOS are at much higher risk for developing endometrial overgrowth (hyperplasia), endometrial polyps, and uterine cancer.

To fend off endometrial uterine abnormalities, a woman should have a menstrual uterine bleed at least every 3 months. If menstruation occurs less often, some form of progesterone replacement is recommended to suppress overgrowth of the endometrial lining of the uterus. Oral progesterone taken every 3 months will induce predictable menstrual bleeding and help protect the uterus from excess estrogen associated with PCOS.

Women with PCOS have low-grade inflammation throughout their system, as well. In addition to increasing the woman's risk for developing diabetes and premature heart disease, this inflammation also stimulates the ovaries to produce more androgens and testosterone. The oral medication, metformin, reduces insulin resistance, thereby reducing ovarian testosterone production. This reduction in masculinizing hormones helps decrease acne and hirsutism, and may help ovaries ovulate again.

During a woman's reproductive years, if ovulation is not occurring on a regular basis, the pituitary gland will not detect progesterone, so it secretes more luteinizing hormone (LH) to try to stimulate ovulation or oocyte (egg) release from the ovary. Elevated LH levels cause a woman's ovaries to secrete more testosterone, as well. This excess testosterone production leads to more acne and hirsutism. Since PCOS patients have functioning follicles in their ovaries, they produce estrogen, so they have normal serum follicle-stimulating hormone (FSH) levels. Women with PCOS have elevated LH to FSH ratios, usually LH: FSH ratios greater than 2:1.

Hormonal imbalances associated with PCOS inhibit ovulation, generate unwanted masculinizing physical features, cause infertility, and dramatically increase a woman's risk for developing diabetes, hypertension, premature heart disease, fatty liver, sleep apnea and depression. Because of problems with ovulation, most women with PCOS have trouble getting pregnant. PCOS is one of the main reasons for infertility in women, and PCOS causes 75% of female infertility linked to ovulation problems. PCOS-associated infertility is treated with the selective estrogen receptor modulator (SERM), clomiphene (Clomid, Serophene, Androxal) pills, which help trigger ovulation. Clomiphene increases a woman's chance of conceiving twins. The chance of conceiving twins naturally is 1 in 88 pregnancies (1% to 2%). There is an 8% chance of conceiving twins while taking clomiphene.

Since PCOS causes ovarian hormone imbalance, treatment has focused on reducing testosterone production by the ovaries. Surgeries such as "wedge resection of both ovaries" or laparoscopic "ovarian drilling," reduces the amount of ovarian tissue pumping out excess androgens and restores ovulation. Both of these surgeries, however, are complicated by post-operative pelvic adhesions and scarring, causing further difficulty getting pregnant or the pregnancy does not implant properly in the uterus.

Menstrual irregularity in a woman suffering from PCOS is effectively and safely treated with hormone preparations found in low-dose monophasic oral contraceptive pills (OCPs) containing a combination of low dose estrogen-plus-progesterone. These OCPs override dysfunctional ovarian hormone production, prevent ovarian cyst formation and suppress polycystic ovaries' production of excess testosterone. By providing a steady balance of progesterone and estrogen in a woman's system, oral contraceptive pills (OCPs) prevent overgrowth and abnormalities of the endometrial lining of the uterus, and help protect her from uterine cancer. OCPs also decrease a woman's risk of ovarian cancer by 50%. Excess androgens, and too much testosterone is the root cause of the PCOS conundrum, so these OCPs are the best overall treatment for a woman with PCOS who do does not wish to get pregnant.

Progesterone-only medications can be used to induce regular menstrual bleeding, but they will not address the other endocrine and metabolic problems associated with PCOS. Untreated endocrine and metabolic dysfunction associated with PCOS causes a woman to develop diabetes, heart disease and hypertension at a much younger age than her contemporaries. Depending on the severity of her PCOS, a woman may need an insulin-sensitizing medication, e.g.-metformin, or an anti-androgen medication, e.g.-the diuretic, spironolactone, added to her oral contraceptive pill (OCP) regimen to reach desired clinical goals.

Metabolic parameters improve and stabilize after a year of medical therapy for PCOS. Of course, it also helps considerably for an overweight or obese PCOS patient to reduce her weight. It takes at least a year of OCP therapy for a PCOS patient to notice a decrease in unwanted hair growth or detect a significant decrease in acne. Medical or hormonal treatments for PCOS do not eliminate established hirsutism. They help slow down the rate of new unwanted hair growth. Electrolysis and laser hair removal will eliminate pre-existing objectionable hairs.

Since PCOS is a chronic medical problem, if medical therapy is discontinued, the endocrine and metabolic problems of PCOS resurface. Fortunately, as long as a woman does not smoke, she can safely stay on the low-dose OCPs until she is menopausal. Coupled with requisite weight loss, these medical therapies significantly improve the appearance and overall health of a woman with PCOS.

PERIMENOPAUSE

In addition to eliminating ovulation pain, alleviating PMS symptoms and treating the hormonal imbalances of PCOS, oral contraceptive pills (OCPs) containing a combination of low-dose estrogen plus progesterone are very helpful during a woman's perimenopausal years. Buffering the chaotic hormonal peaks and troughs generated by declining ovarian function, OCPs foster smooth sailing for a woman experiencing perimenopausal turbulence. By overriding dysfunctional ovaries, OCPs prevent erratic ovulation, modulate waffling estrogen levels and compensate for poor progesterone output generated by aging perimenopausal ovaries.

Oral contraceptive pills (OCPs) help prevent irregular, heavy uterine bleeding, decrease pelvic cramping, curtail ovarian cyst formation, alleviate fibrocystic breast symptoms, reduce the frequency of migraines, blunt uterine polyp formation, and help manage uterine fibroids and endometriosis. Vacillating hormone production from aging perimenopausal ovaries exacerbates these gynecological issues in women. By creating stable estrogen and progesterone levels in a woman's system, OCPs help minimize these "female problems," and decrease the need for gynecological surgeries.

During perimenopausal ovaries' wobbly descent into menopause, hormone production is trending downward, but ovulation still occurs sporadically. In response to decreasing estrogen and progesterone levels, the pituitary secretes more and more follicle-stimulating hormone (FSH) and luteinizing hormone (LH), trying to whip aging ovaries back into action. Women with elevated, but not menopausal, FSH levels can still get pregnant, so a perimenopausal woman should not forget about contraception; otherwise, a "change of life baby" can occur. Repeated measurements of blood serum FSH and LH levels at 4 to 6-month intervals can be helpful in establishing whether the woman is progressing through menopause.

Because the doses of estrogen and progesterone used in menopause replacement therapy are too low to suppress ovulation and overcome ovarian dysfunction during the perimenopausal years, female hormone replacement therapy is not helpful in managing symptoms of perimenopausal ovaries. Once ovarian function winds down to a stop, and perimenopause shifts to menopause, then it's show time for menopause hormone replacement therapy. When a woman experiences 12 consecutive months without a menstrual period, she has achieved menopausal status.

ORAL CONTRACEPTIVE PILLS (OCPs)

After being on oral contraceptive pills (OCPs) containing low-dose estrogen plus progesterone for just 5 years, a woman's risk of ovarian cancer and endometrial uterine cancer decreases by 50%. Her risk of colon cancer decreases by 20%, as well. The longer OCPs are used, the more a woman reduces her risk of developing these cancers. This protective effect lasts for decades after stopping the OCPs.

1 in 70 women will develop ovarian cancer, with only 10-15% of ovarian cancers occurring in women with a predisposing genetic mutation. The overwhelming majority of women diagnosed with ovarian cancer do not have this genetic mutation. Since there is no screening program proven effective for detecting early ovarian cancer, over 70% of women diagnosed with the disease are diagnosed in advanced stages (Stage 3 and Stage 4), with dismal survival rates. Ovarian cancer is the number one cause of death from gynecologic malignancies. For prevention of ovarian cancer, only undergoing major surgery, that is, a total hysterectomy and removal of both fallopian tubes and ovaries, provides better protection from ovarian cancer than taking oral contraceptive pills (OCPs).

The doses of estrogen and progesterone hormones found in the low-dose oral contraceptive pills (OCPs) used today are 1/5th the dose of hormones in older, high-dosed OCPs used in the past. Women on current low-dose OCPs are not plagued by nausea, headaches, breast tenderness or liver growths experienced by their mothers and grandmothers who may have used the higher dosed OCPs. In the 21st century, only the better tolerated and much safer low-dose OCPs are available. Monophasic OCPs contain the same low dose of estrogen plus progesterone in every hormonally active pill. Monophasic low-dose oral contraceptive pills (OCPs) do not increase the incidence of breast cancer. Any slight increased risk of breast cancer associated with OCP use is connected to using OCPs with variable hormone dosing from week to week (triphasic OCPs) or using the higher-dosed OCPs from years ago.

Understandably, whether using low-dose oral contraceptive pills (OCPs) to treat ovulation pain, PMS, PCOS, perimenopause, other gynecological conditions, or just for sheer contraception, most women who are doing well on OCPs want to stay on them as long as possible. Smokers increase their risk for strokes, so smokers over the age of 35 cannot take OCPs. However, as long as a woman does not smoke, she can stay on low-dose OCPs until she is 56 years old.

MENOPAUSE

When a woman finally reaches menopause, her ovaries are depleted of follicles/oocytes (eggs). She no longer ovulates, so she cannot get pregnant naturally. Without oocyte/egg-bearing follicles, her ovaries cannot produce estrogen or progesterone either. If the pituitary gland in the woman's brain is not bathed in estrogen, it secretes more follicle-stimulating hormone (FSH) to try to stimulate depleted ovarian follicles/oocytes (eggs) to generate more estrogen. This causes blood serum FSH levels to become elevated and stay elevated.

Without ovarian oocytes (eggs) to ovulate and produce progesterone, the progesterone-deprived pituitary gland secretes more luteinizing hormone (LH), trying to encourage depleted ovaries to ovulate and produce progesterone. This causes blood serum LH levels to become elevated and stay elevated. Persistently elevated blood serum FSH and LH levels, coupled with very low estrogen levels, are diagnostic of menopause. Ovarian failure means no more menstrual cycles, no more oocytes (eggs) for potential pregnancy, and no more ovarian follicles to produce estrogen and progesterone. Depleted and senescent menopausal ovaries stop reacting to elevated FSH and LH. No other condition raises blood serum FSH levels to the high elevations incurred by menopause. Menopausal FSH levels may rise more than LH levels because the kidneys are more effective in eliminating LH from the bloodstream.

ANDROGEN ANTHOLOGY

So, where's testosterone in all this? A woman's adrenal glands and ovaries produce a steroid hormone known as androstenedione. As an intermediary hormone used in the biochemical pathway for producing sex hormones, androstenedione can be converted to either testosterone or estrogen. In premenopausal women, half of her androstenedione is produced by the adrenal glands, and her ovaries generate the other half. Androstenedione is converted to testosterone by the woman's ovaries and her adrenals, as well as by other tissues in her body.

1/3 of a premenopausal woman's circulating testosterone comes from her ovaries; 1/3 is manufactured by her adrenals; and the remaining 1/3 is made from the peripheral conversion of androstenedione to testosterone by other tissues in her body. Generally, a woman's testosterone level is one-tenth of a man's. Testosterone production at multiple sites explains why menopausal women experience variable testosterone levels.

Androgens are masculinizing hormones because they generate male characteristics. Despite persistently elevated LH levels, follicle/oocyte (egg)-depleted menopausal ovaries cannot ovulate. Elevated LH, however, may still stimulate some aging ovaries to manufacture a little testosterone. The amount of androgenic juice left in menopausal ovaries varies from woman to woman. For some menopausal women, ovarian testosterone production shuts down simultaneously with its loss of estrogen and progesterone production. For other women, testosterone continues to trickle out from menopausal ovaries for several years.

When aging ovaries eventually become incapable of manufacturing any testosterone, a woman depends on her adrenal glands to continue some androgen production. A woman's global testosterone levels drop by 50% during menopause. When this dip is compared to her 90% drop in estrogen levels due to menopause, her system is exposed to a relative excess of testosterone. No longer modulated by estrogen, what little testosterone a menopausal woman has is now free to roam her body. Unfortunately, this is not as good as it sounds. Instead of enjoying the confidence boosting and libido enhancing properties of testosterone, most menopausal women cope with rogue facial hairs, acne's resurgence, and shape-shifting, with fat deposition displaced from hips and thighs to the waist and abdomen. These are not the joys or charms of uninhibited testosterone, but rather its troublesome side effects.

Since menopausal ovaries are no longer producing estrogen, a woman's adrenal glands are called upon to outsource estrogen precursors. The androstenedione secreted by the adrenals is not only converted to testosterone, but some androstenedione is converted to estrogen by aromatase enzymes residing in the woman's adipose (fatty) tissue. As a postmenopausal woman continues to age, however, her aging adrenals' contribution of precursor androstenedione for estrogen production diminishes, and eventually proves inadequate. Unfortunately, at these meager estrogen levels, there is not enough estrogen to maintain a woman's residual secondary sex characteristics.

As elderly men and women are drained of their sex hormones, their masculine and feminine gender-defining facial and physical characteristics recede, and they appear to resemble each other. Biologically, this is analogous to how it all started. Cute and cuddly in their bassinets, swaddled newborns in a nursery are indistinguishable, so pink and blue caps are used to identify their gender. From a distance, hormone-depleted elderly men and women parked in the activities room of a nursing home also appear similar. Aging without sex hormones is an androgynous free-fall.

Sadly, many hormone-deprived older women end up confused and barely shuffling across the hallway to the bathroom, while others are sidelined and languish in wheelchairs. The symphony of ovarian hormones does not have to end on such a wretchedly sour note. Appropriately timed and properly managed female hormone replacement therapy helps a menopausal woman sustain her vitality, maintain her spirit and, at any age, dance to the music.

HORMONES: LET'S GET BIOCHEMICAL

Hormones are chemical messengers produced by endocrine glands in the body. Unlike exocrine glands, such as sweat glands, salivary glands, and breast tissue, which secrete their juices to nearby organs through a duct system, endocrine glands release hormones directly into the bloodstream. These signaling molecules then hitch a ride on protein carriers in the blood and travel to distant target cells. Once it reaches its destination tissue, the hormone latches onto its designated receptor in the target cell to bring about cellular responses.

Hormones enable organs to function properly and keep the body healthy. They help control metabolism, utilize sugar, fats and protein appropriately, maintain salt and water balance, support muscles and bones, modulate inflammation and immunity, develop and sustain sexual characteristics, perpetuate reproduction, and allow the body to recover from illness and heal from injury. With so much at stake, an inadequate amount of any hormone is damaging.

There are two types of hormones, steroids, and non-steroids. All steroid hormones are made from cholesterol, so they all possess the characteristic chemical backbone of their cholesterol precursor. Although they have different impacts on various tissues, all steroids resemble each other. Non-steroidal hormones such as insulin, thyroxin, prolactin, adrenalin, etc. are not made from cholesterol, so their biochemical structures vary dramatically from each other.

Although the adrenal glands, ovaries, and testicles are the primary steroid producers of the body, the liver, skin and fat cells can also generate some steroids; in particular these "peripheral," non-glandular tissues can manufacture estrogen and some testosterone from precursors provided by the adrenals. Brain cells and nerves also have enzymes for the synthesis of neurosteroids, which modulate nerve cell excitability and transmission of nerve impulses, as well as temper responses to anxiety, stress and depression. These steroids promote neuroplasticity, which are cellular changes required for learning, memory and recovery from brain trauma. Steroids are found in animals, plants and fungi, so steroids are necessary for life at many levels.

Steroid hormones are grouped together by the type of receptors that they bind to when they reach their target tissue. There are glucocorticoid steroids, e.g.-cortisol, required for nutrient metabolism, inflammation, immunity, and heart function, and they are critical for maintaining the body's internal stability. The mineralocorticoid steroids are required for salt and water balance in the body. Estrogen, progesterone and testosterone round out the trinity of sex steroids. Some steroids allow us to survive, e.g.-glucocorticoids and mineralocorticoids, while others, e.g.-sex hormones and neurosteroids, determine how we live. Although testosterone is the male hormone, and estrogen is the female hormone, men and women have just a little bit of each other's sex hormones circulating in their system. A man's estrogen levels are the same as a postmenopausal woman's paltry estrogen levels, and women have only 10% of the testosterone levels found in men.

CHOLESTEROL: WHERE it ALL BEGINS

Steroids are made from life-sustaining cholesterol. Because cholesterol is an essential building block of every one of our billions of cells, Nature did not leave cholesterol acquisition to chance. The liver manufactures 85% of our body's cholesterol, and the rest comes from dietary intake. The cholesterol consumed in our diet has very little impact on our blood cholesterol levels.

While the brain represents only 2% of our body weight, 25% of the cholesterol in our body is found in the brain. Every brain cell and every nerve fiber is coated with cholesterol-rich myelin. Myelin not only nourishes and protects these cells, but it also facilitates the passage of electrical messages throughout the brain and nervous system's circuitry. Multiple sclerosis, a nervous system disorder of unknown cause and with no known cure, involves the degradation of this myelin sheath, which is so critical to nerve function.

Cholesterol circulates in the blood attached to its lipoprotein carrier, and because of this bulky lipoprotein carriage, cholesterol cannot cross the blood-brain barrier. The blood-brain barrier prevents large molecules from entering the brain; therefore, all of the cholesterol present in the brain must be produced locally within the brain. Cholesterol is the basic building block for all steroids manufactured by the brain and body. If cholesterol is aggressively trampled down to very low levels with cholesterol-lowering drugs, it can cause marked disruption in the production of pivotal steroids.

Statins are prescription drugs that interfere with the body's production of cholesterol and are used to lower blood cholesterol levels. Apart from water-soluble pravastatin (Pravachol) and rosuvastatin (Crestor), all other cholesterol-lowering statin drugs are fat-soluble and can cross the blood-brain barrier. On statin packaging labels, the FDA warns that some patients have developed memory loss or confusion while taking statins. Degenerative diseases, such as Alzheimer's dementia, are being linked to imbalances in brain cholesterol. Also, statins can cause muscle pain, weakness, muscle damage and liver damage. Statin use significantly increases the risk of developing diabetes by 50%.

Resembling their biochemical parent, all steroid hormones are organic compounds with cholesterol's characteristic molecular backbone of four fused rings: three of the rings are 6-carbon rings (hexagons) linked together to a fourth 5-carbon ring (pentagon). These rings are labeled A, B, C and D. Steroids vary by minor alterations of attachments to this cholesterol backbone or by the oxidation of carbon atoms within the rings. These slight chemical differences lead to striking alterations in biochemical activity. For example, by simply removing a single carbon attachment and hydroxylation of an $=O$ to an $-OH$ on the A ring, testosterone becomes estrogen. Obviously, estrogen's influence on the body is very different from testosterone's impact.

Through a series of enzymatic changes, cholesterol is transformed into estrogen, testosterone or progesterone. While keeping cholesterol's chemical backbone intact, the first chemical step involves docking off cholesterol's tail to form pregnanes. Pregnanes serve as the precursors to all other human steroids. Pregnanes can be converted to either progesterone or dehydroepiandrosterone (DHEA). DHEA is converted to androgens, whereas versatile progesterone can be converted to glucocorticoids (cortisol), mineralocorticoids (aldosterone) or androgens (androstenedione). Androstenedione can then be converted either to testosterone or estrogen. Based on biochemical conversions, progesterone gives rise to estrogen and testosterone. Testosterone can then be modified into estrogen, but estrogen can only be styled into another estrogen. Powered by cholesterol-based steroids, these hormones make love, sex and reproduction possible.

STEROID RECEPTORS

Since steroid hormones are derived from cholesterol, they are lipid or fat-soluble, so they travel easily across lipid-laden cell membranes of their target organs. Once inside, the steroid hormone connects up with its specific receptor found within the target cell. The receptor bound steroid hormone travels to the cell's control center, the nucleus, to direct the cell's genetic DNA to produce hormone-driven cellular changes, such as secondary sex characteristics.

Oil and water don't mix, so fat-soluble steroids don't travel well in the salt-water based bloodstream. Once an endocrine organ secretes a steroid hormone, the hormone binds to a specific protein carrier and then cruises through the bloodstream to get to its destination. For example, sex hormones travel attached to their companion sex-hormone binding globulin (SHBG). Once they reach their target cell, the steroid disembarks and then easily crosses through the lipid-laden cell membrane to enter the cell and meet up with its steroid receptor within the cell. Although sex hormones may ride the same SHBG ferry to get to their target destinations, cells have different receptors or docks for estrogen, testosterone, and progesterone.

TRIO of ESTROGENS + One

From the Greek word *oistros* meaning "frenzy, sting, gadfly" and Lithuanian *aistra*, meaning "violent passion," and adding the suffix *-gen* meaning "producer of," estrogens were named for their importance in producing estrus cycles. Estrus is the periodic state of sexual excitement in female mammals that immediately precedes ovulation, during which time she will accept mating with the male. Obviously, humans have monthly menstrual cycles, as opposed to estrus cycles, but estrogen is the name given to female steroid hormones that develop and maintain female sexual characteristics, and influence the female reproductive system.

Estrogens play decisive roles in puberty, menstruation, sexuality, pregnancy and parturition. Not only does estrogen refine a woman's facial features, but it also develops her female sexual ornamentation, such as a small waist-to-hip ratio, velvety skin texture, and fat deposition in breasts, thighs, and buttocks. Estrogen strengthens and ripens vaginal tissues, and lubricates the vaginal canal for sexual intercourse. Estrogen matures follicles/oocytes (eggs) for ovulation and helps prime the endometrial lining of the uterus for implantation of the developing embryo. Estrogen, along with its cousin steroid, progesterone, is needed to sustain a pregnancy, effect labor and delivery, and trigger the breasts for milk production. Estrogen helps testosterone fuel a woman's sex drive.

The three main estrogens found in a woman's body are estrone, estradiol, and estriol. There is a fourth estrogen, estetrol, but it is only detected in a woman's body when she's pregnant. These sister estrogens are very similar structurally, differing from each other merely by the number of hydroxyl (-OH) attachments to their cholesterol chemical backbone. The numerical shorthand used to identify these estrogens reflects these attachments:

- Estrone (E1) has only one hydroxyl (-OH) attachment, thus its E1 designation, and because of its ketone (=O or "-one") attachment, it's named estrone, as in "estr+one."
- Estradiol (E2) has two hydroxyl (-OH) attachments, di- for two. The hydroxyl attachment linked to carbon #17 bends up above the

plane of its cholesterol backbone, so estradiol is also known as 17-beta estradiol.

- Estriol (E3) has three hydroxyl (-OH) attachments, tri- for three
- Estetrol (E4) has four hydroxyl (-OH) attachments, tetra- for four.

All estrogens are derived from androgens, either from the androgen androstenedione or the androgen testosterone. The aromatase enzymes found in ovaries, testicles, adrenals and fat cells convert these androgens to estrogens. Androstenedione is aromatized to estrone (E1), testosterone is aromatized to estradiol (E2), and estrone (E1) and estradiol (E2) can convert back and forth to each other. Both estrone (E1) and estradiol (E2) can be converted to estriol (E3) by the woman's liver, and when she is pregnant, the placenta also converts the DHEA-S androgen generated by the fetus' adrenal glands into estriol (E3). Manufactured by the fetal liver during pregnancy, estetrol (E4) is transported to the maternal circulation through the placenta.

ESTRADIOL

Estradiol (E2) is the predominant estrogen circulating in a woman's bloodstream during her reproductive years, and as the major hormone secreted by the ovaries, estradiol is the strongest and most active form of estrogen. Nearly every cell in a woman's body has estrogen receptors, so estrogen impacts the function of all her organs from head-to-toe.

When estradiol is flowing freely prior to menopause, the prevalence of cardiovascular disease in women is much less than in men. However, after 10 to 15 years of estrogen deficiency, postmenopausal women not only catch up, but they surpass their same-aged male counterparts in their risk of heart attacks and strokes. Levels of estradiol (E2) in men are comparable to the meager amounts of estradiol (E2) found in postmenopausal women. Estradiol (E2) is the workhorse and "golden girl" of the estrogen family. It is the estrogen that is produced by the woman's ovaries during her reproductive years, so naturally, relieving menopausal symptoms and staving off damages associated with estrogen deficiency involves replacing estradiol

(E2). Estradiol (E2) is the "it" hormone when it comes to a woman's menopausal health and beyond. On average, therapeutic levels of blood serum estradiol range around 50 to 150 pg/mL.

ESTRIOL

Estriol (E3) is the predominant estrogen of pregnancy. The placenta (afterbirth) produces large amounts of estriol (E3) from DHEA-S generated by the fetus' adrenal glands. Estriol (E3) levels in non-pregnant women are very low and are equivalent to estriol (E3) levels in men, and these very low levels do not decrease any further with menopause. Any estriol (E3) in a non-pregnant woman is the metabolic waste product of the liver's breakdown of estradiol (E2) and estrone (E1).

Estriol (E3) is considered a weak estrogen because it is only 15% as potent as either estradiol (E2) or estrone (E1). Estriol (E3) does not preserve bone density, does not improve memory, mood or sleep, nor does it deliver the cardiovascular benefits achieved with estradiol. Estriol (E3) simply does not have the same positive benefits for menopausal health as those provided by replacing estradiol (E2). No estrogen does it better than estradiol (E2).

ESTETROL

Estetrol (E4) is an estrogen that is detected in a woman's system only during pregnancy. Estetrol (E4) is manufactured by the fetal liver and reaches the maternal blood circulation via transport through the placenta. Both male and female babies manufacture estetrol (E4) while they are growing in mom's uterus. Once the baby is born, its liver stops producing estetrol (E4). Estetrol's (E4) exact physiological function is unknown, but recent clinical research reveals that it behaves similarly to estradiol (E2) in alleviating hot flashes and improving vaginal tissue health, as well as preventing and treating osteoporosis. Interestingly, estetrol (E4) acts as an estrogen antagonist on breast tissue; similar to the way the selective estrogen receptor modulators (SERMs), tamoxifen (Nolvadex) and raloxifene (Evista), help decrease a woman's risk of breast cancer. Set to be available shortly, estetrol (E4) will be the first bioidentical estrogen found in an oral contraceptive pill (OCP).

Currently, oral contraceptive pills contain the synthetic estrogen, ethinyl estradiol, which resembles estradiol (E2).

ESTRONE

Estrone (E1) is the predominant estrogen in postmenopausal women. Since menopausal ovaries no longer manufacture estradiol, a woman's adrenal glands become her source of trickle-down estrogens. The adrenals secrete the androgens, androstenedione and testosterone, which are converted to estrone (E1) estrogen by aromatase enzymes that are found in the ovaries, testicles, adrenals, and adipose (fatty) tissue. Some of this estrone (E1) is modified to estradiol (E2). The heavier a woman is, the more estrogen producing adipose (fatty) tissue she has, so she possesses a built-in, non-ovarian source of endogenous estrogen. Because she has this estrogen circulating in her body, overweight or obese menopausal woman may experience fewer hot flashes and less vaginal dryness, than healthy weight menopausal women.

Male or female, young or old, regardless of race, creed or color, people who are overweight or obese end up walking around with way too much estrogen in their system. Even though we need oxygen, water, and sugar to survive, the overabundance of any of these life-staining substances proves lethal to our bodies. The air we breathe is only 20% oxygen, excess fluids precipitates seizures or heart failure, and elevated blood sugar (diabetes) is extremely damaging. Likewise, too much estrogen in the human body is harmful. Excess estrogen production in overweight or obese men leads to the development of breasts (gynecomastia), breast lumps and breast cancer, as well as erectile dysfunction, decreased libido, infertility, blood clots, fatigue and mood changes. Excess estrogen generated by excess adipose (fatty) tissue in a woman increases her risk of blood clots, breast cancer, ovarian and uterine cancers. Tipping the scales towards a healthy weight will promote hormone harmony and happy living for men and women of all ages. On average, blood serum estrone levels in premenopausal women range from 30 to 200 pg/mL. In postmenopausal women, estrone levels are between 30 to 70 pg/mL.

ESTROGEN METABOLISM

Any medicine, food, or hormone taken into the body is ultimately processed by the liver for disposition and disposal. In breaking down these materials, chemical reactions in the liver produce byproducts, which are then excreted in the bile. Bile flows into the intestinal tract for disposal or the excreted metabolites flow out in the urine. The medical term for these byproducts is "downstream metabolites."

In the liver, estradiol and estrone are broken down into various downstream metabolites such as 2-hydroxy-estradiol (2-OH-E2), 2-hydroxyestrone (2-OH-E1), 4-hydroxyestrone (4-OH-E1) and 16-hydroxyestrone (16-OH-E1), which the liver then further modifies into estriol (E3) and methoxy (-O-CH3)-metabolites of estrogen. It is theorized that excess levels of the "bad estrogen metabolites," such as 16-OH-estrone and 4-OH-estrone may be associated with a higher risk of breast cancer, ovarian cancer, and uterine cancer; whereas, the "good estrogen metabolites," such as 2-OH-estradiol, 2-OH-estrone, estriol and the methoxy-estrogens, may not increase this risk. For example, having a higher 2-OH-estrone to 16-OH-estrone ratio may indicate a lower risk for estrogen-sensitive cancers.

Each woman's estrogen metabolism is different, so the balance between "good" and "bad" estrogen pathways varies among women. The production of bad estrogen metabolites may be reduced with lifestyle interventions such as healthier eating, exercising and not smoking. Scooting estrogen down a better metabolic pathway is yet another reason for a healthy lifestyle.

WIPING OUT ESTROGEN

By suppressing the aromatase enzyme that converts testosterone to estrogen, aromatase inhibitor (AIs) medications are used to treat breast cancer in postmenopausal women. Because the only source of estrogen in a postmenopausal woman is her adipose (fatty) tissues' conversion of adrenal gland provided androstenedione and testosterone to estrone (E1), aromatase inhibitors abolish virtually any production of estrogen within her body.

Prior to menopause, a woman derives most of her estrogen from her ovaries' secretion of estradiol (E2), so aromatase inhibitors (AIs) are not used in premenopausal women. Aromatase inhibitors (AIs) are used to decrease the risk of breast cancer recurrence in postmenopausal women with estrogen-receptor positive (ER+) tumor types, and may be used to decrease the occurrence of breast cancer in high-risk postmenopausal women, as well.

PROGESTERONE

As its name implies, progesterone is a "pro-gestation or pro-pregnancy" ketone (=O) steroid hormone that exists for gestational purposes only, so the ovary produces progesterone only after ovulation. Progesterone preps the breasts and uterus for potential pregnancy and suppresses ovulation during pregnancy. If conception occurs, the ovary continues to produce progesterone through the first trimester of pregnancy. After about 12 weeks gestation, the placenta is large enough to take over progesterone production from the ovary and carries the pregnancy to term. If conception does not occur, progesterone levels drop; estrogen levels descend, and the endometrial lining of the uterus is shed in a process called menstrual bleeding or "having a period."

Without progesterone to stabilize the endometrial lining of a woman's uterus, estrogen causes this endometrial tissue to proliferate and grow and grow. Sometimes polyps can develop inside the uterus, or this overgrowth, called endometrial hyperplasia, can degenerate into uterine cancer. For women who have not had a hysterectomy, and have estrogen in their system, progesterone needs to be delivered to the uterine cavity to prevent abnormal tissue growth within the uterus. Obviously, if a woman has had a hysterectomy, she does not need progesterone's uterine protection.

There are various progestogens and progestins, but there is only one true progesterone (P4). Progestogen is the umbrella term for hormones or chemicals that can bind to progesterone receptors within a cell to produce progesterone-directed activity. Progestogens include naturally occurring progesterone, bioidentical progesterone, and synthetic progestins. Natural progesterone is the progesterone produced by a woman's ovaries. Bioidentical or "body"-identical progesterone is chemically identical to the natural progesterone produced by a woman's body, regardless of how it was created and irrespective of what raw material it is derived from. Progestins, also known as "synthetics," are chemicals that mimic progesterone's actions, but do not have the same chemical structure as natural progesterone. Progestins, in particular, megestrol acetate (Megace), are used medically to help improve appetite and reduce muscle wasting in people suffering from cancer or AIDS.

For a reproductive aged woman, progesterone, the "pro-gestation" hormone, is mainly involved in sustaining a pregnancy. If the pituitary gland in the brain is bathed in progesterone, it registers the presence of progesterone as a potential pregnancy or an already pregnant state. At this point, there is no need for the pituitary to further stimulate the ovaries to ovulate during an imminent or concurrent pregnancy. Suppressing ovulation using the progesterone feedback mechanism is the reasoning behind hormone-based birth control methods. Pregnancy results in high levels of progesterone, as well as elevated levels of estrogen, so a pregnant woman cannot get pregnant on top of her current pregnancy. After delivering the baby, progesterone and estrogen levels drop, so ovulation occurs. A new mom can conceive during the postpartum period.

When progesterone is circulating in a woman's system, ovulation is suppressed. Progestins suppress ovulation, so they are used in contraceptives such as oral contraceptive pills (OCPs), contraceptive patches and vaginal rings, in emergency contraception pills (Plan B or Plan B One-Step), in contraceptive shots (DepoProvera), contraceptive implants (Implanon and Nexplanon), and IUDs (Mirena/Liletta or Skyla).

BREASTFEEDING

If a new mom exclusively breastfeeds her baby, then the prolactin hormone stimulating breasts' milk production, and the oxytocin hormone stimulating the breasts' let down reflex, suppress ovulation by disrupting the pituitary glands' production of follicle-stimulating hormone (FSH) and luteinizing hormone (LH). Without synchronized FSH and LH levels, ovulatory menstrual cycles do not occur. Lack of menstrual periods during this time is referred to as "lactational amenorrhea," which lasts longer in women who exclusively breastfeed than in those who combine breastfeeding with bottle-feeding. Frequent (at least 8 to 12 times per day) and exclusive breastfeeding of the baby (no bottle supplementation), often referred to as "on-demand breastfeeding," is a relatively reliable method for preventing pregnancy for the first 6 months postpartum.

POSTMENOPAUSAL PROGESTERONE

Once a woman is menopausal, she is no longer fertile, so pregnancy or contraception is a non-issue. Without progesterone, however, estrogen naturally stimulates the endometrial lining of the uterus to proliferate and grow and grow. This tissue overgrowth can lead to endometrial polyps or hyperplasia, which may then deteriorate into uterine cancer. In the realm of menopause hormone therapy, contraception is not the purpose of progesterone's involvement. Progesterone's sole function is to prevent endometrial tissue overgrowth in the uterus of a woman who is taking estrogen replacement therapy.

Menopausal women who have had a hysterectomy, and are taking estrogen replacement therapy, do not need progesterone. For women with a uterus taking estrogen replacement, uterine protection can be achieved with FDA-approved, pharmaceutical-grade, bioidentical progesterone (micronized oral pills or vaginal gels), a synthetic progestin (medroxyprogesterone, norethindrone acetate, etc.), a progestin-containing intrauterine device (Mirena/Liletta IUD) or a tissue selective estrogen complex (TSEC). A TSEC combines estrogen with a selective estrogen receptor modulator (SERM) that acts like progesterone on the uterus.

TESTOSTERONE

Testosterone is an androgenic steroid. Androgens are the hormones that play a role in developing male traits and reproductive activity and include androstenediol, dehydroepiandrosterone (DHEA), androstenedione, testosterone, and dihydrotestosterone.

After cleaving off the tail from cholesterol's classic steroid backbone, newly minted progestogens can be converted to dehydroepiandrosterone

(DHEA) or androstenedione. Either of these androgens can then be converted to testosterone. Androgens are present in both males and females; with the principal androgens being androstenedione and testosterone. DHEA simply functions as a precursor to other androgens. Although men have 10 times more testosterone than women, women produce testosterone as well. Of all the androgens circulating in the body, only testosterone can bind to testosterone receptors to cause any effects on tissues. One of the main functions of androgens is to be converted to estrogen. On a one-way street to estrogen bliss, testosterone can be converted to estrogen, but estrogen cannot be converted back to testosterone.

1/3 of a woman's testosterone comes from her ovaries, 1/3 from her adrenals, and 1/3 from the conversion of precursor androgens into testosterone by the liver, skin and adipose (fatty) tissue. Testosterone helps women maintain muscle mass and bone strength, ponies up a positive outlook on life and contributes to sex drive. By the time a woman is menopausal, she may have only 50% of the testosterone she once had. Some women feel this testosterone slump while others are not too bothered by it. Interestingly, if a menopausal woman is on adequate estrogen replacement and has normal thyroid function, yet she's freezing all the time, she may have low testosterone levels. For women, a touch of testosterone goes a long way. On average, blood serum testosterone levels in women range from 20 to 70 ng/dL.

ANABOLIC STEROIDS

Anabolic steroids are synthetic variants of the male sex hormone testosterone. "Anabolic" refers to the muscle and bone building properties of these steroids, but since these are androgenic hormones, they have masculinizing effects, as well. These steroids can legally be prescribed to treat male sex hormone deficiencies or used in the treatment of diseases that result in loss of lean muscle mass, such as muscle wasting from cancer or AIDS. Alternatively, high-dose synthetic progestins, such as megestrol acetate (Megace) can increase lean body mass in these patients, as well.

Some athletes, body builders and others use anabolic steroids to try to enhance performance and/or improve their physical appearance. When abused in this manner, these powerful steroids can cause profound medical and psychological problems, chemically castrate men and masculinize women. Men experience shrinkage of testicles with low sperm count and infertility, baldness, growth of breasts (gynecomastia), heart problems and an increased risk of prostate cancer. Women sprout facial hair, develop acne, experience greasy hair and male pattern baldness, voice deepening, loss of menstrual cycles and infertility. Stunted growth due to premature skeletal maturation from anabolic steroids prohibits teenagers from reaching their maximum adult height. Impaired judgment and volatile mood swings can also occur, with mania and dangerous "roid rage" leading to violence. Using these steroids beyond physiological replacement levels results in testosterone toxicity.

DHEA

Dehydroepiandrosterone (DHEA) is an androgen steroid hormone produced mainly by the adrenal glands, but some DHEA is manufactured by the skin and brain, as well. Since testicles also produce DHEA, male DHEA levels are 30% higher than in females. DHEA levels peak at about 20 years old, and then gradually decline with age. Aside from being a precursor in the biochemical production of testosterone and estrogen, any other specific physiological role for DHEA in the body remains unclear. DHEA levels decrease with age, and folks with higher DHEA levels have better bone density and respond better to antidepressant medications. DHEA levels are lower in women with systemic lupus erythematous (lupus), and lower DHEA levels may be associated with more rapid HIV/AIDS disease progression.

DHEA has been touted to have anti-aging, anti-depressant, anti-obesity and anti-cancer benefits, while simultaneously improving skin thickness, strengthening bones, improving athletic performance and boosting sexuality. In the United States, DHEA preparations are available as dietary supplements. Most of the claims made about DHEA's benefits are based on results from animal, rather than human, studies. This is problematic, because animals metabolize DHEA differently from humans, so their bodies' response to supplements may vary from ours. Fewer studies have looked at the effects of DHEA on humans, and most of these are short-term, small-scale trials in elderly adults. Clinical results are somewhat inconsistent, so additional research with well-designed, long-term studies involving larger numbers of people is needed.

Any beneficial results or side effects attributed to DHEA supplements are most likely due to its conversion to estrogen and testosterone. Because of DHEA's conversion to testosterone, some women may develop unwanted masculinizing side effects such as facial hair growth, scalp hair loss and deepening voice. Since DHEA can also be converted to estrogen, postmenopausal women may enjoy estrogenic benefits while men may experience breast enlargement, shrunken testicles and decreased sperm production. DHEA supplementation may also have a deleterious impact on hormone-sensitive cancers, such as breast cancer or prostate cancer. DHEA may hold some promise in certain situations, but more research is needed to elucidate its clinical usefulness. Meanwhile, if blood serum DHEA levels are below normal, judicial oral supplementation, fine-tuned by clinical assessments and hormone testing, may be helpful for some women.

VITAMIN D - the SUNSHINE HORMONE

The largest organ in the body, the skin, uses ultraviolet (UV) sunlight to manufacture vitamin D. The UV "B" radiation triggers the conversion of cholesterol to vitamin D3, which is then further modified by the liver and kidneys to its biologically active form of vitamin D. On average, just 20 minutes of sun exposure, three times a week, between the peak UV light hours of 10am to 3pm, will generate healthy levels of vitamin D. In the United States, people living north of the 37th parallel, geographically a line drawn from Los Angeles, CA to Columbia, SC, do not get enough sunlight throughout the year for adequate vitamin D synthesis, so oral vitamin D supplements are recommended.

Vitamins are organic compounds (chemicals that contain carbon), which are needed in small quantities to sustain life. Because the body cannot synthesize these "vital amines," they must be acquired through the diet. Inadequate vitamin intake leads to vitamin deficiency diseases. For example, vitamin C deficiency leads to scurvy. Vitamin D is unique, because it is the only "conditional vitamin," meaning supplementation is conditional and dependent on inadequate sun exposure. Adequate exposure to sunlight can eliminate the requirement for vitamin D to be in the diet; however, when there are conditions precluding adequate sun exposure, then supplemental oral intake of vitamin D is required. The sunshine vitamin's synthesis starts in one location, the skin, and then it is secreted directly into the bloodstream to impact tissue activity elsewhere, so Vitamin D is also categorized as a hormone. Like all other cholesterol-based steroid hormones, vitamin D is fat-soluble and crosses lipid-laden cell membranes easily.

Vitamin D is needed for the body's intestines to absorb calcium from food sources and dietary supplements. From heart rhythms and nerve transmissions to muscle contractions and adequate blood clotting, calcium is vital to every cell's function. Because bones need vitamin D to absorb and use calcium, magnesium, and phosphate effectively, vitamin D is critical for bone mineralization and teeth maintenance. Vitamin D deficiency in adults leads to osteoporosis and tooth loss. In children, vitamin D deficiency results in rickets, growth retardation, and dental problems. If mom is vitamin D deficient, then her breast milk will not contain adequate vitamin D for the baby. If a woman is not getting enough vitamin D through sun exposure, it can be obtained through vitamin D-fortified foods or supplements. Unless blood tests indicate low vitamin D levels, a daily oral supplement of 1000 IU of vitamin D3 should take care of most women's vitamin D needs. It's okay if this vitamin D supplement is in addition to the vitamin D 400 IU found in most multivitamins. Blood tests indicate that healthy levels of 25-hydroxy vitamin D range between 20 to 100 ng/mL.

As the world turns, the sun never sets on these elegant and captivating steroids. From sex steroids to life-sustaining cortisol and vitamin D, these cholesterol-based, well-designed hormones lovingly make the world go round.

HORMONES: BIOIDENTICALS vs. SYNTHETICS

There is a lot of confusion about synthetic hormones versus natural substances, compounded preparations versus off-the-shelf pharmaceuticals, bioidenticals versus imitation hormones. To understand their relevance to menopause hormone therapy, we need to review the terminology.

BIOIDENTICALS, aka "BODY"-IDENTICALS

Steroid hormones produced by a woman's body are considered "natural," and since they are generated within her system, they are also referred to as "endogenous" hormones. What may be natural and endogenous to one creature may be alien to another. For example, the 10 different estrogens found in conjugated equine estrogen (Premarin), which is made from pregnant mares' urine, are natural to a pregnant horse, but they are exotic and unnatural to a woman.

Conversely, regardless of where they come from, hormones that are chemically identical in molecular shape, structure and make-up to hormones naturally endogenous to a woman's body are accurately considered bioidentical or "body"-identical. These bioidentical hormones do not need to be made by a biological organism; they just need to be identical in chemical structure to the hormones produced naturally by the woman's body. It's not the source; it's the structure that makes a hormone bioidentical.

All hormones distributed for human consumption are produced or synthesized in a lab somewhere. Raw materials for the synthesis of bioidentical hormones are mainly derived from plants, usually extracted from wild yams, soybeans, peanuts, canola and pine trees. These substances then undergo chemical processes to become a hormone product prescribed for therapeutic purposes. Whether distributed by the commercial pharmaceutical industry or compounded by a pharmacist, as long as the final hormone formulation is chemically and structurally identical to a hormone produced by a woman's body, it is a bioidentical hormone.

There are FDA-approved, pharmaceutical-grade bioidentical hormones for estrogen, progesterone and testosterone available in a variety of doses and formulations. Oral micronized estradiol (Estrace), estradiol vaginal tablets (Vagifem), oral micronized progesterone (Prometrium), progesterone vaginal gel (Crinone/Prochieve) and topical testosterone gel (AndroGel or Testim) are some of the bioidentical hormone preparations prescribed for replacement therapies. Micronized means that small particles of the bioidentical hormone are used to formulate the preparation, which improves the hormone's absorption and bioavailability within the body. Not only are these FDA-approved, pharmaceutical-grade bioidentical preparations tested for potency, purity, efficacy and safety, the chemical structures of the hormones in these prescriptions are identical to the hormones naturally produced in a woman's body.

Compounded bioidentical hormones, on the other hand, are mixed or compounded at the pharmacy level, so they are not governed by the same type of production oversight required of commercial pharmaceuticals. The FDA allows legitimate preparation of compounded formulations to be regulated by state boards of pharmacy. Traditionally, compounded medications are used when a patient is allergic to an ingredient in a commercially available preparation or if the patient requires an alternative form of medication delivery. Custom-blending commercially available drug products do not render compounded hormones any safer, or more natural, than their FDA-approved, pharmaceutical-grade, bioidentical counterparts.

In menopausal women, hormone levels in the saliva do not represent what is circulating in the bloodstream, nor do they necessarily correlate with response to treatment. Saliva testing is analogous to relying on urine dipsticks to manage insulin hormone therapy in a diabetic patient. Hormones are transported to their target organs via the bloodstream, so therapeutic levels need to be assessed through blood tests.

For menopausal health and happiness, hormone therapy should achieve therapeutic blood serum estradiol levels between 50 to 150 pg/mL. No matter what the estrone or estriol levels are, any menopause hormone therapy needs to reach adequate levels of estradiol to be effective. Blood serum levels of 30 to 50 pg/mL of estradiol are the lowest estradiol levels women ever experience during their reproductive years. This is level of estradiol that occurs during the uterine bleeding phase of the menstrual cycle. On day 3 or 4 of a woman's period, the ovaries' production of estradiol starts increasing and eventually the estradiol level peaks at its pre-ovulatory high of 400 pg/mL.

Since bioidentical hormones are identical to hormones naturally produced by the body, they cannot be patented. However, systems for delivering bioidentical hormones into the body, such as transdermal skin patches, topical gels, emulsions, skin sprays, etc., or "micronized" oral hormone preparations, can be patented. Methodology or the process by which bioidentical hormones are manufactured can also be patented. By altering the molecular structure of hormones, synthetic steroids offer patent protection and profitability for 17 years. Predictably then, commercial pharmaceutical efforts are directed more towards creating and marketing synthetic hormones.

Natural progesterone is not well absorbed through the skin's outermost keratin layer, so a woman would need to slather herself all over with progesterone cream to transmit adequate progesterone to her uterus. Although natural progesterone vaginal gels (Crinone/Prochieve) are absorbed well and protect the uterus, many women find them cumbersome for long-term use. There is an FDA-approved, pharmaceutical-grade bioidentical oral micronized progesterone (Prometrium) pill available, and it is made from peanut oil.

A new oral hormone pill for menopause hormone therapy, which contains a combination of bioidentical estradiol and bioidentical natural progesterone (TX-001HR), is undergoing a phase 3 study to evaluate its efficacy and safety compared to placebo. In this REPLENISH clinical trial, the natural progesterone in the combo gelatin capsule is not derived from peanuts, so it will give women with a peanut allergy an option for natural oral progesterone.

SYNTHETICS

"Synthetic steroid hormones," also known as, imitation hormones, are man-made steroids formulated or synthesized to resemble and act like hormones produced by the human body. This is accomplished by simple alterations to the chemical attachments linked to the fused four-ring cholesterol backbone common to all steroids.

Although synthetic steroids are not bioidentical, that is, they are not chemically identical to the hormones produced in the human body, they do resemble natural hormones and they produce similar hormonal effects on the body's tissues. When bioidentical hormones are degraded by stomach acid, deactivated by the liver or poorly absorbed, synthetic steroids are required to achieve therapeutic goals. Contraceptive hormones, some menopause hormones (medroxyprogesterone (Provera), anabolic steroids, and steroids used to treat infections, autoimmune diseases or organ transplants, are examples of synthetic hormones.

TIBOLONE – the Multi-faceted Menopause Hormone

Tibolone (Livial) is a unique steroid hormone that combines all the power of estrogen, progesterone and testosterone in an easy to swallow, once a day pill. At a dose of either 1.25mg or 2.5mg, it alleviates menopausal hot flashes, night sweats, vaginal dryness, disturbed sleep and mood swings. Tibolone restores a woman's lost libido while simultaneously preventing osteoporosis, dementia, and urinary incontinence. It does not cause breast tenderness nor does it increase a menopausal woman's breast density on mammograms. Tibolone is not associated with adverse cardiac events, such as heart attacks, or increasing blood clots in deep veins. Tibolone helps decrease a woman's risk of colon cancer, as well. Tibolone accomplishes all this without increasing a woman's risk of breast cancer or uterine cancer.

A synthetic steroid that is structurally related to the progestins found in oral contraceptives, tibolone is classified as a selective tissue estrogen action regulator (STEAR), because it has biologically active metabolites with tissue-specific estrogen, progesterone and testosterone actions. After being swallowed, tibolone is partly activated in the intestines and then released into the bloodstream. Final activation of tibolone's hormonal metabolites occurs in target tissues such as brain, breast, bone, uterus, bladder, skin, etc.

Since 1990, tibolone has been used for menopause hormone therapy in over 90 countries throughout the world, but it is not available in the United States. It is used in Europe, Australia, and Asia, to treat bothersome menopausal symptoms of hot flashes, night sweats, vaginal dryness and painful intercourse. It is also approved to prevent osteoporosis and reduces the risk of osteoporotic hip and spine fractures in older women.

Unlike other oral estrogen hormone therapies, the selective estrogen receptor modulators (SERMs) such as tamoxifen (Nolvadex) or raloxifene (Evista), or the tissue-selective estrogen complex (TSEC) containing estrogen with a SERM (Duavee), tibolone is not associated with an increased risk for blood clots. Like any other oral estrogenic hormone administered to a woman who is at least a decade beyond menopause, when tibolone is introduced to an estrogen-deprived postmenopausal woman 60 years or older, it is associated with an increased risk of strokes. Because aging blood vessels are inherently prone to develop blood clots and strokes, special precautions need to be observed before an older woman considers initiating any type of hormone therapy 10 or more years after menopause.

Tibolone-induced enzyme changes in breast tissue's estrogen metabolism lower the concentration of biologically active estrogen found within breast tissue, so tibolone causes far less breast tenderness than estrogen. Although estrogen-only therapy is not associated with an increased risk of breast cancer, menopause hormone therapy increases breast density on mammography in about 15% of estrogen-only users and 35% of estrogen-plus-progestin users. Breasts are made up of milk-producing glandular tissue and fatty tissue. As women get older, they have more fatty tissue in their breasts, and less milk-producing glandular tissue, so their breasts are less dense. Mammograms are more accurate and easier to interpret in older, fatty breasts as compared to younger, more glandular dense breasts. For a menopausal woman, having dense breast tissue on mammograms is linked to an increased risk of breast cancer compared to women with less dense breasts. Since progesterone prepares the breast for pregnancy and lactation, it is not surprising that progesterone added to estrogen replacement therapy increases breast density. Tibolone, on the other hand, does not increase breast density in menopausal women.

In a clinical trial involving women who had their breast cancer surgically treated, and where 75% of these women were also on tamoxifen or aromatase inhibitor adjuvant therapy, adding 2.5mg of tibolone to reduce their hot flashes was associated with an increased risk of breast cancer recurrence, especially in women with normal bone mineral density. Women with osteopenia or osteoporosis did not encounter a relapse of their breast cancer when tibolone was added to their treatment regimen. All the women experienced improved bone mineral density with the tibolone; nonetheless, at this juncture, tibolone is not recommended for women with breast cancer. Tibolone's ability to lower bioactive estrogen levels in normal breast tissue may be lost on breast cancer cells.

Estrogen stimulates the endometrial lining of the uterus to grow and grow, and this tissue proliferation increases a woman's risk of developing uterine cancer. Therefore, those women who have not had a hysterectomy and still have their uterus require progesterone to help prevent estrogen-stimulated overgrowth of the endometrial lining. Progesterone, especially synthetic progestins, cause increased breast density on mammograms, and this can be associated with a slightly increased risk of developing breast cancer. Tibolone, on the other hand, neither stimulates the endometrial lining of the uterus to proliferate, nor does it increase breast density.

Sex hormone binding globulins (SHBG) not only transport hormones to their target tissues, but they also bind and tie up hormones, as well. By decreasing the liver's production of SHBGs, tibolone increases levels of unbound, free testosterone. Not only does testosterone maintain skeletal muscle mass and balance, but it also elevates mood and improves concentration. A decided advantage of tibolone is that it increases sexual desire and enhances arousal and orgasms, without the androgenic side effects of acne or hirsutism associated with testosterone therapy.

With tibolone (Livial), a menopausal woman safely enjoys the healthy benefits of estrogen, progesterone and testosterone with minimal side effects. Although not bioidentical to the hormones naturally found in a woman's body, tibolone may be considered a multi-purpose hormone option for alleviating bothersome menopausal symptoms, while simultaneously preventing long-term debilitating diseases exacerbated by ovarian hormone deficiency.

HORMONES: PHYTOs, MYCOs, XENOs and DESIGNER NON-STEROIDALS

There are a variety of estrogenic substances out there. Some are the real deal, and some are imitations. Some are strong, and some are weak. Some are steroids, and others are non-steroidals. Some are user-friendly, others, not so much. To understand estrogen's omnipresence, we need to explore the galaxy of estrogens. There are two main categories of estrogen. There are the "classic" estrogen steroid hormones, and then there are the cholesterol-free, non-steroidal substances that are endowed with estrogenic activity.

Estrogen steroid hormones, whether natural, bioidentical or synthetic, all possess the structurally distinctive fused four-ring cholesterol chemical backbone common to all steroids. Examples of steroid hormones include the estrogens found in oral contraceptive pills (OCPs), estrogen patches, vaginal rings, as well as the estrogens in menopause hormone replacement therapy.

By definition, non-steroidal estrogenic substances lack the cholesterol-derived steroid backbone, but they still possess estrogenic powers. These chemicals may come about naturally, or they may be manufactured; some may contaminate our food or environment while others are prescribed as medical therapy for infertility, cancer treatment, and osteoporosis prevention. Because they are not steroids, non-steroidal medications are never bioidentical to the hormones found naturally in a woman's body.

Non-steroidal drugs, such as DES, selective estrogen receptor modulators (SERMs) like tamoxifen (Nolvadex), raloxifene (Evista), clomiphene (Clomid, Serophene, Androxal), do not possess chemical structures resembling a woman's estrogen molecule, but they have estrogenic impact in her body.

PHYTOESTROGENS

Phytoestrogens ("phyto-" meaning plant) are estrogenic substances found in some plants. Isoflavones in soybeans and lignans in flaxseed are examples of phytoestrogens. Consumed in large enough quantities, these phytoestrogens can influence physiology. Back in the 1940s, decreased fertility was observed in sheep that were grazing in pastures with red clover, a phytoestrogen-rich plant. This "clover disease" was due to excess estrogenic compounds disrupting the sheep's reproductive cycles.

Since phytoestrogens come from biological plant sources that exist in nature, they are natural; however, these estrogenic substances are unnatural to a woman's body. A woman's body neither produces these phytoestrogens nor, unlike sheep, does a woman have the enzymes needed to convert phytoestrogens into bioidentical estrogens. However, some women experience relief from their hot flashes with dietary phytoestrogen supplements. There really is no conclusive evidence that these dietary phytoestrogen supplements significantly reduce a woman's risk for heart disease, improve her bone density or reduce her cancer risk. For soy or flaxseed to reduce a woman's risk of breast cancer, consumption of these foods during childhood and adolescence is required. Whether adult soy food intake reduces breast cancer risk is unclear.

MYCOESTROGENS

Mycoestrogens ("myco-" meaning fungus) are estrogenic chemicals found in certain fungi. Some of these fungi contaminate cereal grains and animal feed sources, producing estrogenic compounds that make their way into people's diets.

XENOESTROGENS

Plastic, "the material of a 1000 uses," was invented in 1907, and since then, hundreds of xenoestrogens, ("xeno-" meaning foreign) estrogenic compounds, have been introduced into the environment by industrial, agricultural and chemical companies. These alien estrogenic chemicals are found in herbicides, pesticides, organic solvents and plastics, as well as in general hygiene consumer products, such as toothpaste, lotions, perfumes, cosmetics, deodorants and fabric softeners.

Two of the most prevalent and damaging xenoestroges are phthalates and bisphenol-A (PBA). Phthalates are chemicals that soften plastic, so they render plastic durable and flexible. Shower curtains, toys, IV tubing and IV drip bags, polyvinyl chloride (PVC) products, and plastic food wrappings harbor phthalates. That "new car smell" is a heady blend of phthalates. Bisphenol-A (BPA) is used to manufacture polycarbonate plastic and epoxy resins lining most food and beverage containers. The walls of plastic water bottles containing "healthy" water have BPA. These BPA-based polymers are subject to hydrolysis and may leach into the food or beverage. Just to be on the safe side, it's better to eat from glass, ceramic or stainless steel containers, when possible. To minimize leaching of undesirable xenoestrogens into one's food, do not microwave food in plastic or styrofoam containers; use glass or microwave-safe ceramics, instead.

As endocrine disrupting compounds, xenoestrogens disturb the reproductive physiology of organisms habiting the planet, and this hormonal imbalance has lead to anatomical genital confusion among fish, turtles, mice, and polar bears. Higher up the food chain, xenoestrogens have also been implicated in precocious puberty in children. Precocious puberty is the development of secondary sex characteristics before the age of 8 in girls and before the age of 9 in boys. This results in earlier sexual maturation, earlier closure of bone growth plates and shorter adult stature. Xenoestrogens can interfere with ovulation causing irregular menstrual periods and decreased fertility. Surrounded by unnecessary estrogenic substances everywhere, it's no wonder that men's sperm counts are decreasing, as well. Obviously, the wrong kind of estrogen, at the wrong time, in the wrong person, can be damaging.

DESIGNER NON-STEROIDALS

Over the years, some non-steroidal estrogens have been synthesized for medicinal and therapeutic purposes. Diethylstilbestrol (DES), selective estrogen receptor modulators (SERMs), and tissue selective estrogen complexes (TSECs) are medications that are used in infertility, for the alleviation of bothersome menopausal symptoms, and for the treatment and prevention of breast cancer and osteoporosis. These exotic estrogenic chemicals pose the same increased risk for developing blood clots as any other oral estrogen therapy: from a baseline risk of 1 in 1000 to 3 in 1000. They also increase an older woman's risk of stroke by 30%: from a baseline risk of 3 in 100 to 4 in 100. The actual chance that a particular woman using hormones will have a blood clot or stroke is still very low.

The DES STORY

Diethylstilbestrol (DES) is the first and most potent synthetic form of estrogen ever manufactured. It is a powerful non-steroidal estrogen that was initially developed in 1938, and until the early 1980s, it remained the hormonal treatment of choice for advanced breast cancer in postmenopausal women. When Mayo Clinic's 1981 head-to-head comparison of DES to tamoxifen (Nolvadex) therapy showed similar breast cancer response rates, but with fewer side effects in tamoxifen users, cancer treatment protocols switched to utilizing tamoxifen over DES. DES was also the first effective drug treatment for symptomatic metastatic prostate cancer in men. Until the early 1980s, bilateral testicle removal or DES or both were the standard initial treatment for painful metastatic prostate cancer. Then in 1985, the gonadotropin-releasing hormone (GnRH)-agonist (Lupron) was found to have similar response rates to DES, without DES's estrogenic side effects, so prostate cancer treatment protocols switched to using GnRH-agonists over DES.

From 1938 to 1971, DES was used to prevent miscarriages and premature deliveries in pregnant women. At that time, it was believed that these obstetrical problems occurred because some women did not produce enough estrogen to sustain a pregnancy. In 1971, when DES was identified as a cause of a rare vaginal-cervical cancer in young women exposed to DES before birth, the Food and Drug Administration (FDA) advised physicians to stop prescribing DES to pregnant women. The risk for this clear cell adenocarcinoma of the vagina-cervix in a DES daughter is 1 in 1000 female babies exposed to DES. Most of these cases occur in DES-exposed daughters younger than 30 years of age; however, 1 out 3 women diagnosed with this rare type of gynecological cancer is a non-DES exposed, older woman over the age of 50. Since the risk for a DES-exposed daughter developing this cancer, as she gets older, is currently unknown, screening for clear cell adenocarcinoma of the vagina-cervix has no upper age limit. Any abnormal vaginal bleeding or discharge should be thoroughly evaluated, including rotating the vaginal speculum to view the anterior and posterior walls of the vagina. DES-exposed daughters are also at increased for developing breast cancer.

Infants whose mothers took DES during the first 5 months of pregnancy may sustain reproductive tract abnormalities. A "T-shaped" uterus and atypical cervical shapes with ridges or collars and vaginal adenosis occur in DES-exposed daughters. Since they experience a higher rate of ectopic pregnancies, miscarriages, and premature delivery, pregnancy in a DES-exposed woman is considered high-risk. Despite increased risks for infertility and adverse pregnancy outcomes, most DES-exposed daughters, however, can become pregnant and carry a pregnancy to term. DES-exposed sons may develop benign cysts in the epididymis, the tightly coiled tubes connected to the testicles. So far, research has shown no decreased fertility for these men, even with testicular abnormalities, and a possible relationship for increased risk of testicular or prostate cancer in DES-exposed sons is unclear.

When DES was discovered to be harmful to humans, it was moved to veterinary use. As an estrogen, low-dose DES has been very successful in treating urinary incontinence in spayed female dogs. Currently, DES's use in humans is restricted to clinical trials for the treatment of various hormonally responsive malignancies.

SERMs

Selective estrogen receptor modulators (SERMs) are synthetic chemicals that act like estrogen on some tissues in a woman's body, and act as anti-estrogens in other tissues. Because of this dual action, SERMs are also referred to as estrogen agonists/antagonists. These non-steroidal compounds are used to treat ovulation problems in infertility, low testosterone in men, and to prevent and treat breast cancer. They are also used to treat menopausal issues associated with estrogen deficiency, such as painful intercourse due to vaginal dryness and bone-thinning due to osteoporosis. The most commonly used SERMs are clomiphene (Clomid, Serophene, Androxal), tamoxifen (Nolvadex) and raloxifene (Evista). Newer SERMs include ospemifene (Osphena) and the bazedoxifene found in the tissue selective estrogen complex (TSEC) marketed as Duavee. Women who are pregnant or may become pregnant, as well as nursing mothers, should not use SERMS. SERMs are associated with an increased risk for developing blood clots and strokes.

CLOMIPHENE

Clomiphene (Clomid, Serophene, Androxal)) is a SERM that is utilized in both women and men. It is used to induce ovulation in infertile women suffering from polycystic ovary syndrome (PCOS) or infrequent ovulation. The evidence is lacking for the use of clomiphene in couples where the cause for infertility is unknown. Clomiphene can lead to multiple ovulations, increasing the chance of twins to 1 out of 12 births (8% twin rate). In the general population, the chance of having twins is 1 out of 88 births, and the chance of having triplets is only 1 out of 88^2 (1 out of 7,744) births.

Clomiphene has also been found to be an effective treatment for low testosterone levels in men. Compared to testosterone replacement, not only is clomiphene cheaper and more convenient to take as an oral pill, it does not shrink testicles or cause infertility the way testosterone treatment can. Because of its athletic performance-enhancing effects, clomiphene is included in the World Anti-Doping Agency list of illegal doping agents in sports.

Like tamoxifen (Nolvadex), prolonged use of clomiphene can increase the development of cataracts.

TAMOXIFEN

Tamoxifen (Nolvadex) is the SERM that is used as adjuvant therapy to decrease the risk of recurrence of estrogen-receptor positive (ER+) breast cancer. In women at high-risk for developing breast cancer, tamoxifen can also be used to prevent the disease. Tamoxifen was initially created when scientists were tasked with finding an emergency contraception. Tamoxifen has no contraceptive effect on humans. In fact, tamoxifen is just as effective as the other SERM, clomiphene (Clomid, Serophene, Androxal), in triggering ovulation in women with polycystic ovary syndrome (PCOS). Usually prescribed for 5 years to women over age 35, tamoxifen acts as an estrogen antagonist on breast tissue, while simultaneously exerting estrogenic influence on a woman's uterine tissues. Although tamoxifen increases cataract formation and may cause vaginal dryness, it does help maintain bone density in a woman's spine and hip.

Women on tamoxifen often experience dreadful hot flashes. Selective serotonin reuptake inhibitor (SSRI) antidepressants such as paroxetine (Paxil, Brisdelle), fluoxetine (Prozac) or sertraline (Zoloft) help alleviate hot flashes and anxiety in menopausal women. Because SSRIs inhibit CYP2D6, the liver enzyme that converts tamoxifen into its active form, endoxifen, they interfere with tamoxifen's effectiveness in protecting a woman's breasts. Of all the SSRIs, venlafaxine (Effexor) has the least impact on inhibiting the CYP2D6 enzyme and is the safest choice when taken with tamoxifen. For those women who cannot take venlafaxine (Effexor), citalopram (Celexa) would be the second choice. Bupropion (Wellbutrin, Zyban) is an antidepressant that is prescribed for seasonal affective disorder (SAD) and to help people quit smoking, but it is a strong inhibitor of the CYP2D6 enzyme, as well. Because tamoxifen acts as an estrogen agonist on the uterus, it can cause the endometrial lining to proliferate, thicken and sprout endometrial polyps. The risk of endometrial uterine cancer in postmenopausal tamoxifen users is double that of nonusers, and this increased risk persists for 20 years after stopping tamoxifen. Any time a woman on tamoxifen experiences unusual uterine bleeding, she needs to be evaluated for the possibility of abnormal tissue growth in her uterus.

RALOXIFENE

Raloxifene (Evista) is another SERM that exhibits estrogen antagonist effects on breast tissue and is as effective as tamoxifen in preventing estrogen-positive (ER+) invasive breast cancer in postmenopausal women. Raloxifene does not stimulate the endometrial tissue lining of the uterus, so it does not increase a woman's risk for uterine cancer. It acts like estrogen on trabecular bone, so it prevents and treats osteoporosis of the spine. Although it helps maintain spinal bone density, raloxifene is not effective in reducing osteoporosis-related hip fractures. Like tamoxifen, raloxifene can cause hot flashes, but unlike tamoxifen, raloxifene is unaffected by CYP2D6 metabolism, so SSRIs can be used to help ease raloxifene-induced hot flashes. Although tamoxifen and raloxifene have beneficial effects on a woman's cholesterol lipid profile, both are associated with an increased risk for blood clots and strokes.

OSPEMIFENE

When a woman's vaginal and vulvar genital tissues are deprived of estrogen, they become thinner, dryer and less elastic. This loss of tissue architecture and function is called vulvovaginal atrophy (VVA) or genitourinary syndrome of menopause (GSM). Without some type of estrogen treatment, vaginal tissue integrity deteriorates, so menopausal women suffer from vaginal dryness, scarring and painful sexual intercourse. This can significantly impact the quality of life for many women and may cause relationship issues. Since the vagina is an estrogen-dependent organ, estrogen replacement therapy maintains vaginal tissue anatomy and function, and enhances sexual enjoyment.

Ospemifene (Osphena) is a SERM that is a non-estrogen oral treatment for painful intercourse due to postmenopausal vulvar/vaginal tissue atrophy. As a SERM, ospemifene (Osphena) acts as an estrogen on some tissues and an anti-estrogen on other tissues in a woman's body. Similar to other SERMs, ospemifene causes hot flashes and increases a woman's risk for blood clots and strokes. Similar to fellow SERMs, tamoxifen (Nolvadex) and raloxifene (Evista), ospemifene (Osphena) exhibits anti-estrogen effects on breast tissue while providing estrogen-like bone protection. Unlike other SERMs that don't touch the vagina, ospemifene exerts a strong, estrogen effect on the vaginal tissues, so it is used for the treatment of vulvovaginal atrophy (VVA) and painful intercourse in postmenopausal women unable or unwilling to use estrogen replacement. Although ospemifene does not appear to stimulate the uterus as much as tamoxifen, its package insert prescribing information recommends that physicians consider coupling ospemifene with a progesterone to protect a woman's uterine lining from overgrowth and potential cancerous changes induced by ospemifene.

BREAST CANCER PREVENTION with SERMs

Among postmenopausal women at increased risk of breast cancer, taking either the tamoxifen (Nolvadex) or raloxifene (Evista) SERM for 5 years can reduce their risk of estrogen receptor-positive (ER+) breast cancer by 38%. Since 80% of breast cancers are estrogen receptor positive, SERM's prevention of invasive breast cancer in high-risk women is rather significant.

TSECs

The head-to-toe benefits of menopause hormone therapy are linked to estrogen replacement, and clinical trials have confirmed that estrogen-only menopause hormone therapy is not associated with an increased risk of breast cancer. Taking estrogen-plus-progesterone, particularly a synthetic progestin, does increase a woman's risk for developing breast cancer, but ever so slightly. For example, 4 out of 100 women between the ages of 50 to 79 years old will develop breast cancer during the next 10 years. If all 100 of these women are taking estrogen-plus-progesterone hormone therapy, then 5 out of 100 hormone-taking women will be diagnosed with cancer. This is the 25% increased relative risk of breast cancer that everyone talks about, from 4 women to 5 out of a 100. This is an increased absolute risk of less than 1% (0.8% to be exact). A woman's individual risk of developing breast cancer while taking physiologically based menopause hormone replacement therapy is really quite small.

For menopausal women who have had a hysterectomy, female hormone replacement therapy involves replacing her estrogen. For those women who have a uterus, progesterone needs to be added to temper estrogen's unfettered stimulation of the endometrial lining of the uterus. Without progesterone, unopposed estrogen can increase a woman's risk of developing endometrial uterine cancer.

An alternative to progesterone is using a selective estrogen receptor modulator (SERM) with anti-estrogenic effects on the uterus. A tissue selective estrogen complex (TSEC) is the pleasant union of an estrogen with a SERM. Conjugated equine estrogen (the estrogen found in Premarin) 0.45mg coupled to the SERM, bazedoxifene 20mg, is a TSEC marketed as Duavee. The estrogen component of this hormonal duo provides a woman with the benefits of estrogen replacement therapy, while the SERM component acts as an anti-estrogen on the uterus, preventing endometrial tissue overgrowth. This is accomplished without exposing a postmenopausal woman's breasts to the progesterone hormone. The bazedoxifene also appears to act as an anti-estrogen on the breast, so there is no increase in breast pain or breast density on mammograms. For women with a uterus, Duavee is indicated for the treatment of menopausal hot flashes and night sweats, as well as the prevention of postmenopausal osteoporosis. Similar to other oral estrogens or SERMs, Duavee is associated with an increased risk for blood clots and strokes.

SPRM Detour

Selective estrogen receptor modulators (SERMs) do not resemble estrogen's steroid chemical structure, but act like estrogen in some tissues, and exhibit anti-estrogen impact on other tissues in a woman's body. On the other hand, selective progesterone receptor modulators (SPRMs), such as ulipristal acetate (Ella), mifepristone (RU486) and telapristone acetate (Proellex), are synthetic steroids that possess the distinctive cholesterol chemical backbone common to a woman's natural progesterone, yet act more like anti-progesterone. Unlike progesterone or progestins, selective progesterone receptor modulators (SPRMs) do not stimulate breast cells to proliferate, nor do they increase breast density on mammograms. Although they resemble steroids structurally, SPRMs do not interfere with ovarian hormone production, so a woman's estradiol, progesterone and testosterone levels remain normal.

Emergency contraception acts by inhibiting a woman's ovulation. Compared to the over the counter oral emergency contraception pill containing 1.5mg of the synthetic progestin levonorgestrel (Plan B One-Step), which needs to be taken within 72 hours of unprotected sex or birth control failure, the SPRM ulipristal acetate (Ella) 30mg pill can be prescribed as emergency contraception for 5 days following unprotected sex. This provides extra protection since sperm can live for 5 days in a woman's reproductive tract.

Mifepristone (RU486) is a synthetic steroidal anti-progesterone pill approved by the FDA for non-surgical abortions within the first 63 days of pregnancy. It is also used for the treatment of Cushing's syndrome, an adrenal disorder. Treatment for uterine fibroids (leiomyomas) and endometriosis in women consists of surgery, hormonal contraception, or short-term treatment with gonadotropin-releasing hormone (GnRH)-agonist shots. GnRH-agonists induce a wicked menopausal-like state and promote bone loss, so their use is not recommended for more than 6 months. Once treatment stops, the uterine fibroids may grow back, and the endometriosis symptoms return. Telapristone acetate (Proellex) is an oral SPRM that alleviates symptoms of heavy bleeding and pain associated with uterine fibroids and endometriosis while maintaining a woman's estrogen balance.

Since the root cause of menopausal difficulties is estrogen deficiency, nothing alleviates bothersome menopausal symptoms as holistically and effectively as estrogen therapy. Nothing takes care of postmenopausal estrogen loss as safely and naturally as FDA-approved, pharmaceutical grade, bioidentical hormones. These hormones are structurally and chemically identical to the estradiol, progesterone and testosterone molecules once produced naturally by a woman's ovaries. Alternatively, for women who have personal or medical issues that deter them from taking menopause hormone replacement therapy, designer estrogen compounds, such as selective estrogen receptor modulators (SERMs) and tissue-selective estrogen complexes (TSECs), provide alternative therapeutic options.

PROGESTERONE: PILLS, VAGINAL GELS or IUD

Estrogen replacement therapy was introduced in the early 1940s to counteract menopausal symptoms of hot flashes, night sweats, vaginal dryness, and depression. In the 1970s, progesterone was added to estrogen to reduce the risk of uterine problems associated with estrogen-only therapy. Since then, we have learned that exposing the rest of a postmenopausal woman's body to synthetic progesterone can be problematic, especially when it comes to slightly increasing her risk of breast cancer and blood clots in her lungs. Let's investigate these issues in more detail and introduce some alternatives to body-wide exposure to synthetic progesterone.

Within the holy trinity of ovarian hormones, estrogen is the principal force of womanhood, progesterone promotes pregnancy, and testosterone is the tantalizing motivator. Since estrogen receptors exist in all organs throughout a woman's body, estrogen is important for maintaining her health and happiness. When a woman loses estrogen, she develops a range of menopausal symptoms, some more bothersome than others, but all leading to tiresome aging. Estrogen performs over 400 functions in the body. With prolonged estrogen deficiency, the body's infrastructure breaks down, tissues dry out, metabolism shifts and organs malfunction. All things considered, aging without estrogen is an unpleasant affair for most women. Quality of life improves significantly with appropriate menopause hormone therapy.

PROGESTERONE'S PURPOSE

In a reproductive aged woman, the "pro-gestation or pro-pregnancy" progesterone hormone prepares the breasts and uterus for pregnancy. If there is no potential for pregnancy, progesterone is simply not around. In a menopausal woman on hormone replacement therapy, progesterone's sole purpose is to protect the uterus. Estrogen stimulates the endometrial lining of the uterus to proliferate and grow and grow. This tissue overgrowth can lead to abnormalities such as endometrial hyperplasia, polyps, and endometrial uterine cancer. Progesterone modulates estrogen's impact on the uterus and prevents endometrial tissue overgrowth.

1 out of 3 women has had a hysterectomy by the time she is 65 years old, so she does not need to bother taking progesterone with her estrogen replacement therapy. On the other hand, menopausal women who still have a uterus need to couple their estrogen therapy with progesterone, or a substance that acts like progesterone, for uterine health. Without progesterone's action on the uterus, "unopposed estrogen" stimulates the endometrial lining of the uterus to proliferate, and this uninhibited tissue overgrowth may degenerate into uterine cancer.

Progestins are synthetic progesterones that chemically resemble, but are not identical to the progesterone produced by a woman's ovaries. Oral progestins used in menopause hormone therapy are designed to resist enzymatic degradation in the gastrointestinal tract, so they can remain biologically active in their mission to suppress estrogen's proliferative action on the endometrial uterine lining. About 15% of women using synthetic progestins experience weight gain, hair loss, and depressive symptoms.

Compared to synthetic progestins, most menopausal women who need to take progesterone with their estrogen replacement therapy fare better with bioidentical natural progesterone. Identical in chemical structure to the progesterone found naturally in women, "body"-identical or bioidentical progesterone is associated with fewer side effects when compared to synthetic progestins. FDA-approved, pharmaceutical grade, bioidentical progesterone is available as an oral pill, micronized oral progesterone (Prometrium) or as a vaginal progesterone gel (Crinone, Prochieve). Bioidentical progesterone in topical creams is poorly absorbed through the skin's outermost keratin layer, so a woman's endometrial uterine lining may not receive enough progesterone to counter estrogen's stimulation of the uterus. This could lead to problematic uterine bleeding, endometrial polyps and uterine cancer.

Progesterone prepares breasts for potential lactation by plumping up the milk-producing glandular tissue within the breasts. This increases breast tissue heterogeneity and breast density on mammograms and makes mammograms more difficult to interpret. Because young, perky breasts have more milk-producing glandular tissue than postmenopausal breasts, mammograms are not as reliable in younger women. As women age, the milk-producing glandular tissue is replaced by less dense, fatty breast tissue. By design, mammograms are more accurate in older, fatty breasts. Heterogeneously dense breast tissue visualized on older women's mammograms is linked to increased risk of developing breast cancer. Breast density may increase in a postmenopausal woman receiving synthetic progestin with her estrogen.

Estrogen replacement therapy does not increase a woman's risk of breast cancer; in fact, women taking estrogen have a 23% reduced risk of breast cancer compared to women taking a placebo (sugar pill). When it comes to issues of breast cancer and hormone replacement therapy, progesterone is the "bad boy" of menopause hormone therapy. Estrogen-plus-synthetic progestin use for more than 7 years slightly increases a woman's individual risk of breast cancer by less than 1% (0.8% to be exact). So, where does the 25% increased relative risk for breast cancer that we keep hearing about come from? Well, 4 out of 100 women between the ages of 50 to 79 years old will develop breast cancer during the next 10 years. If all 100 women are on estrogen plus synthetic progestin hormone therapy, then 5 out of 100 hormone-taking women will be diagnosed with breast cancer. From 4 to 5 is a relative risk increase of 25%. Although a woman's individual risk of developing breast cancer while taking estrogen plus synthetic progestin is quite small, even that less than 1% (0.8% to be exact) slight absolute increased risk can be minimized further by replacing the synthetic progestin with a bioidentical progesterone.

One of the ways estrogen helps protect a woman from heart disease is by increasing her "good" HDL-cholesterol ("H" for hurray) and lowering her "bad" LDL-cholesterol ("L" for lousy). Synthetic progestins decrease estrogen's positive effect on a menopausal woman's cholesterol lipid profile.

Oral estrogen therapy increases a woman's chance for developing a blood clot from 1 in 1000 in non-estrogen users to 3 in 1000 women taking estrogen. 10% of the time, a piece of this clot breaks off and travels through the bloodstream and lodges in the lungs, causing a blockage, called pulmonary embolism. Untreated, a pulmonary embolism can be fatal. When comparing menopausal women on estrogen-only therapy to women taking estrogen-plus-progestin, the risk for pulmonary embolism is not significantly increased for women on estrogen-only therapy. The synthetic progestin may be playing a role in a blood clot drifting off from a leg vein or pelvic vein to become lodged as a pulmonary embolism. All in all, exposing a postmenopausal woman's body to synthetic progestins can be problematic.

Medroxyprogesterone acetate (Provera) is the most commonly used synthetic progestin in menopause hormone therapy, and it is the progestin coupled to conjugated equine estrogen (Premarin), marketed as Prempro or Premphase. The medroxyprogesterone is either taken as 2.5mg swallowed every day or 5mg to 10mg taken daily for 2 weeks of each calendar month. Other preparations where estrogen is coupled to synthetic progestins include:

- Estradiol plus norethindrone (Activella-oral pill, CombiPatch-skin patch)
- Estradiol plus norgestimate (Prefest)
- Estradiol plus drospirenone (Angeliq)
- Estradiol plus levonorgestrel (Climara Pro skin patch)
- Ethinyl estradiol plus norethindrone (Femhrt)

FDA-approved, pharmaceutical-grade, bioidentical progesterones, such as oral micronized progesterone (Prometrium) and sustained-release vaginal progesterone gel (Crinone/Prochieve), are dependable progesterone delivery preparations that reliably protect the uterus. Prometrium is made from peanut oil, so women with a peanut allergy should avoid it. When used as the progesterone in menopause hormone therapy, the 100 mg dose of Prometrium can be swallowed daily, or the 200mg dose can be taken daily for 2 weeks of each calendar month. The bioidentical vaginal progesterone gels, Crinone or Prochieve, are available in 4% (delivering 45mg of progesterone per application) or 8% (delivering 90mg of progesterone per application) strengths. The 4% strength can be used intravaginally daily for 2 weeks of each month or the 8% strength can be used intravaginally twice a week year round. Since progesterone administered vaginally is directly transported into the uterus through the "uterine first-pass effect," effective protection of the endometrial uterine lining is achieved despite low blood serum levels of progesterone. This exposes the rest of the woman's body to less progesterone.

Menopause hormone therapy regimens using 14 days of progesterone each calendar month generate predictable monthly uterine bleeding. The alternative approach to progesterone, which is a daily intake or a continuous daily exposure to progesterone can cause irregularly irregular uterine bleeding or spotting for up to a year after initiating menopause hormone therapy. After 6 months on the daily combined estrogen plus progesterone therapy, 60% of women no longer experience uterine bleeding. As time goes by, bleeding tends to get lighter and lighter, so that after a year of being on this regimen, over 90% of women stop having any uterine bleeding. The daily or continuous progesterone regimen protects the endometrial lining of the uterus more effectively than intermittent progesterone exposure. Some women prefer the predictability of scheduled uterine bleeding, so they opt for the regimen that induces a monthly period. If uterine bleeding occurs at off-schedule times, the abnormal bleeding needs to be evaluated. Other women would rather deal with unpredictable bleeding for the initial year of hormone therapy, to reach a point of no more uterine bleeding. For these women, any uterine bleeding beyond a year needs to be evaluated.

The recommended doses of progesterone or progestin are usually coupled to the standard dose of estrogen replacement therapy used in

50-something menopausal women. That daily estrogen dose equivalency is: 1 mg of micronized oral estradiol or 17beta-estradiol (Estrace) = 0.625mg of oral conjugated equine estrogen (Premarin) or synthetic conjugated estrogen (Cenestin, Enjuvia) = 0.75mg estropipate (Ogen 0.625) = 5 mcg of oral ethinyl estradiol (Femhrt) = 0.05mg/day of estradiol in estrogen skin patches (Vivelle-Dot) = 0.05mg/day of estradiol acetate in a vaginal ring (Femring).

TSEC

There are synthetic chemical alternatives to progesterone developed for endometrial uterine protection. Coupled to the conjugated estrogen found in Premarin, bazedoxifene is a selective estrogen receptor modulator (SERM) found in the tissue selective estrogen complex (TSEC) marketed as Duavee. The estrogen component alleviates hot flashes, decreases vaginal dryness and helps prevent bone loss, while the SERM, bazedoxifene, counters estrogen's stimulation of the endometrial lining of the uterus. Like other oral estrogens and other SERMs, Duavee increases a woman's risk for blood clots and strokes. For women who have a uterus, this once a day pill is a progesterone-free method of using estrogen replacement therapy.

PROGESTERONE IUD

When applied to menopause hormone therapy, the only purpose of even having progesterone, progestin or a progesterone-like chemical on board is to modulate estrogen's stimulation of uterus. Because a menopausal woman is no longer reproducing, the "pro-gestation or pro-pregnancy" hormone serves no physiological function at this stage of her life. Exposing her non-uterine parts, particularly her postmenopausal breasts, to progesterone is problematic.

So, it makes sense to limit delivery of progesterone to the only organ that requires it, the endometrial lining of the uterus. This is effectively and safely accomplished using the progestin-impregnated Mirena/Liletta IUD (intra-uterine device). The T-shaped flexible IUD has been used in Europe since 1991, and it received FDA approval in the United States in

2000. The progestin IUD contains 52 mg of levonorgestrel progestin. Levonorgestrel is found in various oral contraceptive pills (Alesse, Nordette, Seasonale, Triphasil), emergency contraception (Plan B One-Step, Preven) and the menopause hormone patch (Climara Pro). The FDA has approved the progestin-containing IUD for contraceptive purposes and the treatment of heavy uterine bleeding. With this IUD, pelvic cramping decreases and menstrual blood flow is reduced by at least 50%. In fact, the progestin IUD is as effective as endometrial ablation for the treatment of heavy menstrual bleeding. In carefully selected women, it may be beneficial for the treatment of endometriosis, adenomyosis, uterine fibroids, and endometrial hyperplasia. Progestin IUDs may also prevent endometrial uterine problems associated with tamoxifen (Nolvadex) therapy used to treat breast cancer.

Obviously, a menopausal woman does not need the IUD for contraception. For a woman on estrogen replacement therapy, the progestin IUD is simply a means of delivering progesterone to the target organ that needs it, the endometrial lining of the uterus. Meanwhile, the rest of her body is spared from unnecessary progesterone exposure. The Mirena/Liletta progestin IUD releases 20 micrograms of the levonorgestrel progestin into the uterus daily. Very little, less than 10%, of the very, very low dose progestin released into the uterine cavity by the IUD is ever absorbed into the bloodstream. Compared to the synthetic progestin medroxyprogesterone (Provera) 2.5mg pill swallowed every day or the bioidentical micronized progesterone (Prometrium) 100mg pill swallowed every day, a woman's exposure to the IUD's progestin is miniscule. The Mirena/Liletta IUD needs to be replaced every 5 to 7 years. During a 10-minute procedure in the gynecologist's office, the spent IUD can be removed, and the new progestin IUD inserted on the same day. The procedure is comfortable when the prostaglandin, misoprostol (Cytotec), is used to help soften and dilate the cervix. For women with a normal uterus, the risk of uterine perforation with an IUD is minimal, occurring in less than 1 out of 1000 insertions.

Unfortunately, women who have undergone endometrial ablation in the past are not candidates for any uterine protection system utilizing the convenience of an IUD. Regardless of the surgical technique used to achieve endometrial ablation, whether laser, freezing, ultrasound, balloon, rollerball, etc., the internal uterine scarring caused by an ablation procedure prevents the uterus from housing an IUD.

With the progestin IUD delivering progesterone only to the target organ that needs it, i.e.- the uterus, a menopausal woman garnishes the many benefits of estrogen replacement therapy without exposing her breasts or the rest of her body to progesterone or any other synthetic chemicals with progesterone-like actions. It's an easy, breezy progesterone delivery system, and a hormonal win for a menopausal woman who has not had a hysterectomy.

When it comes to menopause hormone therapy, women who have had a hysterectomy do not need progesterone in any shape or form. Thanks to a variety of progesterone preparations, menopausal women with a uterus have safe, effective and personalized options for uterine health maintenance. Now, all menopausal women, with or without a uterus, can capitalize on the numerous health benefits of estrogen replacement therapy.

HOT! HOT! HOT!

The hallmark of menopause is hot flashes, also known as hot flushes. These thermal disruptions are characterized by a sudden sensation of intense heat or burning in the face, neck and torso, followed by skin redness (flushing) and drenching perspiration. As the sweating dissipates, a cold and clammy feeling lingers. The hot flash may be associated with heart palpitations or an anxious feeling. Sometimes women experience weakness, fatigue, faintness or vertigo with their hot flashes, as well. A few menopausal women experience cold flushes, as opposed to hot flushes. Because these uncomfortable temperature shifts are associated with blood flow changes to the skin, perspiration and heart palpitations, clinically they are referred to as vasomotor symptoms. The average length of a hot flash is about three minutes, and their frequency is unpredictable and variable from woman to woman and varies from day to day within an individual woman. On average, menopausal women suffer half a dozen of these daytime, nighttime, anytime thermal intrusions daily.

85% of menopausal women experience hot flashes, night sweats or heat waves, and on average, they occur for about 7 to 10 years. 1 out of 3 women weathers hot flashes for more than 10 years after menopause, and 15% suffer from hot flashes for over 15 years. That's a lot of thermal turbulence. Only a fortunate few make it through menopause without breaking a sweat. Women who are rendered menopausal at a younger age tend to have more severe hot flashes and for more years, than older women who go through menopause naturally. Some perimenopausal women experience hot flashes and night sweats for years prior to their final menstrual period. Aging ovaries produce erratic peaks and troughs of estrogen, which can confuse the body's thermostat.

Although hot flashes are usually considered a menopausal woman's problem, men can also develop hot flashes if their level of testosterone drops suddenly. Hot flashes occur in men who have had their testicles removed or who take medication to decrease testosterone levels for the treatment of advanced prostate cancer.

HYPOTHALAMIC THERMOSTAT

When the brain is no longer bathed in estrogen, there is narrowing of the thermal neutral zone in its hypothalamus. This thermal neutral zone is the body's physiological thermostat and allows body temperature to remain stable even though the room or ambient temperature changes. When this hypothalamic zone is narrowed, sweating or shivering thresholds decrease. Hot flashes appear to be triggered by a sudden lowering of the thermostat in the hypothalamus. As a consequence, heat loss mechanisms are activated to cool the body down. The body perspires, the capillaries in the skin expand or vasodilate, causing flushing and increased heart rate; meanwhile, there is decreased blood flow to the brain that may cause dizziness and apprehension. This helps explain a menopausal woman's inability to continue her tasks during a severe hot flash. When sleep is interrupted by night sweats, it's difficult for her to get back to sleep.

When a woman's thermostat is malfunctioning, not only is she uncomfortable, her body is signaling that something's awry. Rapid heating and cooling episodes inflict oxidative and inflammatory damage to a woman's body. Hot flashes and night sweats are more than mere annoyances; they compromise a woman's physical and psychological well-being and markedly decrease her quality of life. Hot flashes are not power surges; they're energy drainers. The greater the severity and frequency of hot flashes and night sweats, the worse the woman feels, the lower her overall health status and work productivity, and the more she utilizes healthcare resources. Night sweats and waking episodes during the night cause profound sleep disturbances, which then provoke mood disorders and memory problems. Higher risks for heart disease, diabetes, and strokes are found in women who suffer from hot flashes compared to women without them. Women with more hot flashes have quicker bone turnover, so they experience more bone thinning and osteoporosis. On the other hand, menopausal women who suffer from hot flashes have half the risk of developing breast cancer, compared to women not experiencing menopausal symptoms.

When coping with menopausal hot flashes, certain practical lifestyle changes are helpful. These include:

- Drinking a glass of cool water at the beginning of a hot flash.
- Avoid consuming food and beverages that can trigger hot flashes. For some women caffeine sets off a hot flash. Red wine and aged cheeses contain tyramine, and chocolate has phenylethylamine. These are chemicals that can trigger hot flashes by affecting the brain's hypothalamus temperature control center. These vasoactive (blood vessel stimulating) amines can also trigger migraines.
- Avoid tobacco smoke. Smoking can make hot flashes worse.
- Wear loose, comfortable clothing made of cotton, to help absorb perspiration. Dress in layers, so clothing can be removed quickly when hot flashes flare up.
- Keep environments cool – lower thermostats, open windows, set up fans.
- Engaging in daily exercise increases endorphin production. Nature's built-in pain and stress fighters, endorphins are morphine-like, feel-good chemicals produced within the body. In general, physical activity helps a woman feel better and improves her overall health.

COMPLEMENTARY & ALTERNATIVES

Complementary and alternative therapies for managing menopausal hot flashes include dietary supplements such as black cohosh, ginseng, vitamin E, St. John's wort, flaxseed, evening primrose oil, and activities such as acupuncture, yoga, magnetic therapy, paced breathing and chanting daily.

Soybeans and red clover contain isoflavone phytoestrogens. The isoflavones may provide weak estrogenic activity in some women, so they report milder hot flashes.

Although scientific support for complementary and alternative modalities does not equal their popularity, many menopausal women try these strategies in hopes of alleviating their suffering. There is a high placebo effect rate of 50% to any treatment used for coping with hot flashes. These remedies may help some women feel better, but clinical trials have not shown that these modalities are superior to placebos in providing sustained and consistent relief from hot flashes or menopausal symptoms.

Relizen is one of the few non-prescription products that has a randomized controlled trial (RCT) showing that it significantly reduces hot flashes and night sweats in menopausal women. Relizen, also known as Femal or Serelys, is a purified pollen extract dietary supplement harvested from plants in southern Sweden. It has been available in Europe since 1999, has no reported adverse side effects, nor does it interfere with the efficacy of other medications. In particular, it does not reduce the therapeutic potency of tamoxifen (Nolvadex), a selective estrogen receptor modulator (SERM), which is used in the treatment and prevention of breast cancer.

OTHER PRESCRIPTIONS

For women who cannot or will not take estrogen, there are non-hormonal prescription drugs that may help decrease hot flashes, but they are not as effective as estrogen. Antidepressants such as paroxetine (Paxil, Brisdelle), venlafaxine (Effexor), fluoxetine (Prozac), and sertraline (Zoloft) are helpful in treating hot flashes, with venlafaxine and paroxetine being the most effective. These are selective serotonin reuptake inhibitors (SSRI) and serotonin and norepinephrine reuptake inhibitors (SNRI), which act to increase the availability of serotonin and norepinephrine chemicals in the brain. Antidepressants can cause nausea, sleep disturbances, decreased libido and blunted orgasms. They may also increase suicidal thoughts, increase bleeding risk, and increase the risk for serotonin syndrome (rapid onset of muscles contracting, hyperreflexia, eye muscles twitching and increased body temperature). It also appears that SSRI anti-depressants are associated with a reduction in bone density and an increased risk for falls and osteoporosis-related fractures.

The SERM drug, Tamoxifen (Nolvadex), acts as an anti-estrogen on the breast, so it used to treat breast cancer, as well as reduce the risk of developing breast cancer in high-risk women. Tamoxifen seems to act as an anti-estrogen on the brain's hypothalamus thermostat because tamoxifen brings on wicked hot flashes. The SSRI, paroxetine (Paxil, Brisdelle) inhibits the CYP2D6 enzyme the body uses to convert tamoxifen to its biologically active metabolite, endoxifen so that paroxetine may reduce the therapeutic effectiveness of tamoxifen. Venlafaxine (Effexor) does not appear to inhibit CYP2D6 to any significant degree, so it would be the preferred SSRI to use for women taking tamoxifen.

Gabapentin (Neurontin) is an anti-seizure medication that is also used to calm nerves for pain management. At high doses gabapentin appears to be moderately effective in treating hot flashes, but often causes drowsiness. Clonidine (Catapres) is a medication that acts in the brain to lower blood pressure and is available as an oral pill or a skin patch. Clonidine effectively relieves hot flashes in some women but is completely ineffective in others, and harbors side effects such as dry mouth, constipation, and sleep disturbances.

Menopausal hot flashes are caused by the withdrawal of estrogen from the brain's hypothalamic thermostat, so the most logical and effective treatment for alleviating hot flashes, night sweats or cold sweats is simply replacing a woman's estrogen. No other intervention, therapy or medication treats the root cause of these intrusive thermal disruptions. Only estrogen naturally restores the brain's thermal neutral zone in the hypothalamus and normalizes the body's thermostat. Cooled and calmed by appropriate estrogen replacement therapy, a menopausal woman avoids damaging thermal turbulence, sleeps better and safely maintains her quality of life.

SLEEP, GLORIOUS SLEEP

A woman living into her 80s has devoted 28 years of her life to sleeping. For sustained survival, humans need to spend a third of their lives sleeping, resting their bodies and rebooting their brains. Healthy adults are built for 16 hours of wakefulness and need an average of 8 eight hours of sleep a night. Restful sleep allows the brain to consolidate memories, drift into dreams, and form pathways to learning and retaining information.

Chronic sleep deprivation kills brain cells. Sleep deprivation is used as a weapon of torture, inducing hypnagogic hallucinations, altered reality perceptions and psychosis. A person can survive three times longer without food than they can without sleep. 11 days without sleep and death comes knocking; whereas, it takes about 3 to 4 weeks to starve to death.

A person suffers from insomnia when they experience problems with the initiation, maintenance, duration or quality of sleep. Inadequate sleep leads to significant deficits in concentration, perception and motivation. Lack of sleep causes emotional and psychological problems such as forgetfulness, poor decision-making, irritability, and apathy. Mental health problems such as depression, mania, attention deficit disorder and schizophrenia are exacerbated by sleep disturbances.

In addition to daytime fatigue and drowsiness, sleep deprivation creates microsleep episodes, which are brief moments of sleep that occur when one is normally awake. One cannot control the occurrence of microsleep, and they are not aware of the incident until afterwards. While listening to someone's narrative, one suddenly notices that they missed part of the story, or after having driven somewhere, one may not remember traveling that distance. These are examples of microsleep episodes. Microsleep impacts others since it is can be responsible for traffic accidents and industrial mishaps. The human brain desperately seeks sleep, so it will try to acquire it any which way it can.

The body's resilience, stamina, and physique are maintained through peaceful slumber. Chronic sleep deprivation causes weight gain by disturbing how the body processes and stores carbohydrates, as well as skewing levels of hormones that affect one's appetite. A sleep-deprived woman craves calorie dense foods. Her agitated metabolic machinery alters the balance between the satiety hormone (leptin) and the hormone that makes one feel hungry (ghrelin), causing her to eat more. Lack of sleep ages a woman's skin, as well. Sleep deprivation causes the adrenal gland to release more cortisol, the "chronic stress hormone." Cortisol breaks down skin's collagen and elastin proteins, causing skin to droop and wrinkle. A mirror's reflection of puffy dark rimmed eyes with lackluster rumpled skin is a face begging for more sleep.

Merciless night sweats will jerk a menopausal woman awake from her sleeping serenity. After cooling herself down by throwing off bed sheets, increasing fan speeds and opening windows, the thermally traumatized woman usually finds it difficult to get back to sleep. Frequent trips to the bathroom from an estrogen-deficient twitchy bladder also conspire to deprive a menopausal woman of adequate sleep. Also, menopausal sleep disturbance increases the occurrence of sleep apnea and restless leg syndrome.

Even if she is not dealing with drenching night sweats or coping with a spastic bladder, menopausal drops in estrogen levels disrupt a woman's fundamental sleep architecture. Eight hours of sleep usually involves 5 sleep cycles; each sleep cycle lasts 1 ½ to 2 hours and is composed of 4 stages of sleep. The stages in the sleep cycle are organized by the changes in specific brain activity, e.g.- shallow sleep with alpha brain waves or deep dreamy sleep with slow-wave (delta) brain waves and rapid eye movements (REM), etc.

Menopause alters sleep architecture by decreasing slow-wave deep sleep, decreasing rapid eye movement (REM) sleep, and increasing the number of cyclic spontaneous arousals. Between less quantities of sleep coupled to poor quality of sleep, the menopausal woman never fully reaches sleep nirvana. Operating with a perpetual sleep deficit, she keeps pushing and pulling herself along, trying to compensate for diminished energy and declining spirits.

Inadequate sleep increases inflammation and pain perception while impairing immune function and hampering the body's fight against cancer. 20% of working women are involved in night or evening shift work, which is usually scheduled as night shifts rotating with day shifts, or working the "graveyard shift" into the early hours of the next morning. Women working these nocturnal hours are more likely to develop breast cancer. Interestingly, blind women experience fewer cancers. This dichotomy may be the result of differing melatonin levels between these groups of women.

Melatonin is a hormone produced at night by the tiny pineal gland in the brain, and it is involved in maintaining a person's circadian rhythm, which is the body's biological 24-hour clock determining when we fall asleep and when we wake up. Melatonin levels are not decreased by light exposure in people with total blindness. The incidence of breast cancer in blind women is less than in sighted women. Since melatonin hinders cancer cell proliferation, it may help reduce a tumor's growth. On the other hand, when a person stays awake at night and is exposed to light, melatonin levels drop. Sleep deprivation prevents the body's nocturnal immunological surveillance crew from performing its custodial duties.

Lack of estrogen renders restorative sleep elusive in menopausal women. Some women indulge in a nightcap to help them fall asleep, while others resort to sleeping pills or sedatives. These medications can be addictive and have side effects, such as dizziness, dry mouth, constipation, and morning grogginess. Sleep deprivation is debilitating and dangerous. A woman needs sleep to stay healthy and lucid, and her brain cells need sleep to survive and function. Estrogen deficiency is the cause of menopausal night sweats drenching a woman out of any hope of restful sleep. An irritable and leaky bladder keeps a menopausal woman tethered to the bathroom all night long. Estrogen deprivation is the cause of buckled sleep architecture reducing the critical time needed for deep sleep and dreaming. Only estrogen replacement therapy safely and simultaneously eliminates night sweats, calms a twitchy bladder, and restores rejuvenating sleep and nocturnal tranquility to a menopausal woman.

MIRROR, MIRROR - SKIN, HAIR, and SHAPE-SHIFTING

Hormones not only determine how a woman looks, but they influence how her looks evolve as she ages. Unlike extrinsic aging, where external factors such as excess sun exposure, pollution, smoking or other unhealthy lifestyle habits cause deep wrinkles and leathery skin, intrinsic skin aging is governed by the internal goings-on within a woman's body, her genetic constitution and her hormonal make-up. Thyroid function is involved in skin health and hair growth cycles. Too much thyroid hormone and skin becomes warm, sweaty and flushed. Too little, and skin becomes dry, coarse, thick and pasty. Thyroid malfunction leads to thinning hair and eyebrow loss. Excess cortisol, the "chronic stress hormone," produced by the adrenal glands, destroys skin's collagen and elastin proteins, so skin becomes thinner and wrinkles easier. The relative excess testosterone compared to estrogen that occurs with menopause or ovarian dysfunction causes a woman to sprout whiskers and spawn acne. As female hormones spiral downward, altered metabolism and tissue degradation gain momentum. Along with these unwelcome skin and hair changes, a menopausal woman's "new normal" become obvious in her pear-to-apple shape-shifting silhouette.

WRINKLES

Since estrogen receptors exist throughout a woman's body, it's not surprising that estrogen is involved in maintaining skin integrity and keeping tissues supple. The number of estrogen receptors is highest in facial skin, followed by the skin of the breasts and thighs.

Estrogen strengthens and moisturizes skin while staving off flakes and wrinkles. Generalized tissue thinning, loss of elasticity and dwindling resilience causes aging skin to droop and sag. These changes are particularly prominent in skin areas exposed to light. Obviously, a woman's face, neck, and hands give her age away.

Without estrogen, degeneration of collagen crosslinks and tangling of elastin fibers accelerate, blood circulation to the skin decreases, and hyaluronic acid for fluid balance evaporates. Silky, smooth skin and a woman's tactile allure depend on estrogen. Although menopause hormone therapy slows down tissue degradation exacerbated by estrogen deficiency, it does not alter the reality of genetic aging. Some women come from parents who aged well while others reveal their years early on. 25% of ultraviolet damage associated with premature skin aging occurs prior to age 18, so hormone therapy cannot repair skin already damaged by past sun exposure or smoking. Estrogen has no impact on a woman's risk of skin cancer, either.

Since estrogen has anti-inflammatory and anti-oxidant properties, estrogen withdrawal can lead to increased skin sensitivities. A menopausal woman's skin may appear red and blotchy, and chronic skin conditions such as eczema, psoriasis and rosacea are exacerbated by the loss of estrogen. Despite using moisturizers, an estrogen-deprived woman still experiences dry, itchy, even crawly skin. From the inside to the outside, and across subcutaneous, dermis and epidermal tissue layers, estrogen replacement therapy works from within, to strengthen and stabilize menopausal skin.

NEEDLES & KNIVES

In their endeavor to turn back the hands of time, women pay premium prices and subject themselves to painful processes such as facial peels or face and neck injections with botulinum toxin (Botox), fat or tissue filler du jour. When these tactics fail, they subject themselves to the risks of cosmetic surgical procedures to counter aging and lift sagging skin. Without hormonal support, the durability of these painful and lavish endeavors will not be long lasting in an estrogen-deprived menopausal woman. The dermatological reality is that without estrogen to sustain collagen and elastin cross-links and conserve skin's infrastructure, cosmetic procedures can only go so far and last only so long.

Estrogen replacement therapy preserves connective tissue integrity, limits collagen and elastin loss, improves skin's firmness and elasticity, shrinks pore sizes and decreases wrinkle depth. Estrogen improves wound healing and decreases inflammation, so better surgical results are achieved in a well-estrogenized woman, compared to her estrogen-deprived counterpart. Quite frankly, to get the most out of cosmetic interventions, a menopausal woman should be on adequate hormone replacement therapy prior to being injected, going under the knife or having a laser beamed at her. With estrogen, a woman takes care of her skin from within.

APPLES & PEARS

With menopause, a woman's estrogen levels drop by over 90% and testosterone levels drop by 50%. This sex hormone imbalance leads to markedly reduced estrogen levels relative to testosterone levels. Unfortunately, for most menopausal women, toned muscles, energy highs or lusty libidos do not accompany this surplus of testosterone circulating in their system. Instead, this unbridled testosterone manifests as unwelcome shape-shifting and undesirable hair growth patterns.

Menopausal estrogen deficiency can cause distressing reflections in the mirror. Between the night sweats, frequent nocturnal bladder breaks, and altered sleep cycles, a menopausal woman is perpetually sleep-deprived, so she ends up fatigued, stressed and too tired to exercise. Without estrogen, muscle performance declines, and although her menopausal metabolism has slowed down, her residual testosterone boosts appetite. Excess fat deposition shifts away from thighs and buttocks, and finds its way into the abdominal (visceral) area, so waistlines disappear and muffin tops appear. It is a struggle for an estrogen-deficient menopausal woman to prevent her hourglass or pear-shaped figure from morphing into an apple-shaped barrel.

Vanity sizing can cover up only so much, but this shape-shifting is more than just a problematic wardrobe issue. Once a woman's waistline increases beyond 35 inches, she is at much greater risk for heart disease, strokes, diabetes and breast cancer.

HAIR

Unlike other tissues of the body, hair is not essential to physiological function. Loss of scalp hair does not make one ill, yet thinning hair is distressing to women and balding is disturbing to men. Hair is a part of a person's identity and is one of the principal presentations of a person's "self" to the world. Most individuals have a strong connection between their crowning glory and self-esteem. It's not surprising then that hair enhancement is a multi-billion dollar industry, and over a lifetime, the average woman spends $50,000 on her hair.

Hairs are wispy, yet extraordinarily strong, fibers made up of keratin, a protein substance that grows from hair follicles located in the skin's dermis. The average human scalp has between 100,000 to 120,000 hairs. At any given time, 90% of these hairs are growing while the remaining 10% are resting. The growing hairs continue to do so for about 5 years, at a rate of ½ inch per month. Scalp hair growth in women is slightly faster than in men. This hair-growing period is known as the "anagen" phase. After years of growing, the hair shaft idles in a non-growth holding pattern called the "catagen" phase for a couple of weeks. From this transition phase, the hair shaft shifts into its resting or "telogen" phase. During these several months of resting, the telogen hair shaft detaches itself from the bulb from which it originated, and the hair strand is shed. Meanwhile, the hair follicle's bulb is generating a new hair to replace the shed strand, so the cycle starts all over. Since resting hairs are shed to make way for newly growing hair, one normally sheds 50 to 100 hairs a day.

Soaring estrogen levels during pregnancy prolong the anagen or growing phase of the hair growth's cycle, and contribute to an expectant mom's cascading tresses. After delivering the baby, plummeting estrogen levels cause hair to fall out post-partum. The sudden stress of losing estrogen propels more hair follicles into the telogen or resting phase. The result is an extensive shutdown of the growing hair follicles, with subsequent loss of mounds of hair for one to three months after the baby is born. Since reproductive-aged women's ovaries still produce estrogen, all of this postpartum hair loss will be replaced.

Menopausal estrogen loss, however, is permanent, so hormonally depleted hair follicles are not replaced. Usually a considerable amount of hair, about 50%, can be shed before hair loss becomes an issue. Most menopausal women notice some unwanted change in the pattern of their body hair, with less scalp hair and more facial hair. Menopausal shifts in estrogen-testosterone balance allow testosterone to lay claim to hair follicles' roots and oil glands. Testosterone increases the growth and coarseness of rogue hairs on a woman's chin, upper lip and elsewhere. Also, since testosterone is involved in skin sebum production, menopausal women experience flashbacks of oily skin, acne, and body odor. Everyone ages, but when an estrogen-deprived woman looks in the mirror, she sees more wrinkling, more sagging, more blotchy skin, and more whiskers than her same-aged, well-estrogenized counterpart. Her clothes don't fit right anymore, either.

Menopause hormone therapy cannot neutralize decades of skin damage linked to sun exposure, medical problems or detrimental lifestyle choices. Estrogen replacement therapy does, however, slow down tissue degradation accelerated by declining estrogen levels. Initiating hormone therapy years after menopause has become a distant memory will not reinstate skin's long lost tissue turgor or restore a woman's svelte figure. A menopausal woman can help delay the visible signs of aging with appropriately timed and well-applied estrogen replacement therapy.

WHAT about WEIGHT?

In 1942, while the world was at war, a statistician working in New York City was putting a chart together. He grouped four million people, predominantly healthy, white and middle-classed individuals insured by Metropolitan Life Insurance Company, into categories. These categories were based on height, weight and body frame (small, medium or large). He discovered that, barring any war inflicted casualties or maiming, people who lived the longest were the ones who maintained their body weight at the average level of a healthy 25-year-old. This data gave birth to the Metropolitan Life's charts for "healthy weights" for adult men and women.

For a medium-framed woman, once she reaches a height of 5'0," healthy weight would be around 100 pounds. For every inch above 5'0" her weight would increase by around 5 pounds per inch. For example, a 5'5" woman should weigh 125 pounds, simply calculated by adding 100 pounds for reaching 5'0," plus 5 inches above 5'0" multiplied by 5 pounds for each inch above 5'0" = 25, totaling 125 pounds. If she were 5'8" tall, then her healthy weight would be 140 pounds, and so on.

Just for comparison, because men have heavier bones and more skeletal muscle mass (muscle weighs more than fat), once a medium-framed man reaches a height of 5'0", his healthy weight would be around 106 pounds. For every inch he is taller than 5'0" his healthy weight increases by around 6 pounds per inch. A 5'11" man's desirable weight would be 172 pounds, calculated by 106 pounds for reaching 5'0," plus 11 inches above 5'0" multiplied by 6 pounds for each inch above 5'0" = 66, totaling 172 pounds.

Weight issues have been a concern since sedentary living became more prevalent with the comforts brought on by the Industrial Revolution. Back in the early 1800s, a century prior to the Metropolitan Life height and weight tables, a Belgian mathematician devised a method detailing how much an individual's body weight departs from what is healthy for their height. This equation became known as the body mass index (BMI), and it is a method of categorizing people's weight. BMI provides a simple numeric measure of "relative fatness," by which health care professionals can discuss weight problems more objectively with their patients.

Body mass index (BMI) is calculated by taking a person's weight (kilograms) and dividing it by the square of their height (meters)^2 or by taking a person's weight (pounds) and dividing it by the square of their height (inches)^2 and then multiplying this number by 703.

A BMI of 18.5 to 24.9 is considered healthy

A BMI of 25 to 29.9 is considered overweight

A BMI of 30 to 34.9 is considered obese

A BMI of 35 to 39.9 is severely obese.

A BMI of 40 or above is morbidly obese.

Most women know how tall they are, so the "5' equals a 100 pounds added to 5 pounds per inch taller than 5' guide," is a quick, chart-free, tech-free way to determine desirable, healthy weights. Overweight is being more than 10% above a healthy weight, and obese is being more than 20% or more above a healthy weight.

SUBCUTANEOUS vs. VISCERAL FAT

Subcutaneous fat is the adipose (fatty) tissue lying directly under the skin. It's the fat that can be pinched or grasped with fat calipers. It contains fatty tissue, blood vessels that supply the skin with oxygen and crucial sensory nerves. Not only does fat store energy, which the body mobilizes during periods of physical activity or starvation, but subcutaneous fat also helps insulate our body and acts as a shock absorber cushioning us against trauma. Obviously, we all need some fat to survive, but not that much.

Visceral fat is deposited deep inside the abdomen and chest cavity, out of our reach. This thickened fat accumulates around the bowels, surrounds internal organs, accumulates within the liver (fatty liver), expands the omentum, and even finds its way to the heart. Visceral fat around the heart, also known as pericardial fat, damages the blood vessels supplying the heart, contributing to heart attacks.

When a woman's waist circumference exceeds 35 inches, she has an unhealthy and uncomfortable build-up of abdominal or visceral fat. For men, this occurs when their waist size exceeds 40 inches. This abdominal (visceral) adiposity problem is not just limited to the obliteration of 6-pack abs or the unsightly development of muffin tops and expanded love handles. There is a correlation between abdominal (visceral) fat accumulation and the development of serious metabolic diseases, such as diabetes, heart disease, hypertension, strokes, blood clots, and cancers.

When excessive fat is gained, fat cells expand to four times their original size before dividing into new cells. Adipose (fatty) tissue is more than a source of stored energy. Fat acts as a gland, or endocrine organ, producing hormones and other bioactive substances that can damage our overall health. Visceral fat cells are more biologically active than subcutaneous fat cells in producing unfriendly chemicals, called adipocytokines. Adipocytokines cause system-wide inflammation and irritation and dramatically increase a person's risk for heart disease, diabetes, strokes, blood clots, and cancers.

BODY FAT COMPOSITION

In the healthy weight person, about 10% of total body fat is visceral, while 90% is subcutaneous. In obese individuals, that ratio changes, so that 25% of total body fat is visceral and 75% is subcutaneous. In a healthy weight man, fat makes up 15-18% of his total body weight. In a woman, 20-25% of her ideal body weight is made up of fat. Muscle-bound bodybuilding men have less than 10% body fat. Female athletes, no matter how much they exercise unless they starve themselves or their hormones are unnaturally manipulated, cannot drop their body fat percentage below 15% of their total weight. In order to support a pregnancy, Nature intended that women have more padding than men. During times of famine, a pregnant woman's subcutaneous fat supplies needed calories for fetal growth and development.

DETRIMENTAL BMIs

One-third of American adults are overweight (BMI= 25 to 29.9) and another third are obese (BMI= 30 and above). This leaves only 1 out of 3 voting age Americans sporting a healthy weight. Contrary to holiday cartoons, being overweight or obese does not render one jolly or jovial. Carrying excess weight is not merely a cause for dismay when looking in the mirror. Obesity causes low self-esteem, depression, sexual difficulties, and a litany of other medical problems.

Obesity is associated with elevated glucose levels and diabetes. Elevated blood sugars are teratogenic, meaning excess glucose circulating in a woman's bloodstream causes birth defects. To reduce the chance of having a baby with a birth defect, a woman's fasting blood plasma sugars should be less than 100 mg/dL, and any random plasma glucose should measure less than 200mg/dL, for several months prior to getting pregnant. Once a woman is pregnant, obesity endangers the pregnancy itself. It increases her risk for gestational diabetes, strokes, preeclampsia, and seizures. If an obese woman gets pregnant, her risk for miscarriages, having a baby born with birth defects or delivering a stillborn is much higher than for a healthy weight mom. Obesity increases a woman's chance of having a caesarean section (C-section), and compared to a vaginal birth, having a C-section doubles her risk of damaging and deadly blood clots.

Obesity begets obesity. Babies born to obese parents are bigger, and they tend to grow up to become obese, as well. Sadly, this is not a healthy or happy legacy to pass on to future generations. By causing numerous debilitating diseases, cancers, surgical complications, physical disabilities, psychological and sexual problems, excess adipose (fatty) tissue maims the spirit, destroys the body and damages future generations. Heart disease, diabetes, strokes and blood clots escalate with increasing weight. Urinary incontinence, pelvic organ prolapse, sleep apnea, back problems, and arthritic hips and knees requiring joint replacements weigh obese people down even further. Heavier people experience more gallbladder problems, fatty liver, heartburn or gastroesophageal reflux disease (GERD), and chronic cough than healthy weight individuals. If one cannot see their toes over their gut or potbelly, they are not having much of a sex life either.

OBESITY & CANCER

Where one carries their extra weight makes a difference in what health problems are more likely to occur with increasing poundage. A pear-shaped body with hefty hips and thighs results in mechanical arthritic problems of the hips, knees and feet; whereas, an apple-shaped body with midriff bulge or potbelly suffers more from metabolic, cardiovascular and immunological diseases. Any which way excess fat is accumulated or located, being overweight or obese increases an individual's risk for all types of cancer. 1 out of 3 cancer deaths is linked to excess weight.

Adipose (fatty) tissue houses the aromatase enzyme, which converts androgens and testosterone to estrogen. The more adipose (fatty) tissue one is carrying around, the more excess estrogen is circulating in their system. For men, this excess estrogen can lead to breast development (gynecomastia), which increases a man's risk of breast cancer. Since adipose (fatty) tissue is siphoning off a man's raw testosterone for estrogen production, overweight and obese men experience erectile dysfunction, decreased libido and increased risk of prostate cancer.

When a menopausal woman is 40 pounds above her healthy weight, she doubles her risk of breast cancer. This doubled risk is equivalent to the increased risk associated with having a first-degree relative (mother, sister or daughter) with breast cancer. A simple wardrobe change raises breast cancer risk in menopausal women. An increase in just one skirt size, e.g.- from a size 10 to a size 12, is associated with a 33% greater risk of developing breast cancer. A woman who is 40 pounds above her healthy weight has a five-fold increased risk of developing endometrial uterine cancer. Excess adipose (fatty) tissue leads to cancer.

Since adipose (fatty) tissue converts testosterone to estrogen, excess adipose (fatty) tissue floods a woman's body with excess estrogen. This helps explain why many overweight or obese menopausal women may not suffer from hot flashes to the degree normal weight or thinner women do. Although excess weight may take the edge off menopausal hot flashes, it puts a woman at greater risk for cancers. Too much of a good thing is bad, so excess estrogen produced by excess adipose (fatty) tissue increases a woman's risk of breast cancer, uterine and ovarian cancers. Pancreatic cancer and colon cancer risk also increase as a woman puts on pounds.

CELLULITE

Collagen and elastin protein fibers that connect fat to the skin may stretch, break down or pull tight. This causes subcutaneous fat to bulge out and collect in pockets just below the skin, giving the area an "orange peel" dimpled look. This dreaded cellulite tends to form around the hips, thighs and buttocks. 90% of women will eventually develop cellulite at some point in their lives. Even women who are in shape or are thin have cellulite. Cellulite is not harmful to one's health, but because women are bothered by how it looks, they seek a variety of treatments for it, everything from topical creams to liposuction. Unfortunately, once cellulite appears, there is no effective therapy to eliminate this vexing cosmetic problem.

APPROACHING WEIGHT GAIN

As a woman approaches menopause, weight gain is common, but not inevitable. There is no magic pill or single food that will make one lose weight quickly. Practical lifestyle changes can mobilize excess adipose (fatty) tissue and keep it at bay. Eating healthier, nutrition-rich food, cutting portion sizes, and regular physical activity help melt the waistline away. In fact, the safest and most successful way to lose weight is to lose weight slowly- one pound a week. Because it can be difficult to get all the necessary micronutrients while dieting, taking a multivitamin pill designed for menopausal women several times a week will cover any gaps. Unless otherwise clinically indicated, the daily oral intake of 1000mg of calcium and 1000 IUs of vitamin D should be maintained, as well.

EAT LESS, MOVE MORE

Weight gain occurs when more calories are consumed while fewer calories get burned. Exercise, both aerobic and strength training, helps burn calories. Decreasing caloric intake and increasing physical activity is the most effective strategy for weight loss. Although regular exercise is invigorating, fends off pounds, and elevates spirits, diet and exercise are not 50:50 equal partners when it comes to weight management. In fact, 80% of weight loss is what we eat and drink, and 20% relates to exercise. A 400-calorie slice of cheesecake that takes just 5 minutes to eat commands hours on the treadmill to burn off.

Mediterranean Diet

One of the healthiest, tastiest and most satisfying diets on the planet is the Mediterranean diet. Long enjoyed by people living in the countries bordering the Mediterranean Sea, this high-fiber, high antioxidant, low-glycemic diet consistently and significantly decreases the incidence of heart disease, strokes, diabetes, breast cancers, Alzheimer's and Parkinson's diseases. Surprisingly, despite all their sun exposure, these folks even have a lower incidence of skin cancer and melanoma.

Additional Elements of Healthy Eating Include:

- Reading food labels. Many foods that are low-fat or fat-free replace the fat with sugar or starch to achieve taste equivalence. When we crave food, it's the fat that satisfies us. When we want something salty, we don't sprinkle it out of the saltshaker; we go for chips, fries or cheese balls. When we want something sweet, we don't spoon sugar or cocoa powder; we go for cakes, cookies or chocolate. What our body needs for satiety satisfaction is the fat associated with the salty or sweet food. It's better to eat just a little bit of a gourmet treat than to double or triple up on sugary or salty junk food.

- Practice portion control. Our stomach is the size of our two fists put together. It doesn't take that much food to sustain life, boost energy, release excess fat stores, look great and feel better. Eat slowly, drink fluids and chat liberally during a meal to savor every morsel of food eaten. Meals should be an enjoyable event. The taste and sensual pleasure of the food last longer that way.
- Balance the contents of the meal to approximate the 40% protein, 30% complex carbohydrates and 30% fat ratio. This creates a satisfying meal and helps stabilize blood sugar levels.
- Chat about fat. A gram of fat, any kind of fat, contains 9 Calories. A gram of sugar or a gram of protein contains 4 Calories. Because fat is a more concentrated source of energy, it takes more activity to burn off fat. Some dietary fats are better for us than others, and some should be avoided.

Saturated fat means that every carbon atom in the fat molecule has a hydrogen atom attached to it, so it's saturated with hydrogen. Saturated fats have high melting temperatures, so they are solid at room temperature. Animal fats, butter, and dairy products are saturated fats. By increasing LDL-cholesterol ("L" for lousy, bad cholesterol) and triglycerides lipids in our bloodstream, saturated fats can increase our risk for heart disease and strokes.

Unsaturated fats are not saturated with hydrogen, so they tend to be liquid at room temperature. Plant-derived oils are unsaturated, do not raise LDL-cholesterol and may increase HDL-cholesterol ("H" for Hurray, the good, heart-protecting, cholesterol). People who preferentially eat unsaturated fats instead of saturated fats have less abdominal (visceral) fat.

Monounsaturated fat means that there is only one double bond between two carbon atoms in the fat molecule; so one bond is not saturated with hydrogen. Nuts, seeds, avocados, black and green olives contain monounsaturated fats. *Polyunsaturated fat* means that there are many (poly) double bonds between carbon atoms in a fat molecule, so there are even fewer carbon atoms saturated with hydrogen. Unsaturated fats include the plant-derived extra-virgin olive oil, peanut, canola, sunflower, corn and sesame oils.

The *polyunsaturated fats, omega-3 and omega-6 fats, are* numbered by the location of their double bond on the fat molecule. They are considered "essential fats," because the human body cannot manufacture them, but they are important to the body functioning properly. They need to be an essential component of dietary intake. Both types of omega fats are found in soybean oil, and omega-3 is plentiful in seafood, walnuts, and flaxseed.

Partially hydrogenated fats, also known as *trans fats,* should be avoided. Usually, they are a nice vegetable oil that has been corrupted. The process of manufacturing these fats starts out by heating up a vegetable oil, often soybean oil, and then bubbles of hydrogen are forced into the liquid oil at high pressure. As the hydrogen atoms bond to the carbon atoms in the heated oil, the newly synthesized substance, now a partially hydrogenated fat, becomes more solid. If one keeps forcing more hydrogen bubbles into the heated oil and creates a fully hydrogenated fat, it would become hard as a rock. Partially hydrogenated fats or trans fats are creamy and much cheaper than butter or olive oil, and they have a much longer shelf life than other fats. Solid shortening and stick margarine are examples of trans fats. These manufactured trans fats or partially hydrogenated fats are found in packaged foods, so anything contained in a cellophane wrapper is suspect.

Partially hydrogenated or trans fats increase "bad" or "L" for lousy, LDL-cholesterol while simultaneously decreasing good or "H" for hurray, HDL-cholesterol. This is the perfect recipe for causing cholesterol plaque build up on arteries throughout the body. Arteries supplying the heart, the brain, the intestines, the genitals and the legs then become narrowed and hardened by these cholesterol plaques. This artery-damaging process is known as atherosclerosis. Atherosclerosis compromises blood flow, so organs supplied by these damaged arteries malfunction. When a necrotic plaque cracks apart, a blood clot forms on the crack. If this clot blocks off blood flow, this arterial blockage can cause a heart attack or a stroke or other deadly vascular disasters.

- Cave into cravings, a little. Cravings are often the body's way of letting you know about nutritional deficiencies. Eat a little bit of whatever your body is asking for.
- Be kind to yourself, and make your splurge calories really count. If you want something sweet, by pass the dry donut or last morsel left in the cookie jar. Treat yourself to a gourmet dessert- just eat half of it today, and save the other half for another time.

GO, WHOLE EGGS, GO!

Ob-Gyn doctors are well tuned to the power ovarian eggs (follicles/oocytes) bring to a woman's health and happiness, so it's not surprising to us that poultry eggs would be one of the healthiest foods on earth. Because nuts or seeds germinate a whole plant, these handy snacks pack a powerful nutritional punch. Similarly, amazing nutrients are packed into a poultry egg, as well. In addition to high-quality proteins and good for you fats, whole eggs contain small amounts of every vitamin and mineral required by the human body. Almost all the nutrients are contained in the egg yolk; the egg white contains protein. When hard-boiled, all this awesome goodness comes in a portable, cheap package containing only 80 calories. Although yolks contain cholesterol, eggs improve our cholesterol profile and do not raise the risk for cardiovascular diseases. Eggs tend to raise the good, HDL-cholesterol ("H" for hurray), and eggs change the bad, LDL-cholesterol ("L" for lousy) to a large subtype molecule, which is not associated with an increased risk of heart disease.

The most common cause of age-related blindness is macular degeneration of the retina. One can no longer drive, identify faces or read words. Such loss of vision affects 1 out of 8 older people, and it occurs twice more often in postmenopausal women than in same-aged men. Unfortunately, there is no cure for this progressive blindness, so the focus is on prevention. Egg yolks are loaded with two antioxidants, lutein, and zeaxanthin, which accumulate in the macular region of the eye's retina, keeping the macula pumped up for visual clarity. Hard-boiled, scrambled or sunny side up, eggs are a satisfying and economical super food.

WALK THIS WAY

Good old-fashioned walking is one of the easiest ways for a menopausal woman to get moving and stay moving. It is one of the best things she can do for her body, her beauty, and her long-term health. Humans are built for walking, so it naturally fits into our activities of daily living. Whether walking outdoors or on a treadmill, of all the fitness workouts, walking is the aerobic activity that women, particularly middle-aged and older women, can stick with. Walking promotes heart and bone health just as effectively as jogging or running, without grinding a woman's knees down, damaging her hips or injuring her feet.

Because of anatomical and biomechanical gender differences, women are far more likely than men to suffer sports injuries from running or jogging. Men's legs project straight down from their hips. For the miracle of childbirth, a woman's pelvis is wider relative to her knees, so her thigh bones angle inward more sharply from hip to knee, making a woman's knees less stable. Her kneecaps wander around more, as well. Women's hip bones tend to rotate towards the midline when running, so over time repetitive stress to hip muscles causes bursitis, and eventually the hip joint is permanently damaged. Differences between the way men and women land on their feet when they run or jump contribute to women suffering from more foot problems, as well. Although running burns about 2 ½ times more calories than walking, step by step, walking is a kinder, gentler and more sustainable way for menopausal women to keep moving.

10,000 STEPS

Walking 10,000 steps a day is roughly equivalent to managing 30 minutes of activity most days of the week. Walking is an aerobic activity that burns calories, reduces a menopausal woman's risk for chronic metabolic diseases, and helps her lead a longer, healthier life. The average American woman takes about 5,000 steps a day; so taking a 30-minute walk adds another 3000 healthy steps to the day and burns 150 calories. 8,000 steps a day isn't bad, 10,000 steps a day is better.

Let's Walk Through a Few More Numbers...

To lose one pound, we need to burn 3500 calories. To lose weight sensibly, we should lose one pound per week. Through diet alone, one needs to decrease their caloric intake by 500 calories per day. 500 calories per day x 7 days a week leads to a 3500 calories deficit per week, which sheds one pound a week. By combining dietary changes with walking, we don't need to cut calories as much to achieve the same weight loss. Decreasing caloric intake by just 250 calories a day and burning 250 calories a day merely by walking, we can still lose a pound a week.

Taking into account variations in stride length, on average it takes 2000 steps to walk a mile. Walking 2000 steps burns 100 calories. Since it takes 20 steps to burn 1 calorie, taking 5,000 steps on a walk burns 250 calories. 250 calories burned per day through walking x 7 days = 1,750 calories burned per week, plus reducing intake by 250 calories per day x 7 days = 1,750 calories deficit per week. Added together, 1,750 + 1,750 = a 3,500 calorie deficit per week which sheds a pound per week. This means a woman will lose 25 pounds in just 6 months. By the end of 6 months, these life enhancing, lifestyle changes will be life-long sustainable habits that will keep a woman healthier and happier longer. It's easier to shed pounds through a combination of diet and exercise.

MENOPAUSE & WEIGHT

Once a woman turns 50 years old, she needs 200 fewer calories a day than she did in her 30s and early 40s. An average American woman burns 1700 calories a day. To maintain her weight, a menopausal woman usually needs to limit her caloric intake to 1500 calories a day. If a middle-aged woman continues to eat as she always has but does not increase her exercising, the extra calories will be stored as fat, mainly in her abdominal midriff area. To lose weight through diet alone, a menopausal woman needs to decrease her caloric intake to 1200 calories per day. Without a doubt, metabolic and hormonal changes associated with estrogen deprivation conspire to make it difficult for a menopausal woman not to gain weight. The average woman gains 2 to 5 pounds during menopause, and some women gain as much as

15 pounds. Estrogen loss causes a woman's body to metabolize calories and manage fat differently. A natural decline in energy expenditure coupled to a lower resting metabolic rate, along with an increase in appetite-related signals, all contribute to menopausal weight gain.

As her estrogen level declines a menopausal woman's appetite increases, especially for less nutritious sugary and fatty foods. This is similar to the PMS-related food cravings many women experience with their menstrual cycles. These premenstrual and menopausal food cravings are linked to lower estrogen levels depleting serotonin and acetylcholine chemicals in a woman's brain, so the body seeks foods to restore these neurotransmitters. Women tend to become more sedentary as they get older, as well. They take the elevator instead of the stairs, they have others load the groceries, they use drive-thru pharmacies, banking and car washes, etc. Menopausal symptoms of fatigue, apathy and depression may drag them away from the treadmill or pull them off the dance floor.

As middle age approaches, women lose skeletal muscle mass and gain more fatty tissue. A pound of muscle at rest burns 3 times more calories than a pound of fat. Declining estrogen levels decreases resting metabolic rate in a menopausal woman by 40-70 calories a day. These calories add up if she does not compensate for them by reducing food intake or increasing exercise. Even when an estrogen-deficient menopausal woman exercises, however, loss of skeletal muscle and decreased aerobic lung power result in burning fewer calories per effort compared to her well-estrogenized counterpart. To maintain the same calorie burn, an estrogen-deprived menopausal woman requires more frequent and more intense exercise.

One might think that more hours spent awake, drenched in night sweats would sizzle away more calories. But, the opposite occurs. Metabolism slows down the morning after a sleepless night. Sleep deprivation compounds any situational life stressors, so adrenal glands produce more cortisol, the "chronic stress hormone." This stimulates a woman's body to cling even more to calories, which packs on more abdominal (visceral) fat. Because of hormone losses and physical slow downs, a menopausal woman's body preferentially deposits fat in the abdominal (visceral) area. More than an inconvenient wardrobe issue, shape-shifting from an hourglass silhouette to a heavy pear-shape and then to an apple-shape renders a woman far more vulnerable to the deadly consequences of heart disease, diabetes and cancer.

By reinstating a menopausal woman's healthy metabolic environment, appropriate estrogen replacement therapy can help curb the tide of weight gain. On its own, estrogen cannot resurrect a woman's svelte figure, but coupled with sensible dietary changes and reasonable exercises, menopause hormone therapy goes a long way to keeping unhealthy pounds away.

SEX REVISITED

Sparked by sight and sound, sexuality is an intrinsic part of humanity. It takes less than 2 minutes to decide if one fancies someone. 60% of the decision is based on appearance and body language, and 40% percent on the tone and speed of the other person's voice. Hence, the global reach of the cosmetic and fashion industries, and the universal practice of small talk. Prompted by reactions and driven by instinct, a heady cocktail of hormones and brain chemicals fuels sexual attraction. Sex is a pleasurable mechanism of conception, and sexual activity is an interactive source of recreation and helps fortify long-term romantic attachments. The need for closeness, caring and companionship is a lifelong human trait.

Sex is vital to the survival of the human species. Compared to animals that produce many offspring, human reproduction is relatively inefficient. During fertile ovulation time, the chance of a 20-something couple, in tip-top baby-making condition, getting pregnant after a single sexual encounter is 10%. To offset this reproductive handicap, sexual activity is immensely pleasurable to humans, so they keep doing it over and over and over. Frequent sex improves the chance of conceiving. Within a year of unprotected sexual intercourse, over 90% of fertile couples will become pregnant.

ZOOLOGY SIDEBAR

Most egg-laying creatures are polygamous, and the female leaves her fertilized eggs to fend for themselves. Birds also lay eggs, but birds are monogamous and most exhibit biparental care of their young. Mammals give birth to their babies, and with their larger, milk-producing mammary glands, females monopolize the feeding of newly born young. Most male mammals do not look after their offspring. They did their part in donating sperm, so they tootle off to impregnate another female. Interestingly, from a total of 4000 mammalian species, only 3% are mutually monogamous – gibbons, prairie voles, and wolves, to name a few. Like most mammals, humans are not strictly monogamous either, but their offspring are helpless and vulnerable for a relatively long time. Cooperative child rearing maximizes the youngster's chance of survival, and Nature planned for this human circumstance, as well. In addition to pleasure chemicals released during orgasms, sexual intercourse floods the brain with hormones that encourage pair bonding and long-term attachment.

THE MECHANICS

The skin is the largest organ of the body, and touch is the most frequent method of sexual arousal, with the most direct effect on sexual response. While men tend to focus on the physical stimulation involved in sexual contact, the key to female sexuality seems to be liberation from fear and anxiety. The male model of sexual arousal and response is basic hydraulics - blood flow to the penis, leading to erection, and then orgasmic ejaculation.

A woman's sexual arousal and climax are more complex, and events do not always occur in a predictable sequence. Her arousal includes emotional experiences and a variety of physiological processes. Events that are part of arousal include mental sexual excitement, pleasure from stimulation of non-genital areas of the body, vaginal lubrication, increased blood flow to vulvar and vaginal tissues, and pleasure from stimulation of the clitoris and the anterior wall of the vagina, the so-called G-spot. The entire ring of tissues that surround the vaginal opening and the outer third of the vagina are all connected by nerves and blood vessels to the clitoris, which is connected to the brain. A purely sexual organ, the clitoris has more than 8,000 sensory nerve endings. These pelvic tissues, together with the woman's psyche, are responsible for the excitation leading to sexual climax. A combined clitoral and vaginal orgasm is the most powerful orgasm a woman can experience.

The best of both worlds, this blended orgasm is triggered by clitoral stimulation and then amplified by vaginal contractions during sexual intercourse. Unassisted penile thrusting is less efficient at generating female orgasms, so two out of three women "fake it till they make it." Only 30% of women reliably climax through intercourse alone, no matter how long it lasts, no matter what size the penis, and no matter how the woman feels about her partner. As always, location and timing are all part of the magic.

Unfortunately, medical problems and medications can undermine a couple's sex life. Medical conditions or treatment that damage the blood supply or nerves to the pelvis, such as diabetes, high blood pressure, pelvic radiation, alcoholism or smoking, extinguish sexual arousal and orgasms. Neurological conditions, such as multiple sclerosis, Parkinson's disease, amyotrophic lateral sclerosis (ALS) or spinal cord injury, impair sexual responsiveness. Hormonal imbalances from thyroid disease, adrenal problems or a prolactin-secreting pituitary brain tumor (prolactinoma) inhibit sexuality, as well. Medications such as antidepressants, anticonvulsants, antianxiety pills, sleeping pills, antipsychotic meds, muscle relaxants, blood pressure pills, cholesterol-lowering medications, narcotics, and any other mood or mind-altering drugs, such as cocaine, alcohol or marijuana, can all stifle sexual arousal and squelch orgasms.

PLEASURE CHEMICALS

Love makes the world go round, and hormones make it all happen. Orgasmic sex releases a constellation of hormones and a host of neurotransmitters that affect the mind and body in a very pleasurable way.

These Chemicals of Content include:

- *Adrenaline (epinephrine)* increases heart rate, blood pressure, and breathing rate. Pupils become dilated, and blood flow to the skeletal muscles increases during sex. Body heat rises and capillaries in the skin expand, so for a woman it's very typical for her cheeks and chest area to flush red, the "sex flush." Adrenaline makes one feel exhilarated.

- *Serotonin* is a *"satisfaction chemical,"* and creates a sense of bliss and tranquility after sexual intercourse. Both the brain and intestines manufacture this mood regulator. When we crave comfort food or retail therapy, what we're really craving is serotonin satisfaction. Chocolate and sunshine stimulate our brain to release serotonin, as well. Orgasm releases serotonin, which is one of the reasons we relax after an orgasm feeling content and satisfied. Serotonin is the same chemical released by heroin, morphine, alcohol and antidepressants.
- *Dopamine*, the *"happiness hormone,"* is a feel-good chemical released in the reward center of the brain. It acts as a stimulant and dopamine levels keep increasing until orgasm is reached. Dopamine stimulates desire and reward by triggering an intense rush of pleasure. Drugs that increase dopamine levels, such as levodopa for Parkinson's disease, can cause spontaneous erections in some patients. Dopamine is the same chemical released by cocaine and methamphetamines.
- *Endorphins* decrease pain, relieve stress and enhance pleasure. As their name implies, endorphins are morphine-like substances originating endogenously from within the body. They are chemicals that bind to opiate receptor sites in the brain to relieve pain. Endorphins are also released during sex, skydiving, exercise, spicy food consumption, yoga, and acupuncture. Endorphins bring a sense of security and serenity and make us feel relaxed after sex.
- *Prolactin* release is linked to feelings of sexual satisfaction, and also makes us feel sleepy after orgasmic sex. For both genders, the magnitude of post-orgasmic prolactin release following penile-vaginal intercourse is 4 times greater than that following masturbation. This suggests a more physiologically satisfying sexual experience when both partners tango. Prolactin relieves sexual arousal after orgasm and allows for sleepy recovery time after sex. This refractory period is the time after an orgasm during which it is physiologically impossible to have another orgasm. This hiatus usually lasts 20 minutes for most men, but can last for 20 hours in some. All the

blood drains away from the spent erection, and any attempts to get blood flow back into the limp, hypersensitive penis are uncomfortable and downright painful. Albeit much shorter in duration than men's, women also experience post-orgasmic clitoral hypersensitivity, in which further sexual stimulation does not produce excitement, but discomfort. A woman's refractory period lasts just one to two minutes after climaxing, and then she's ready to go again, so most women can have multiple orgasms. Sustained orgasms are possible for some women if they can withstand being continuously stimulated after their first orgasm.

- With orgasmic sexual activity, the pituitary gland of the brain releases oxytocin and vasopressin (antidiuretic hormone). Nearly identical in chemical structure, these love hormones are pivotal relationship enhancers. They promote post-orgasmic sleepy spooning and help bond the relationship. The more sex, the greater the bond.

The *"cuddle hormone," oxytocin,* and the *"monogamy molecule," vasopressin,* flood the brain during sex. Both men and women produce these bonding brain chemicals, but oxytocin plays a stronger role in women, whereas vasopressin has more influence in men. Oxytocin is the chemical basis for our craving and capacity for romantic attachment, and it promotes love and trust between people who are intimate with each other. As orgasm subsides, waves of oxytocin flood their systems, fear and stress are blocked out, and it's cuddle time. Women produce more oxytocin than men, and it lasts for two days in her system.

A couple of hours after sex, a man's oxytocin is wearing off, but his vasopressin has already kicked into overdrive. Vasopressin released after intercourse creates a desire to stay with his sexual partner and inspires a protective sense, even jealousy, about their relationship. Orgasmic vasopressin surges are associated with the formation of long-term monogamous relationships. Fear of commitment may be due in part from genetic variation in vasopressin receptors located in the reward centers of the brain.

Powerful feel-good chemicals, along with bonding hormones, discourage us from quickly hopping out of bed to immediately seek out another playmate. Instead, satisfying sex renders folks drowsy, so they drift off to sleep together. It's no surprise that the shorter days and longer nights of autumn and winter result in more pregnancies. More babies are born in the month of September (conceived in December-January) than in any other month, followed by August, July and June (autumn conceptions).

Sexual activity plays a significant role in the way partners relate to each other. Because lovemaking generates pleasure and intimacy, it often results in stronger emotional bonds. Not just through intercourse alone: each touch, each embrace, and each kiss strengthen sexual attraction. Sexual interaction is influenced by the strength of a couple's relationship and the physical condition of each partner. As long as the brain is marinated by sex hormones, and the genitals possess functioning nerve circuitry and adequate blood supply, that is, electric and plumbing are up to code, sex can be enjoyed for decades beyond one's reproducing years.

SEXUAL FEELING

A happy and engaging sex life is associated with health benefits for everyone. Improved cardiovascular health, increased psychological well-being, lower levels of depression, and a better overall quality of life, are some of the dividends of remaining sexually active. Estrogen and testosterone are the quintessential aphrodisiacs. Without these sex hormones fueling desire and capability, attempts at sexual activity become a painful exercise in frustration. Male erection and female lubrication may be triggered by direct stimulation, but it's the brain that interprets the experience. Orgasmic sex releases an array of hormones and a host of neurochemicals that affect the mind and body in very pleasant ways. As things are happening between the legs, 30 different parts of the brain are activated during an orgasm, including those responsible for emotion, touch, joy, satisfaction and memory.

Obviously, sexual desire involves more than hormones. Relationship quality, how one feels about their body, cultural and religious issues, family upbringing, past sexual trauma, stress, medical conditions, fatigue and sleep deprivation, all impact one's desire for sexual activity. Any mood or mind-altering drugs such as alcohol, antidepressants, narcotics, anti-anxiety pills, sleeping pills, cocaine or marijuana, suppresses sexual desire and curbs orgasms. A few women riding the perimenopausal roller coaster of hormonal peaks and troughs may experience waves of sexual interest. Although a woman may be having irregular menstrual periods, she still ovulates intermittently, so she can still get pregnant well into her early 50s. Contraception should be a consideration during the perimenopausal years of erratic ovulation; otherwise, a "change of life baby" can occur.

Once the last ovarian follicle/oocyte (egg) has been spent, and the final menstrual period has come and gone, the perimenopausal carnival ride of sex hormones slides to a stop. With menopause, there are no more worries about potential pregnancy, but plummeting ovarian hormone levels tug away at sexuality and sexual enjoyment. A menopausal woman sustains a 90% drop in her estrogen levels, and her testosterone levels decrease by 50%. Waning libido, diminished orgasms and painful intercourse sabotage sexual encounters. No wonder sex slows down for women with ovarian hormone deficiency.

Menopausal women are not alone in their mid-life sexual dilemmas. 50% of middle-aged men have low testosterone levels and experience low libido and erectile dysfunction. Unlike menopausal women's dramatic loss of estrogen, men do not battle a sudden drop in testosterone levels when they hit 50. Instead, since the age of 30, a man's testosterone level has been steadily decreasing by 1 to 2% every year. In addition to laconic libido and inopportune impotence, men with low testosterone notice diminished physical strength from reduced muscle mass and thinning bones. They also encounter breast tissue development (gynecomastia), increased abdominal (visceral) fat, difficulty concentrating, wandering motivation, insomnia, and depression.

BLUE for BOYS

Simple solutions can help revive a man's broken sex life. Penile hydraulics is helped with drugs classified as phosphodiesterase-5 (PDE-5) inhibitors. Sildenafil (Viagra), tadalafil (Cialis) and vardenafil (Levitra) are PDE-5 inhibiting drugs that increase blood flow to the genitals to produce and sustain an erection.

Any testosterone deficiency, as defined by blood serum testosterone levels below 300 ng/dL, is treated with testosterone shots, sprays, patches, pellets or gels. Like any other hormone deficiency treated medically, testosterone replacement should be administered in physiologic doses and monitored appropriately. Judicious clinical management will prevent the unhealthy and dangerous consequences associated with recreational anabolic steroid use. Normal blood serum testosterone levels for men range between 300 to 1000 ng/dL, and adequate testosterone levels help the PDE-5 inhibitor drugs work better. With his libido restored by testosterone therapy and erections resurrected with a PDE-5 inhibitor, a 21st century male can now enjoy sexual activity well into his golden, now considered platinum, years.

PINK for GIRLS

What about "pink Viagra" for women? Back in 2004, after years of research, Viagra's manufacturer announced that they were ending their attempts to develop a feminine version of Viagra. Sildenafil, the active ingredient in Viagra, relaxes the smooth muscles around the clitoris and increases blood flow to the genitals. In clinical trials, however, most women did not associate these physical changes with subjective feelings of sexual arousal and desire. In fact, there was no difference between the genital engorgement experienced by women complaining of low arousal and those without sexual problems. Since sildenafil (Viagra) is neither an estrogen nor a testosterone hormone, it is not surprising that sildenafil (Viagra) is no more effective than the placebo (sugar pill) in boosting women's libido.

Although the FDA has not approved Viagra for females, women have been known to sneak one of their partner's little blue pills and feel it works for them. When loss of genital congestion or loss of pleasure from direct stimulation is caused by nerve damage associated with medical conditions such as diabetes, multiple sclerosis, pelvic radiation or radical hysterectomy for cervical or uterine cancer, off-label use of sildenafil (Viagra) or other PDE-5 inhibitors can be considered.

Off-label use allows physicians to legally prescribe FDA-approved medications for a purpose not listed on the product's packaging label. This is commonly done, as 20% of prescriptions written in the United States are for off-label therapies. Based on sound scientific evidence or medical opinion, off-label use of a drug or device may represent the standard of care for certain treatments.

PINK VIAGRA?

Because female sexual desire involves interactions among multiple brain neurotransmitters, sex hormones, and psychosocial factors, addressing only the plumbing issue with PDE-5 inhibitors, e.g.-sildenafil (Viagra), would not be enough to restore a woman's desire to engage in sexual activity.

In August 2015, the FDA approved flibanserin (Addyi) for premenopausal women with hypoactive sexual desire disorder (HSDD), also known as female sexual interest/arousal disorder (FSIAD). Flibanserin (Addyi) is a prescription drug that alters brain chemicals that affect sexual desire. It is a 5-HT1A receptor agonist and 5-HT2A-receptor antagonist medication, which had initially been investigated as an antidepressant. Flibanserin (Addyi) preferentially targets receptors in certain areas of the brain and helps restore the balance between the sexual excitatory effects of dopamine and norepinephrine (adrenalin) neurotransmitters over the sexual inhibitory effects of serotonin. In its three registration clinical studies, flibanserin (Addyi) increased the number of satisfying sexual events by only one (1) event per month, compared to placebo (sugar pill). This is merely a marginal improvement.

Unlike sildenafil ("blue" Viagra), which is a PDE-5 inhibitor that works on genital vascular plumbing, marketing endeavors are inaccurately touting flibanserin (Addyi) as the "pink Viagra" for women. Unlike sildenafil (Viagra), which is taken before each sexual encounter, the flibanserin (Addyi) pill needs to be taken daily. Flibanserin's (Addyi) adverse side effects, such as lowering blood pressure, fainting and fatigue, are significantly worsened when the medication is used with alcohol, so FDA-approval of this pill includes the addition of several safety restrictions. Pregnant women should not take this drug. Patients must sign a form acknowledging the risks associated with taking this drug, particularly fainting and extreme sleepiness. Problems associated with using flibanserin (Addyi) are considered so significant that, unlike most other medications, doctors will have to take a special training course to be certified to prescribe the drug.

GO, ESTROGEN!

Nothing takes care of a woman's sexuality like estrogen. Estrogen provides lubrication and keeps her genital parts in working order. Estrogen allows her testosterone to be a positive influence instead of a hormonal handicap. Estrogen helps maintain a woman's most powerful sex organ, her brain. Not only does the brain interpret the sights, sounds, smells, tastes and touches of sexuality, but it also sparks all those feel good and bonding hormones released with orgasmic sexual intercourse. In other words, a woman just can't get any sexual satisfaction without estrogen.

With the onset of menopause, the ovaries stop producing estrogen, so not only does a woman sustain a 90% drop in her estrogen levels, her testosterone levels are reduced by 50%. The adrenal glands, which sit on top of her kidneys, continue to produce testosterone and androstenedione androgens. Androstenedione can be converted to testosterone and estrogen in adipose (fatty) tissue. Some of the testosterone is further modified into more estrogen, so heavier menopausal women tend to have some estrogen percolating through their system. This variable availability of sex hormones explains why sexual issues vary among menopausal women. For some, hormonal downshifts vaporizes libido and genitals dry up quickly. For others, their adrenal glands' trickle of testosterone is enough to keep them coasting for a while.

Although vaginal aging occurs at different rates for women, menopause brings on the inevitable decline of ovarian hormones in every woman. When sex hormone levels dip below certain levels, neither the mind is interested, nor is the body capable of sexual activity. It's a simple numbers game of estrogen plus testosterone. If a woman's blood serum estradiol levels are below 20 pg/mL, estrone levels are below 30 pg/mL, and total testosterone levels are below 20 ng/dL, then there is "zero sex." Such low hormone levels render a woman physically and psychologically incapable of enjoying orgasmic sexual intercourse. For some women, this is no great loss. For others, lack of sexual dimension to their existence is unacceptable to themselves or their partner.

Since testosterone fuels sexual interest and estrogen enables enjoyment, a woman needs a balance of both hormones to maintain her sexual mojo.

If only testosterone is administered to a menopausal woman, the results are neither healthy nor appealing. Estrogen-deficient, but loaded with testosterone, she'll sprout whiskers while peppered with acne, her breasts shrink while her abdominal (visceral) girth increases, and her hair thins while her voice deepens. Meanwhile, her cholesterol, blood pressure, and aggression increase, while her insomnia and irritability worsen. Regrettably, despite being pumped up with testosterone, an estrogen-deficient woman is all dressed up with nowhere to go. This testosterone-infused makeover may not be attractive to others, and although the desire is restored, her sexual anatomy is not fully operational without estrogen. Without estrogen, dried out vaginal tissues, bladder blunders, decreased blood flow through pelvic vessels, and faulty nerve endings in the genitals, tarnish any sexual rejoicing. For a menopausal woman, even if the sun, the moon, and the stars are all aligned, sex is not enjoyable without estrogen. In a woman, any testosterone replacement therapy requires adequate estrogen levels to work its magic.

If all other stressors inhibiting sexual activity and enjoyment have been resolved, and if a menopausal woman on estrogen therapy is still bothered by a lackluster libido, then her hormone levels should be assessed. She may need a little more estrogen or a touch of testosterone added to her hormone replacement therapy. There are different estrogen pills, skin patches, topical gels, skin sprays, and vaginal rings available to supply needed estrogen. Simply switching hormone preparations may be all that's needed to improve her body's estrogen distribution and revive a menopausal woman's sex life. Oral medications that are taken daily tend to drift down to low levels 18 or so hours after taking them. Switching from an oral estrogen pill to an estrogen patch, for example, may maintain more stable estrogen levels during the day and all through the night.

Like any other oral medication, estrogen pills are absorbed through the intestine, delivered to the liver and then distributed to the rest of the body. Transdermal estrogen delivered topically through skin patches, gels or sprays are absorbed directly through the skin, avoiding the first-pass through the liver. Oral estrogen pills stimulate the liver to produce more sex hormone binding globulin (SHBG). SHBG binds testosterone, and takes it out of action. Since transdermal estrogen initially bypasses the liver, estrogen skin patches do not increase the liver's production of SHBG. The lower the SHBG, the more testosterone is free to do its thing. On the other hand, in hot humid climates, where just walking down the street a woman breaks into a sweat, or if a woman is a frequent hot tub or Jacuzzi user, her estrogen patch may not be adhering to her skin as efficiently, thus lowering the delivery of estrogen into her system. To ensure adequate estrogen levels in this situation, it may be more practical to take oral estrogen pills instead of fussing with peeling patches.

TESTOSTERONE for WOMEN

Once a woman's estrogen levels are adequate, if her testosterone levels are below normal then replacing some of her lost testosterone may revive her sexual interest and energy.

Interestingly, if a menopausal woman's thyroid function is normal, and she's on adequate estrogen replacement, yet she's still having problems feeling cold, her testosterone levels may be too low. A touch of needed testosterone may warm her up.

A man's testosterone levels are 10 times higher than a woman's. Although production is at a fraction of a man's testosterone output, a woman's ovaries and adrenals have been manufacturing testosterone since puberty. Testosterone is part and parcel of a woman's natural hormone make-up and contributes to her overall well-being. Testosterone modulates mood, memory, energy, as well as sexual interest. Lean muscle mass, bone health and the production of oxygen-carrying red blood cells are helped by testosterone. With menopause, a woman's testosterone levels drop by 50%. Some women notice this drop while others are not bothered by testosterone's decline. If menopause is brought on swiftly, as with the surgical removal of ovaries, then the dramatic and rapid loss of ovarian hormones may require adding testosterone to a women's estrogen replacement therapy sooner than later.

In the United States, there is no androgen preparation that has been specifically approved by the FDA for the treatment of low libido or the treatment of testosterone deficiency in women. Testosterone therapy, however, has been used off-label to treat low libido and sexual dysfunction in well-estrogenized women for over 50 years. Replacing needed testosterone in a menopausal woman already on estrogen replacement therapy should not be confused with the deleterious practice of female athletes taking anabolic steroids as performance enhancing drugs. Supplementing any steroid or hormones above and beyond physiologic levels is patently harmful, and therefore, clinically inappropriate.

For adequately estrogenized women with inadequate testosterone levels, appropriately managed testosterone replacement therapy is safe. There is no evidence from randomized controlled trials (RCTs) that testosterone replacement therapy, in formulations and dosages designed for women, adversely affects lipid levels, carbohydrate metabolism, blood pressure, blood clotting parameters or hematocrit. Also, there is no evidence that transdermal testosterone therapy influences the risk of breast cancer in postmenopausal women.

A woman's testosterone is restored with creams, gels, patches, pellets and oral pills. Such preparations include:

- A *combination estrogen plus methyltestosterone (E+T) pill* that can be prescribed for menopausal women suffering from estrogen and testosterone deficiency. The amount of methyltestosterone in this combo hormone pill for women is too low to cause liver issues, but patients with an active liver disease should avoid oral hormones. Some women find that taking this E+T combo pill every day may be providing too much testosterone, experienced as unwanted facial hair, acne, and weight gain. Staggering the use of the E+T to only certain days of the week should eliminate these problems. Blood serum hormone levels help guide dosing adjustments to estrogen and testosterone replacement, thereby achieving appropriate and healthy levels for each woman.
- *Tibolone (Livial)* is a selective tissue estrogen action regulator (STEAR) steroid that has biologically active metabolites with tissue-specific estrogen, progesterone and testosterone actions.

Structurally, it is related to the 19-nortestosterone progestins found in birth control pills. Tibolone helps maintain lean muscle mass, and interestingly, the number of falls in tibolone-treated women is 25% less than in their same-aged untreated counterparts. Tibolone's testosterone metabolite improves mood and memory and increases libido, arousal, and sexual satisfaction. Its estrogen metabolite improves vaginal tissue health and lubrication, relieves hot flashes and night sweats, and prevents osteoporosis. Women experience less breast tenderness and mammogram density changes with tibolone than they do with estrogen-only or estrogen-plus-progesterone replacement therapies. Similar to oral estrogen or selective estrogen receptor modulators (SERMs) like tamoxifen (Nolvadex), raloxifene (Evista) or ospemifene (Osphena), tibolone does increase the risk of strokes in elderly women who are started on the medication after the age of 60. Unlike other oral hormones; however, tibolone does not increase a woman's risk of blood clots, and it has no impact on her risk of heart disease. Tibolone's progesterone metabolite protects the endometrial lining of the uterus, comparable to that achieved with continuous combined estrogen-plus-progesterone regimens. An impressive therapeutic agent, available as a 1.25mg or 2.5mg oral pill taken daily, tibolone performs multiple beneficial functions with minimal risk. Tibolone is truly a multi-tasking hormone for a multi-tasking menopausal woman. Unfortunately, it is not available in the United States, but since 1990 it has been successfully used by millions of postmenopausal women in over 90 other countries.

- *AndroGel* and *Testim* are topical testosterone gel preparations marketed for men. Women can also use these testosterone gels, but in very small amounts. Women's dosing of 0.25cc to 0.5cc applied daily represents a delivery dose of 0.25mg to 0.5mg of testosterone per day. Testim is probably easier to use, because it comes in a small tube that can be resealed. A small pea-sized amount is applied to the inner wrist each morning, so one tube will last a woman about six weeks.

- *AndroFeme 1%* is a testosterone cream manufactured in Australia specifically for women. Each 1 ml of cream applied to the skin of the lower torso or outer thigh daily provides 10mg of bioidentical testosterone for 24 hours. The cream contains almond oil, so people allergic to almonds should not use it. Each 50ml tube contains 500mg of testosterone, and the starting dose is 0.5ml (5mg) per day.
- The application of *compounded testosterone cream* to the vulva has not been studied in randomized controlled trials (RCTs), but some women find that this improves their sexual arousal and orgasms.
- A *testosterone pellet* that is easily inserted under the skin of the lower abdominal wall or upper buttocks releases a small amount of testosterone over four months. The bioidentical testosterone is compounded in doses ranging from 30mg/pellet to 100mg/pellet. Bioidentical hormones are chemically identical to the hormones produced by our bodies, so naturally they are compatible with our system. There are estrogen and progesterone pellets, as well. These pellets are the size of apple seeds, and because they totally dissolve, similar to absorbable sutures used in surgery, they disappear, so there is no removal or extraction process.
- *Intrinsa* is a testosterone patch made by Proctor & Gamble, specifically for women and was available to patients in Europe. Unfortunately, the company that held the rights to market Intrinsa took the unusual step of voluntarily withdrawing its product license "for commercial reasons." This ladies' testosterone skin patch was applied just below the navel and changed twice a week. The amount of testosterone in the patch was 300 micrograms or 0.3mg per 24 hours, which is an amount 10 times lower than testosterone patches for men. Androderm patches for men, on the other hand, deliver either 2mg or 4mg of testosterone per 24 hours and the patch is applied nightly. The way hormone patches are imbibed with testosterone, a woman cannot simply snip a piece of a man's testosterone

patch for herself. It's an integrated system, so any cuts or tears may cause testosterone to leak out.

- *DHEA* is the acronym for dehydroepiandrosterone, which is an androgen hormone produced by the adrenal glands. It's production peaks in our mid-20s and then steadily declines, so that by the time we reach 80, our DHEA levels are down by 80%. DHEA acts as a "parent hormone," which is converted into its offspring hormones of estrogen and testosterone. Some women take DHEA supplements in hopes of improving their energy and libido. Any positive impact may be due to a placebo effect, or their body may be converting the DHEA supplement into either estrogen or testosterone, giving them the hormone boost they need. Because DHEA is sold as a dietary supplement in the United States and not considered a medication, the FDA does not monitor its safety or effectiveness, so there can be variable quality in DHEA preparations. DHEA should not be taken without clinical supervision. Because of peripheral conversion of DHEA to other hormones, estrogen, testosterone and DHEA hormone blood levels need to be monitored closely. If a woman with normal levels of DHEA consumes DHEA supplements, she may experience unwanted side effects, such as facial hair, acne, and weight gain.

Love makes the world go round; hormones power the passion, and sex is how it all comes together. A many splendored activity, not only is sex vital to the survival of the human species, but making love also brings intimacy and comfort to a relationship. Sexual feelings and sexual activity help bond a couple together, physically, emotionally and spiritually. For women, ovarian dysfunction translates into sexual dysfunction, and menopausal hormone loss renders sexual activity tiresome and painful. No matter how harmonious the orchestra, a romantic fiddle can't play without its bow. For sexual symphony ovarian hormone deficiency needs menopause hormone replacement therapy.

VAGINAL WOES

When estrogen levels diminish, blood flow to the genitals subsides and sexual organs recede. Reduced blood flow decreases sustenance to these organs, so a woman's pelvic tissues lose support, lose elasticity, dry out and function poorly. Degradation of tissue anatomy and decreased organ functionality is known as atrophy, from Greek *a-*, for "not" and *trophia*, meaning "nourished." One of the earliest signs of vulvovaginal atrophy (VVA) or genitourinary syndrome of menopause (GSM) is the loss of lubrication. Vulvar tissues are the outer lips of the vaginal opening. The mucosal lining of the vaginal canal, as well as the tissues supporting the vagina, depend on estrogen for health and happiness. With estrogen's support, the vagina is robust, pink and juicy. Without estrogen, the vagina becomes dull, pale and dry, fading into a feeble ghost of its former self. Not only is the vaginal canal compromised, but the entire genital area also becomes parched, withered and less pliable. Friction and thrusting during sexual intercourse traumatizes these weakened vaginal tissues, causing pain, tears, bleeding and infections. Plagued by arid and shrinking vaginal tissues, sexual intercourse becomes so painful and traumatic that it eventually becomes impossible.

Pelvic tissues, nerves, and blood vessels contain high levels of estrogen receptors, so when estrogen dwindles, sexual reactivity decreases. Estrogen loss compromises blood circulation to the genitals and diminishes pelvic nerves' responsiveness. A menopausal woman may not detect weakened genital sensations, decreased lubrication, and reduced blood flow as distinct symptoms, but collectively, they will lead her to perceive that she is less sexually responsive. Within five years of menopause, 50% of women suffer from vaginal dryness and uncomfortable intercourse. For others, it may take a decade of estrogen deprivation before vaginal wasting and bladder blunders become problematic. Unlike other menopausal symptoms that may resolve after a few years, vaginal atrophy and painful sex just get worse and worse as the years go by. The vagina becomes narrower, shorter and inelastic. Because of vaginal pain or inopportune urine loss, a woman who formerly enjoyed sex may avoid intimate situations in which she feels compelled to engage in sexual intercourse. Vaginal woes, bladder mishaps, and bland orgasms undermine a postmenopausal woman's desire for intimacy.

VAGINAL ECOSYSTEM

Without estrogen to support a healthy vaginal ecosystem, the nature of the vaginal environment changes. The vaginal acid-base balance shifts from lactic acid and hydrogen peroxide producing, good microbes, flourishing in a healthy, acid pH habitat, to disease generating bacteria, populating a hostile, alkaline vaginal canal. Opportunistic bad microbes can now propagate much easier in this weakened and dry vaginal tundra. The postmenopausal woman suffers from bouts of vaginal burning and inflammation, as well as recurrent vaginal and bladder infections.

When thin, fragile and chapped vaginal walls housing bad microbes rub against each other, they produce a rainbow of vaginal discharges, ranging from clear, white, yellow, green, and burgundy to brown, and even bloody spotting. Only 1 out of 3 women correctly diagnose what she thinks is a yeast infection, another third have more than one infection, and the rest have something else, like vulvar psoriasis or a sexually transmitted disease (STD). Whenever a postmenopausal woman develops any vaginal bleeding, discharge, itching or irritation "down there," she should be evaluated by a gynecologist.

Although most of these postmenopausal vaginal symptoms are due to atrophic vaginitis, infections, or vulvar skin problems, they could be a harbinger of gynecological cancer. An itchy patch could be vulvar dysplasia.

177

One-third of all cervical cancers occur in women over age 65. 1 in 70 women will develop ovarian cancer with its peak incidence occurring around age 65. The most common type of gynecological cancer is endometrial uterine cancer, which can present with postmenopausal bleeding or vaginal discharge. Bleeding from the bladder or bowel can sometimes be confused with bleeding from the vaginal area, so a thorough diagnostic evaluation is warranted.

LUBRICANTS & MOISTURIZERS

Nothing takes care of the vagina like estrogen, but for women who are not candidates for estrogen therapy or are not comfortable using hormones, lubricants and moisturizers may help relieve pain during intercourse.

Vaginal lubricants are not absorbed by the skin or mucosa and are immediate-acting, so they are applied to the vagina right before sex. Water-based lubricants are non-staining. Silicone-based lubricants are insoluble in water, so they can be used in the hot tub, shower or pool; however, removing silicone residue requires washing with soap and water. Oil-based lubricants, such as baby oil, mineral oil or petroleum jelly (Vaseline), should be avoided, as they can cause vaginal irritation and weaken latex (made from rubber) condoms. Polyurethane (made from plastic) condoms do not break with oil-based lubricants. Warming lubricants are marketed as enhancing sexual response and function. These products cause a warming sensation on the skin that's triggered by menthol or capsaicin, a component of chili peppers.

Vaginal moisturizers, on the other hand, not only reduce the painful friction associated with atrophic vaginal tissues, they cling to the vaginal lining in a way that mimics natural secretions. Moisturizers can be applied before sex, but they work better when applied regularly every 3 to 4 days. Moisturizers may help normalize vaginal pH to a healthy acidic environment, which helps decrease vaginal irritation. Replens, Rephresh and Luvena are vaginal moisturizers. Some postmenopausal women who use a moisturizer regularly may still need to add a lubricant for vaginal comfort during sexual activity.

OSPEMIFENE (OSPHENA)

Ospemifene (Osphena) is a non-estrogen oral treatment for painful sex due to menopausal atrophic vaginal tissues. As a pill taken daily, its oral route is advertised as an advantage over other products that are applied topically in the vaginal canal. It is not an estrogen hormone, but it is an estrogen agonist/antagonist medication, also known as a selective estrogen receptor modulator (SERM). When a SERM attaches to estrogen receptors on certain tissues, it acts like estrogen (agonist), but when the same SERM attaches to estrogen receptors on other tissues, it acts as an anti-estrogen (antagonist). Ospemifene (Osphena) acts like estrogen on vaginal tissues and causes cellular changes that improve vaginal tissue turgor and elasticity, making sex less painful. Similar to other estrogenic therapies in a menopausal woman who has a uterus, Ospemifene (Osphena) stimulates the endometrial lining of the uterus to grow and grow, thus increasing a woman's risk of uterine cancer. The package insert recommends that a progesterone agent be added to ospemifene (Osphena) therapy to protect the uterine lining. Ospemifene (Osphena) increases the risk for blood clots and strokes, as well. Unfortunately, ospemifene's (Osphena) anti-estrogen action on a woman's brain hypothalamic thermostat precipitates hot flashes and excessive sweating.

TSEC

The tissue selective estrogen complex (TSEC) drug marketed by its trade name, Duavee, is a combination oral pill that pairs conjugated estrogen (the same estrogen found in Premarin) 0.45mg with the SERM, bazedoxifene 20mg. This medication is taken daily to treat menopausal hot flashes and prevent osteoporosis in women with a uterus. Estrogen stimulates the endometrial tissue lining of the uterus to proliferate, thicken and potentially degenerate into uterine cancer. The bazedoxifene SERM component of Duavee acts as an anti-estrogen on the uterus, so it prevents the uterine tissue from proliferating in response to estrogen's stimulation. This is similar to the uterine protection provided by progesterone used in traditional menopause hormone therapy. However, unlike progesterone, which contributes to breast problems in menopausal women, the bazedoxifene SERM component has no impact on breast tissue, so it does not cause breast tenderness or breast density changes. While alleviating menopausal hot flashes, the estrogen component maintains healthy vaginal tissues and bone density. Since it is a combination pill of oral estrogen plus a SERM, this medication does increase a woman's risk for blood clots and strokes. Women who have had a hysterectomy have no need for uterine protection, so they would not be prescribed Duavee.

VAGINAL ESTROGEN

Vaginal estrogen, whether delivered as an estrogen cream, a tiny vaginal suppository or a vaginal ring, restores the vaginal ecosystem, reestablishes the healthy vaginal pH environment, resurrects the thickness and elasticity of the vaginal tissue, and improves vaginal blood flow. During embryological development, the lower urinary tract structures come from the same tissue origins as the vagina, so vaginal estrogen preparations help decrease urinary frequency and urinary incontinence, as well as prevent recurrent urinary tract infections in postmenopausal women. Very little estrogen is absorbed through the vaginal walls into the bloodstream, so vaginal estrogen impacts only the local pelvic anatomy, not the rest of the body.

Estrogen vaginal creams (Estrace or Premarin, 0.5-1.0g dose) or the tiny estrogen vaginal suppository (Vagifem-10mcg estradiol tablet) are inserted into the vagina twice a week to maintain vaginal tissue health. The low-dose estrogen-infused vaginal ring (Estring- 2mg estradiol) is inserted into the upper third of the vagina, like a tampon, and remains there for three months before being taken out and replaced. The flexible 2" silicone vaginal ring does not interfere with sexual intercourse.

It takes a couple of months for vaginal estrogen therapy to do its magic and restore vaginal tissue architecture and function to its previous glory. About 20% of women who are taking oral estrogen or using the estrogen patch to alleviate menopausal symptoms may still have vaginal or bladder issues. This is due to downshifting of estrogen receptors within the vaginal walls, as well as increased breakdown of estrogen by vaginal enzymes brought on by menopause. Both estrogen receptor-alpha (ER-alpha) and estrogen receptor-beta (ER-beta) are present in a premenopausal woman's vaginal canal, whereas estrogen receptor-beta (ER-beta) is absent from vaginal tissue in a menopausal woman. These receptor and enzyme changes explain individual variability in the severity of menopausal atrophic vaginal changes, as well as the vagina's response or non-response to oral or transdermal estrogen in some women. When vaginal estrogen is added to their hormone replacement therapy, the pelvic symptoms resolve, and there is no worry that the medications interfere with each other.

The root cause of menopausal vaginal symptoms is estrogen deficiency. Estrogen replacement therapy is the most natural and effective way to preserve tissue architecture and maintain vaginal health, as well as enable sexual arousal and orgasmic pleasure for menopausal women. When estrogen therapy is discontinued, pelvic tissue integrity is lost, so the vagina and bladder revert to their parched and weakened state of atrophy, painful intercourse and bladder irritability. Both the vagina, and its embryological and anatomical neighbor, the bladder, need estrogen replacement for a menopausal woman's genitourinary health, sexuality, and happiness.

BLADDER BLUNDERS - DRY, but LEAKY

Estrogen keeps a woman's pelvic organs moist, supple, healthy and happy. An estrogen deprived menopausal woman dries out vaginally, yet she has a leaky bladder, and sometimes leaks stool. There are estrogen receptors in the vagina, the bladder and the urethra (the tube that drains the bladder to the outside world), as well as the pelvic floor muscles. Estrogen preserves a woman's pelvis. Estrogen deficiency results in drying, thinning and atrophic deterioration of a woman's vulvar, vaginal, bladder and pelvic tissues. Atrophy means organs shrink, tissues lining the organs thin, supportive tissue breaks down, elastic fibers slacken, and blood flow to these structures decreases.

Without estrogen, rosy resilient pelvic tissues deteriorate into pale and weak disrepair. 50% of postmenopausal women between ages 50 and 60, and 70% of women over age 70 suffer from urinary incontinence or vaginal atrophy. 20% of postmenopausal women endure accidental bowel or stool leakage, as well. Without estrogen, women end up depending on incontinence pads and adult diapers. Bladder control problems in women occur when pelvic muscles supporting the bladder are too weak (stress urinary incontinence) or when the bladder muscle itself is too active (urinary urge incontinence). Estrogen deficiency amplifies these symptoms, so many postmenopausal women suffer from a mix of both stress and urge urinary incontinence.

STRESS URINARY INCONTINENCE (SUI) &
PELVIC ORGAN PROLAPSE (POP)

Involuntary loss of urine that occurs when a woman laughs, coughs, sneezes, exercises or has sex is considered stress urinary incontinence (SUI). She may even leak urine when she climbs stairs, gets out of a car or simply stands up from a chair. Although this is usually an anatomical problem that originated with pregnancy and childbirth damaging the muscles and nerves in the pelvis, prolapse problems progress and get worse during menopause. The bladder and urethra eventually lose traction from supporting muscles, so urethral hypermobility occurs and stress urinary incontinence sets in. Urethral hypermobility obliterates the pressure gradient between the bladder and the urethra that is needed to prevent involuntary urine loss. When the pressure in the abdomen exceeds the closing pressure of the bladder's urethra, the woman loses urine. Being overweight or obese increases intraabdominal downward pressure on the bladder, and exacerbates urinary incontinence problems.

Pelvic organ prolapse (POP) occurs when a woman's anatomy becomes distorted by a dropped bladder, vaginal walls collapsing, the uterus slipping, or bowel buckling against the vagina. 50% of all postmenopausal women suffer from pelvic organ prolapse, which further compounds bladder and bowel control problems.

The BLADDER-BONE CONNECTION

Menopausal women suffering from pelvic organ prolapse (POP) are at increased risk of developing bone-thinning diseases like osteopenia and osteoporosis. Estrogen loss leads to ruptured collagen cross-links and disorderly elastin connections within tissues supporting organs throughout a woman's body. This suboptimal tissue architecture not only weakens support of pelvic organs, but it also distorts bone's infrastructure, so bones wither, as well. Conversely, menopausal women with osteoporosis-related vertebral body fractures of the spine are at increased risk of developing urinary incontinence and pelvic organ prolapse (POP). Without estrogen, bones crumble and organs prolapse.

Osteoporosis-related spine fractures occur without trauma and are due to postural stresses alone, such as sitting, standing or walking. These compression spine fractures cause spinal deformity (dowager's hump) and height loss. Getting shorter in the thoracic (chest) area increases intraabdominal downward pressure. Sustained downward pressure on pelvic structures increases the risk of developing urinary incontinence and pelvic organ prolapse. By preventing osteoporosis-related spine fractures, menopause hormone therapy helps a woman's pelvic organs stay put and function better. Estrogen therapy also prevents recurrent urinary tract infections in postmenopausal women.

POP TREATMENT

Treatment options for pelvic organ prolapse (POP) span from pelvic muscles exercises, biofeedback, vaginal cones and pessaries, to antidepressants and pelvic reconstructive surgery. These include:

- Kegel pelvic floor muscle exercises may help with mild to moderate prolapse problems. Kegels involve tensing, lifting and drawing up the muscles around the vagina and anus. A woman needs to work up to 50 to 100 squeezes a day, every day for several months, for these exercises to be effective.
- Physical therapy focusing on pelvic muscles may involve biofeedback and electrical stimulation of targeted muscles. Progressively heavier vaginal cones can be placed inside the vagina, and pelvic floor muscles are then exercised to hold the cone in place and prevent it from slipping.
- Vaginal pessaries can be inserted into the vagina, where they reposition a dropped bladder, sagging rectum or prolapsed vaginal wall. Pessaries must be fitted by a medical professional, and every three months the patient has to return to the doctor's office to have the pessary removed, the vaginal tissues inspected for erosions, and then the cleaned pessary is replaced.
- The antidepressant duloxetine (Cymbalta) is used in Europe to treat stress urinary incontinence (SUI). Cymbalta is a serotonin-norepinephrine reuptake inhibitor (SNRI), so it increases the amounts of serotonin and norepinephrine neurotransmitters, which are thought to play a role in the modulating the nerves that support the bladder

muscles. Increased neurotransmitter activity stimulates closure of the bladder's urethra, and decreases urine loss.

- For stool incontinence, there is a vaginal bowel control device that reduces fecal incontinence episodes. It is a silicone pessary-like device inserted into the vagina with a posteriorly directed balloon. The woman controls the inflation pump through a tube in the vagina. When the balloon is inflated, it compresses the rectum shut and interrupts stool passage. The balloon can then be deflated to allow for stool evacuation. The device can be inserted and removed by the woman as she wishes. It should be taken out once or twice a week for cleaning.

Unfortunately, estrogen therapy cannot repair muscles and nerves damaged from pregnancy and childbirth decades ago, nor can estrogen counter years of increased abdominal weight bearing down on pelvic structures or compensate for smokers chronic cough pumping down on a woman's bladder. As time goes by, pelvic organ prolapse (POP) gets worse and worse, so these anatomical issues require surgical correction, such as slings, suspensions, and realignment procedures. Nearly 20% of postmenopausal women will need specialized pelvic reconstructive gynecological surgery to correct pelvic organ prolapse, and 30% of these women will undergo two or more of these types of pelvic surgeries during their lifetime.

URINARY URGE INCONTINENCE (UUI)

Not only is urinary and stool incontinence from pelvic organ prolapse exacerbated with menopause, overactive bladder problems and urinary urge incontinence (UUI) worsen with estrogen deficiency, as well. Spastic bladder muscle contractions cause urinary frequency, urgency, leaks, and dribbles, even when the bladder is not full. Urinating more than eight times in 24 hours is too frequent. Waking up more than once a night to urinate is too often. This nocturnal urinating is referred to as nocturia. The "gotta go, gotta go" bladder with urge incontinence curtails a menopausal woman's activities, restful sleep, social interactions and travel plans. Limiting intake of caffeine, alcohol, and other bladder irritants, along with bladder retraining tools, such as timed voiding, distraction and relaxation, are somewhat helpful. Despite these behavior modifications, most menopausal women continue to experience bladder accidents if they don't make it to the bathroom on time.

There are non-hormonal pills that may help calm a confused or overactive menopausal bladder, and decrease episodes of urinary urge incontinence. These medications act to either relax the bladder muscle or tighten the urethra, the tube draining the bladder to the outside world. These include:

- Anticholinergic drugs, like oxybutynin (Ditropan), tolterodine (Detrol), and solifenacin (Vesicare), relax bladder muscles and increase bladder filling. The antidepressant imipramine (Tofranil) makes the bladder muscle relax while causing the muscles of the urethra to constrict, thereby decreasing urinary incontinence. Common side effects of these types of medications are a dry vagina, dry mouth, and constipation. They can also cause drowsiness, blurry vision, heartburn, flushed skin, blocked sweating, rapid heartbeat, and cognitive side effects, such as impaired memory and confusion.
- The beta-three adrenergic agonist pill, mirabegron (Myrbetriq), relaxes the bladder muscles and increases bladder filling. Its side effects include headaches, dizziness, hypertension and heart palpitations. Mirabegron can increase blood levels of other medications such as digoxin or warfarin (Coumadin), so these medications need continued blood level monitoring.
- Alpha-adrenergic drugs like the appetite suppressant ephedrine (Ephedra) or the nasal decongestant pseudoephedrine (Sudafed) stimulate the bladder's urethra to constrict and prevent urine leakage. Alpha-adrenergic medication can cause agitation, insomnia, and anxiety.

Due to bothersome side effects, 80% of patients discontinue any type of "gotta go, gotta go" bladder medications after just one year of use. Alternative therapies for an overactive menopausal bladder or urinary urge incontinence (UUI) include interventions such as neuromodulation of the bladder and botulinum toxin (Botox) shots into the bladder's muscle.

Neuromodulation or nerve stimulation techniques may help synchronize bladder muscle contractions by interrupting abnormal reflex arcs that cause bladder dysfunction. These involve:

-   The percutaneous tibial nerve stimulation (PTNS) therapy sends an electrical impulse along a nerve by the woman's ankle. The nerve impulse is then transmitted up to the pelvic sacral nerve plexus controlling bladder function. These 30-minute sessions occur on a weekly basis for three months, and maintenance treatment is rendered when bladder symptoms recur. Improved bladder function dissipates once treatment sessions cease.
-   Another neuromodulation therapy involves a vaginal probe transmitting electrical impulses to the bladder nerves. These 20-minute sessions are done once or twice a day for a couple of months, and maintenance therapy involves sessions three times a week.
-   A more invasive neuromodulation technique involves surgically implanting a battery-powered sacral nerve stimulator device, which may help both urinary and bowel incontinence. The battery needs to be surgically replaced every 5 years.
-   All these nerve stimulation modalities are successful 50% of the time. Women with a cardiac pacemaker are not candidates for electrical neuromodulation therapies, and women with a sacral nerve stimulator device cannot have magnetic-resonance imaging studies (MRIs).
-   Alternatively, botulinum toxin (Botox) can be administered to relax the bladder muscle. Every 3 to 6 months, under anesthesia, a cystoscope is threaded through the woman's urethra to inject Botox

directly into her overactive bladder muscle. Sometimes these Botox injections calm the bladder so much that it can't empty on its own, so the woman needs to have a catheter inserted into her bladder to empty the urine. Until her bladder wakes up again, this self-catheterization may need to occur repeatedly.

Although it may take 5, 10 or 15 years, menopausal hot flashes and night sweats eventually subside and disappear. On the other hand, atrophy and degradation of pelvic organs due to estrogen deficiency is relentlessly progressive, causing more and more misery and humiliating infirmity. Between a twitchy bladder, stress urinary incontinence, and organs prolapsing, it's no wonder that many menopausal women end up governed by their bladder.

Loss of bladder control and accidental bowel/stool leakage are embarrassing hardships condemning many postmenopausal women to adult diapers. Sadly, because of urinary or bowel incontinence, many women end up housebound or parked in a nursing home. Urinary incontinence is 1 of the top 3 diagnoses resulting in a woman's terminal admission into a nursing home. The other two are Alzheimer's dementia and hip fracture. These infirmities could have been prevented with appropriately timed and properly managed menopause hormone therapy.

A woman's pelvic anatomy depends on estrogen for tissue integrity and optimal functioning of all her moving parts "down there." Genitourinary symptoms of menopause (GSM), such as vaginal dryness, vulvar irritation, and painful intercourse, as well as bladder blunders, accidental stool leakage, and urinary incontinence aggravated by estrogen loss, are effectively treated with appropriate estrogen replacement therapy. Just a little bit of estrogen goes a long way towards pleasant and dignified aging in a menopausal woman.

WITHERING SENSES

Sensibility is bound by the senses, and sensuality is dominated by sensitivity. Hormone logic explains why these terms are derived from the same Latin root word *sensus*, meaning "faculty of feeling." For women, these sensations flow from smooth and silky estrogen. Without estrogen, all of a woman's moisture-producing glands malfunction. Faulty fluid production occurs at different rates for different women, but all menopausal women will experience dryness here, there, and eventually, everywhere.

From head-to-toe, a menopausal woman's estrogen-deprived body dries out. Her hair, her eyes, her ears, her nasal passages, her mouth, her airways, her intestines, her skin, her nails, her bladder and her vagina lose the tissue hydration needed for organs to function properly. Her blood vessels harden, her brain tissue shrinks, and her bones become brittle. The only "wet" an estrogen-deprived menopausal woman experiences is a leaky bladder. All these parched and damaging tissue changes are minimized with estrogen replacement therapy. Nothing compares to estrogen's natural and holistic power for maintaining cellular hydration, tissue architecture, and optimal sense and sensitivity in a menopausal woman.

EYES

Eyes may be considered the windows to the soul, but the person views reality through the lens of vision. The most important sensory organ of humans, 80% of a person's impression of the world around them is derived from visual perceptions. As a means of establishing contact with other people, and as an integral part of facial expression, eyes are tantalizing means of communication. As a woman ages, intact vision enables continued independence, along with the pursuit of new adventures. Favorite activities such as reading, writing, crafts, hobbies, watching movies, and actually seeing friends and family depend on vision. Obviously, losing sight profoundly and adversely affects one's quality of life.

Eye problems with deteriorating vision affect older women more frequently than same aged older men. The exact cause of the gender difference is not clear, but it is probably related to the divergent mid-life hormonal environments experienced by men and women. Menopausal women sustain a damaging hormonal hit when estrogen levels plunge around age 50; whereas middle-aged men meander along with their gradual 1 to 2% annual testosterone decline that started back in their 30s. Men do not sustain a precipitous drop in testosterone when they cross the 50-year threshold.

From the surface of the eye to within the eyeball, estrogen affects a woman's sight and vision. The number one cause of blindness in people over the age of 60 is age-related macular degeneration (AMD). The second cause of blindness in this age group is glaucoma. There is no cure for either of these blinding conditions; however, a postmenopausal woman's eyesight fares so much better with appropriate estrogen replacement therapy.

DRY EYE

Tears are fluids that keep eyes moist and healthy, and crying is part of being human. Tears are generated by glands in the eye that produce the watery layer of fluid for cleaning and moisturizing the eye, the oily layer for reducing evaporation, and the mucus layer for lubricating and protecting the eye. The cornea is the clear, dime-sized dome covering the front of the eyeball, through which light initially enters the eye on its path to vision. To remain transparent, the cornea does not have any blood supply, so it is kept nourished and cleansed by tears. Most people blink every 4 seconds, so blinking regulates tears and keeps the cornea's surface smooth and healthy. This protective tear film layer is needed to guard the cornea against damaging dryness and infections and helps the cornea heal from abrasions or trauma.

As a woman moves through menopause and beyond, estrogen loss decreases and alters tear production, so her eyes become drier. Dry eye leads to inflammation and irritation, so it becomes more difficult to read, work at a computer, drive a car or go out in the sunlight. It may also make it unsuitable for her to wear contact lenses. Since tears contain antibodies, when tear volume is down, eyes are more vulnerable to infections, such as keratitis or conjunctivitis (pink eye). Estrogen replacement therapy helps maintain the glands that generate eye-protecting fluids and supports the flow of vision preserving tears.

CATARACTS

Clear vision involves light traveling from the object through the transparent cornea in front of the eye, through the black hole (pupil) in the center of the colored iris, through the transparent optic lens that focuses the light onto the retina. The optic lens is an M&M sized and shaped structure located behind the colored iris of the eye. Like the cornea, the lens has no blood supply and is made mostly of water with some protein. The protein is arranged in a precise lattice to keep the lens clear for light transmission. As one ages, the proteins in the lens break down and clump, so the lens becomes cloudy. A cataract is this clouding of the lens of the eye.

Cataracts grow slowly, so they may not impede vision early on. Eventually, one notices dimming or foggy vision with a decrease in visual clarity that is not correctable with eyeglasses or contacts. Cataracts also cause poor night vision, muted color perception and sensitivity to glare. Streetlights and headlights may seem to be surrounded by a halo, making it dangerous to drive at night. Common risk factors for cataracts are aging, smoking, alcohol, excess ultraviolet (sun) exposure, and diabetes. By age 60, over 90% of people have a cataract, and half the population over age 75 has lost some vision due to cataracts. Once vision-compromising cataracts have formed, the only treatment is surgical removal of the damaged lens, and replacing it with an artificial lens. This is the most common eye surgery performed, and millions of Americans have cataract surgery every year.

Cataracts are more prevalent in postmenopausal women than in similar-aged men. Since estrogen receptors have been detected in the eye's lens, estrogen helps protect the eye from cataracts.

Certain medications that exhibit estrogenic effects on some tissues and anti-estrogen effects on others, known as selective estrogen receptor modulators (SERMs), may increase cataract formation. For example, tamoxifen (Nolvadex), a SERM that is used in the treatment of breast cancer works by acting as an estrogen antagonist on breast tissue, yet it acts like estrogen on a woman's uterus and bones. Tamoxifen also acts as an anti-estrogen on eye tissues, causing visual disturbances and cataract formation.

LIGHT, MACULA, ACTION!

The leading cause of blindness in people over age 60 is age-related macular degeneration (AMD). To understand how estrogen helps prevent AMD in women, let's review what goes on inside our eyes. Light rays travel through the eye's cornea, go through the pupil, and travel through the lens, which focuses light rays onto the retina. The retina is a light-sensitive layer of tissue lining the back of the eyeball. The retina contains photoreceptor rods and cones that turn light into electrical signals that travel up the optic nerve to the brain, where they are translated into visualized images. The rods are located in the edges of the retina and are responsible for peripheral and night vision, black and white sight. Cones are located near the center of retina and are responsible for seeing during the day, in color and in detail.

The retina's macula is a small spot near the center of the retina, and as the most sensitive part of the retina, the macula is responsible for high-resolution, central vision. Macular vision allows a person to read, identify faces and see objects straight ahead. Sensory input from the macula occupies a substantial portion of the brain's visual capacity. As its name implies, age-related macular degeneration (AMD) means that the macular tissue in the center of the retina deteriorates with age. Although AMD may not lead to total blindness; it results in smudging and blurring in the center of one's vision. Over time, the blurred spot gets bigger and darker. This blurring interferes with simple everyday activities, such as reading, writing, cooking, crafts or any close work. Also the ability to recognize faces, drive a car or watch a movie is lost.

Age-related macular degeneration (AMD) starts as "dry" macular degeneration, in which lipid (fat)-laden retinal pigment and cellular waste products form deposits, called "drusen," under the retina. Large drusen lead to thinning and drying out of the macula, causing the macula to lose function. Without a functioning macula, central vision is lost. Over 90% of patients with AMD have this dry variety. As the years go by, they experience slow, but continual, vision loss. Although dry macular degeneration progresses slowly, there is no known cure or treatment. About 10% of people with dry AMD go on to develop a more severe form called "wet" macular degeneration. Wet AMD is characterized by the abnormal growth of blood vessels beneath the retina's macula. These abnormal blood vessels leak and bleed, causing swelling and scarring of the macula. The resulting macular damage may come on rapidly and be severe, with a dramatic loss of vision.

Long-term monthly intraocular injections with medications that block vascular endothelial growth factor (VEGF) may slow down the growth of these abnormal blood vessels. Unfortunately, 30% of patients have an incomplete response to these shots, despite multiple anti-VEGF injections into the eye month after month after month. Because the abnormal blood vessels keep growing back, laser eye surgery or photodynamic eye therapy may require multiple treatment sessions, as well.

There is no cure for macular degeneration. Once damage to the retina's macula takes root and central vision deteriorates, there is no truly effective treatment. As for prevention, age-related macular degeneration (AMD) occurs less often in people who exercise, avoid smoking, maintain a healthy body weight and eat nutritious foods including lots of fish and green leafy vegetables. Also, taking a supplement containing 10mg lutein and 2mg zeaxanthin carotenoids may promote macula-protecting pigments within the retina.

1 in 20 people over the age of 60, and 1 in 8 people over the age of 80, have AMD severe enough to cause serious visual loss. Twice as many women over the age of 75 have AMD compared to men of the same age.

Estrogen-deprived postmenopausal women are at higher risk of developing AMD than their well-estrogenized counterparts. Looking at data from 75,000 postmenopausal women who were part of The Nurses' Health Study (a large informational 30-year research project that followed nurses from 1980 to 2002), researchers found that the risk for advanced or wet AMD was 48% lower in women who received long-term estrogen replacement therapy after menopause, compared to women who did not take female hormones. Women taking estrogen-plus-synthetic progestin had an increased risk for developing early or dry AMD; however, menopausal women taking estrogen-only significantly decreased their chances for developing either wet or dry AMD. Estrogen replacement therapy lowers a woman's odds of developing large drusen deposits in her retina. Oxidative stress plays an important role in the degeneration of the eye's retina layer, and estrogen works as a potent antioxidant, protecting the eye's retina and macula. When compared with monthly eyeball injections and repetitive laser eye surgeries, estrogen replacement therapy is a kinder, gentler way to help a postmenopausal woman retain her vision.

GLAUCOMA

Glaucoma refers to a group of eye disorders that damage the optic nerve and cause blindness. The optic nerve carries visual information from the eyeball's retina to the brain. Glaucoma is usually, but not always, associated with elevated pressure in the eye (intraocular pressure), and, unfortunately, it does not cause symptoms until irreversible loss of vision occurs. After age-related macular degeneration (AMD) of the retina, glaucoma is the second-leading cause of blindness in the United States. AMD is associated with central vision loss, whereas glaucoma causes loss of peripheral vision, so the person ends up with a narrow, tunnel of central vision, where only objects straight ahead are seen. Glaucoma is not curable, and since it is a chronic condition, it needs to be monitored for life. As with AMD and cataracts, more women than men suffer from glaucoma.

The two major categories of glaucoma are open-angle glaucoma and narrow-angle glaucoma. The fluid in the eye flows through an area between the colored iris and cornea, where it drains through the trabecular meshwork at the edge of the iris. This area is referred to as the "angle." Open-angle glaucoma (chronic glaucoma) progresses very slowly, gradually reducing peripheral vision without other symptoms of eye pain or pressure. By the time visual changes are detected, permanent damage to the optic nerve has already occurred. An eye doctor can use a tonometer to measure intraocular pressure, and other diagnostic tools are used to screen for glaucoma. Usually, eye drops are used to treat open angle chronic glaucoma. Closed-angle glaucoma (acute angle closure glaucoma) can come on suddenly, and the person experiences severe eye pain, nausea, and rapid vision loss. Fortunately, because of pain and discomfort, the alarmed sufferer usually seeks immediate medical help and avoids permanent damage. Treatment for this eye emergency requires preventing the eye's iris from blocking the outflow of fluid. This is accomplished by making a laser hole in the iris, an iridotomy.

Currently, there is no definitive way to predict which open-angle glaucoma patient will develop acute angle closure, but acute angle closure affects older women 50% more often than men. Anticholinergic medications used to help treat an overactive bladder or urge incontinence (the "gotta go, gotta go" bladder) pills, can precipitate acute angle-closure glaucoma.

Normal or low-tension glaucoma is a unique condition that experts do not fully understand. It affects adults in their early 60s, and again, it's more common in women than men. Even though the intraocular pressure is normal, optic nerve damage and vision loss still occurs. Perhaps the optic nerve is over-sensitive, or there is atherosclerosis (hardening and narrowing) of the blood vessel that supplies the optic nerve.

Estrogen regulates intraocular pressure by influencing the eye's aqueous production and outflow systems, and an estrogen-deprived optic nerve is more vulnerable to being damaged, even with normal or low-tension glaucoma. Estrogen replacement therapy keeps the eye fluids flowing properly, maintains the optic nerve's resiliency, and reduces a woman's risk of age-related macular degeneration (AMD), glaucoma and blindness. For a menopausal woman, estrogen is a vision of clarity.

HEARING

Estrogen is known to have a protective effect on a woman's auditory (hearing) system. Until bumping into menopause, women have better high-frequency thresholds than men in virtually all age groups. Age-related hearing decline starts after age 30 in men, but not until after the age of 50 in women. This coincides with the menopausal transition and loss of estrogen in women. Estrogen loss triggers a rapid age-related hearing loss in menopausal women. The health consequences associated with decreased hearing include accelerated loss of brain tissue, increased risk of dementia, and increased risk for accidents and hospitalizations. Diminished hearing diminishes physical and mental health overall.

Menopause-related osteoporosis does not only involve the wrist, spine, and hipbones. Bone thinning in the part of the skull bone housing the inner ear is more pronounced in estrogen-deprived women compared to their well-estrogenized counterparts. Loss of this bone causes an inner ear problem known as the superior semicircular canal dehiscence (SSCD) syndrome, where dizziness and unsteadiness are brought on by loud noises or increased abdominal pressure from bearing down. Similar to patching a hole in the drywall, surgery is required to try to reconstruct the osteoporotic upper bony wall housing the inner ear.

Not only does estrogen support the inner ears' bony carriage within the skull, estrogen helps maintain the middle ears' tiny bones involved in transmitting sound. Estrogen also plays a pivotal role in how the brain extracts and interprets auditory information. Sound-processing cells within the brain need estrogen to maintain sensitivity, and estrogen is required to instruct the brain to lay down memories of sounds. By slowing down hearing loss, estrogen hormone therapy helps menopausal women maintain balance and harmony as they age.

SMELL

Although a human's sense of smell is not as keen as a dog's, a person can distinguish thousands of different odor molecules. The sense of smell (olfaction) is the most primitive of the senses. The smell receptor cells are the only neurons in the nervous system exposed directly to the external environment. Even with touching, neurons (nerve cells) for detecting pressure are located in the dermis of the skin, beneath the epidermal (outermost) skin surface. Smelling allows us to identify food, mates and danger, as well as enjoy sensual pleasures like the aroma of perfume, flowers, and pumpkin pie. When inhaled, odor molecules travel into the nose and interact with odor receptors. These odor receptors then transmit the information to the olfactory bulb, which is an extension of brain tissue that sits behind the bridge of the nose. From the olfactory bulb, odor information is propagated to the brain's limbic system, which is the same part of the brain that affects appetites, emotions, sexuality, memory and creativity.

Estrogen deficiency dries out all the mucus membranes in a woman's body, from her eyes to her vagina, and every cavity in between. The mucous membranes lining her nasal passages are no exception. As the nasal membranes atrophy and blood flow to the nasal passages decrease, odors cannot reach the olfactory receptors, so her ability to detect odor molecules decreases. As part of the "use it or lose it" phenomenon of brain activity, decreased odor input causes deterioration of the olfactory nerve, which results in altered and decreased sense of smell.

80% of what we taste is from the food's aroma, so any joy in eating is lost when we cannot detect appetizing smells. Decreased sense of smell can interfere with the ability to notice potentially harmful chemicals, fumes and gases that may have life-threatening consequences. 80% of women over the age of 80 have a marginal sense of smell, and 50% are anosmic, that is, they have lost their sense of smell. Estrogen replacement therapy preserves a woman's sense of smell by maintaining the mucosal integrity of her nasal passages and allowing smell signals to be transmitted effectively from her nose to her intact brain. The nose knows.

BURNING MOUTH... LOSING TEETH

Hormonal downshifts in a middle-aged woman can precipitate burning mouth syndrome (glossodynia), a frazzling condition of pain and irritation throughout the oral cavity and tongue. There are no visible signs of abnormality, and there is no other cause for these symptoms beyond estrogen loss associated with menopause. The pain comes on spontaneously and can last for several years. The taste buds that detect bitterness are located at the back of the tongue, and they are dependent upon estrogen to remain healthy. These taste buds are surrounded by a basket-like collection of pain neurons that become activated when the taste buds are damaged by the lack of estrogen.

Estrogen plays a part in the production and constitution of saliva, so estrogen loss disrupts the salivary flow needed to maintain tissue hydration within the oral cavity. Not only does this cause problems with bad breath, but the dry dental environment also renders tooth enamel more vulnerable to cavities and decay. Estrogen replacement therapy helps prevent periodontal disease, including gingival inflammation and bleeding gums. These changes reflect the impact of estrogen on the preservation of tissues within the oral mucosa, similar to estrogen's power to protect vaginal mucosal tissues from thinning, drying and trauma.

Menopausal estrogen loss not only weakens the bones in a woman's wrists, spine and hips, but it can also cause bone loss in the jawbone. Dry mouth issues, along with thinning jawbones, make tooth loss more likely. 1 out of 3 women over the age of 65 has no teeth, and older women spend more time in the dentist's chair than older men.

Professional singers use female hormone therapy to prevent what they view as unwanted voice changes associated with menopause. Objective voice analysis has documented deepening of women's voices in the early postmenopausal years, with lesser changes associated in women taking estrogen.

SENSES and SENSIBILITY

As vital tools for perceiving the outside world, a woman's awareness and understanding of her environment depend on her senses. As the years go by, aging leads to fading vision, decreased hearing, diminished smell, and waning taste in an estrogen-deprived postmenopausal woman. Crumbling sensory perception and dwindling sensibilities conspire to restrict an older woman's world and impair her quality of life. Estrogen deprivation worsens and exacerbates these crippling afflictions. Estrogen replacement therapy helps a menopausal woman retain her information gathering faculties and preserves her capacity for functioning independently. With her senses intact, a well-estrogenized postmenopausal woman enjoys her world more fully, while aging with dignified sensibilities.

25

GUT FEELING

To stay alive a person needs air, water and food. This holy trinity of human existence generates the rule of 3's for survival: after 3 minutes without air or 3 days without water or 3 weeks without food, a person becomes ill and dies. We need to eat to stay alive, and our digestive tract makes it happen. Digestion involves the mechanical and chemical breakdown of food we eat into smaller components. This allows nutrients to be absorbed through the intestines into the bloodstream, where they can be taken up by the body's cells and used for energy. Non-nutrient-worthy substances are evacuated out the southern end. The gastrointestinal tract is a series of hollow organs joined in a 30-foot long, twisting and turning tube extending from the mouth down to the anus. From chewing and saliva production, through stomach churning and gallbladder secretion, to intestinal motility and waste removal, estrogen is involved every step of the way.

MOUTH (ORAL CAVITY)

The process of digestion begins in the mouth, where the teeth, along with the tongue's massaging action, chew the food, breaking it down into smaller pieces. Salivary juices and enzymes soften the food for easy swallowing. Without estrogen, saliva's composition changes and salivary flow diminishes, so food seems drier. Due to altered taste buds and decreased saliva, menopausal women experience "burning tongue" sensation (glossodynia), along with decreased taste enjoyment. Teeth need saliva to stay healthy, so dry mouth erodes tooth enamel and teeth are lost. 1 out of 3 women over the age of 65 has no teeth. Tooth loss and the need for dentures are significantly reduced in postmenopausal women on estrogen replacement therapy. Since estrogen-deprived, arid nasal passages no longer process appetizing aromas like they used to, eating is not as pleasant as it used to be. Eventually, limited capacity to enjoy food contributes to nutrient deficiencies among aging postmenopausal women.

STOMACH

Once food is manageable enough to swallow, the food bolus then passes from the mouth down to the stomach through a foot long muscular tube called the esophagus. The locomotive process by which food or liquids or anything is advanced through the esophagus down to the stomach, and then moved from the stomach down through the intestines to the outside world is known as peristalsis. Peristalsis is wavelike synchronized contractions of the muscles within the lining of the digestive tract that keep things moving along. Without synchronized peristalsis, food matter gets stuck, uncomfortable pockets of gas develop, and painful bowel muscle spasms occur.

The stomach is about 1 foot long and 6 inches wide, the size of two fists put together. Any water or alcohol that we drink can be absorbed directly from the stomach into the bloodstream. When food makes it to the stomach, the stomach's hydrochloric acid and juices begin the breakdown of fats and proteins. Stomach acid also kills bacteria that may be swallowed. A mucus barrier protects the lining of the stomach, so it doesn't digest itself. Because stomach acid is so strong (stomach pH is 2, compared to water's neutral pH of 7.0 or blood's neutral pH of 7.4), most carbohydrate digestion takes place in the small intestine where juices are more alkaline, with a pH of 8. The stomach takes about 5 hours to mix and digest solid food. The churned food in the stomach is converted into a semi-fluid state called chyme, which then passes into the small intestine.

SMALL INTESTINE

Only 1 inch in diameter, the small intestine is a 20-foot long, convoluted tube extending from the stomach to the large intestine. The gallbladder and pancreas open into the duodenum, the first part of the small intestine, where the gallbladder contributes bile to aid in fat digestion, and pancreatic enzymes help digest the chyme received from the stomach. The small intestine is lined with thousands of tiny folds and projections called villi. There are even tinier projections on each villus called microvilli. All these many, many folds create a huge surface area for absorbing nutrients. The small intestine absorbs 90% of all the protein, fat and carbohydrates that are eaten, as well as absorbing vitamins and minerals provided by the food or oral supplements. Any undigested or unabsorbed food then passes from the small intestine into the large intestine, also referred to as the colon.

Celiac disease (sprue) is an autoimmune disorder of the small intestine that occurs in about 1 in 100 individuals. When genetically predisposed people ingest foods containing gluten, which is found in wheat, rye, barley, and possibly oats, their immune system reacts by damaging the small intestine's villi. This flattens the surface area required for proper food digestion and nutrient absorption. The person becomes malnourished, no matter how much food they eat. Treatment for this chronic condition is a gluten-free diet. Celiac disease (sprue) affects women more often than men, and the condition is exacerbated by menopausal estrogen loss.

LARGE INTESTINE (COLON)

The large intestine forms the last part of the digestive tract. It's a 5 feet long tube, and because its diameter is wider (3 inches) than the small intestine, the colon is considered the "large" intestine. The colon is where any residual fluids and salts are absorbed. After absorption, the remaining undigested matter is squeezed into a bundle, called feces. Feces is composed of undigested food, cells that slough off the inner lining of the intestines, and bacteria. About 30% of the weight of feces is bacteria. These are probiotic or "good" bacteria, and billions of them live in the colon all the time. As long as these bacteria stay within the lumen of the colon, they are harmless. If they get out into the abdominal cavity or migrate into the bloodstream, they can cause blood poisoning or sepsis. The colon bacteria live off fiber and produce gas. Bowel gas enters the intestinal tract through swallowed air, as well. When the bacteria finish with the feces, it is passed into the rectum, where it is stored until it is passed through the anus as a bowel movement. From entry to exit, digestion takes 24 to 48 hours. Consuming 30 to 35 grams of fiber a day maintains transit time and prevents hemorrhoids. Once the fecal matter is evacuated, it is referred to as stool.

GERD

Gastroesophageal reflux disease (GERD) is a digestive condition where stomach acid or stomach contents flow back (reflux) up the esophagus. Because stomach contents are acidic, reflux irritates and inflames the lining of the esophagus, causing heartburn, chest pain and belching (burping). The acid reflux can make it all the way up to the oral cavity, causing bad breath and dental enamel erosions. Women may experience GERD symptoms differently than men. Women have more problems with GERD-associated coughing, wheezing, hoarseness and sore throat. GERD-induced chronic inflammation can cause scarring and narrowing of the esophagus (stricture), making swallowing very difficult. Persistent irritation of the esophagus by stomach acid can eventually result in ominous cellular changes that lead to Barrett's esophagus, a precancerous condition.

Eating large meals or consuming citrus, fatty or spicy foods, peppermint or chocolate, or drinking coffee, can bring on heartburn. By relaxing the lower esophageal sphincter (LES) muscles that usually prevent stomach contents from splashing back into the esophagus, smoking and alcohol increase the risk for GERD. Obesity aggravates GERD, because abdominal (visceral) adiposity increases mechanical pressures in the stomach-esophageal area, causing the lower esophageal sphincter (LES) to remain partially open, which allows stomach acid to continue refluxing up the esophagus. Pregnant women suffer from GERD because high levels of progesterone relax the lower esophageal sphincter (LES) muscle, which then allows stomach contents to flow back into the esophagus. Pregnancy-associated GERD usually resolves after the baby is born.

Estrogen-deprived menopausal women are more likely to suffer from GERD symptoms than their same-aged well-estrogenized counterparts.

Like many muscles in the body, the lower esophageal sphincter (LES) muscles lose strength with estrogen loss. A menopausal woman's weakened lower esophageal sphincter (LES) makes it easier for stomach contents or acid to stream back into the esophagus. As women age, estrogen-deprived bladders become irritable and overactive, becoming the pesky "gotta go, gotta go" bladder. Anticholinergic medications, such as oxybutynin (Ditropan) and tolterodine (Detrol), which are prescribed for overactive bladder or urinary urge incontinence (UUI), increase acid reflux and worsen GERD.

Osteoporosis is the most prevalent bone disease in America, and 50% of estrogen-deprived postmenopausal women will sustain an osteoporosis-related fracture. In addition to being deadly, these fractures are physically debilitating and lead to a downward spiral in physical and mental health. Oral bisphosphonate medications such as alendronate (Fosamax), risedronate (Actonel) or ibandronate (Boniva), are often prescribed to prevent and treat osteoporosis in postmenopausal women. About 30% of women who take these pills experience stomach upset. If these drugs reflux back up from the stomach into the esophagus, they can cause inflammation and erosion of the esophagus. They can also directly damage the mucosal lining of the stomach. In women who already suffer from GERD, oral bisphosphonate use may increase the risk for Barrett's esophagus, a premalignant precursor to esophageal cancer. For a menopausal woman, healthy weight, healthy lifestyle and a healthy estrogen environment keep GERD at bay.

PEPTIC ULCER DISEASE

A peptic ulcer is an open sore or raw area that develops either in the lining of the stomach (gastric ulcer) or in the upper part of the small intestine called the duodenum (duodenal ulcer). These ulcers develop when digestive juices damage the lining of the stomach or duodenum, resulting in craters averaging between a ¼ to a ½ inch in diameter. Cells within the lining of the stomach and duodenum produce a naturally protective mucus barrier to ward off damage from the stomach's acid. When there is a breakdown of the balance between acid production and the mucus defense barrier, an ulcer develops, allowing acid to injure the lining of the stomach or duodenum. This leads to an ulcer.

Long-term use of non-steroidal anti-inflammatory drugs (NSAIDs), such as aspirin, ibuprofen (Motrin) or naproxen (Aleve, Naprosyn) causes peptic ulcer disease. A stomach infection with Helicobacter pylori (H. pylori) bacteria can cause peptic ulcers, as well. Any bacteria that can survive the stomach's acid environment (pH of 2) would have to be rather nasty. Alcohol consumption causes the stomach to produce more acid, which leads to more problems with gastritis and ulcers, and smoking increases the risk of slow-healing duodenal ulcers. Smoking and drinking lead to belly aching.

Although many people with peptic ulcers have no symptoms, signs that indicate an ulcer may be brewing include upper abdominal pain that may either get better with eating or get worse, nausea, and feeling bloated or full. Someone with an ulcer may vomit red blood or "coffee grounds" (blood mixed with stomach acid), or they may have foul-smelling, bloody stools or develop black, tarry stools (blood mixed with digestive fluids). Complications of untreated peptic ulcers include bowel perforation, internal bleeding, and gastric outlet obstruction.

Prior to menopause, the prevalence of duodenal ulcers is significantly lower in women than in men. Men are 5 times more likely to develop duodenal ulcers compared to well-estrogenized women. Postmenopausal estrogen-deprived women, on the other hand, develop duodenal ulcers at rates equal to men. Moreover, a duodenal ulcer follows a more serious course in a postmenopausal woman. Although GERD frequently occurs in pregnant women, active symptoms of peptic ulcer disease are rare during pregnancy. Pregnant women, or women on estrogen-containing oral contraceptive pills (OCPs), are less likely to develop peptic ulcers. Mucosal cells lining the duodenum secrete bicarbonate to neutralize the damaging gastric acid that may spill into the lumen of the small intestine. Prior to menopause, women have significantly higher duodenal bicarbonate secretion than age-matched men. An estrogen deprived menopausal woman's lackluster bicarbonate production renders her duodenum more vulnerable to stomach acid damage. Estrogen keeps mucosal linings juicy, happy and healthy, throughout a woman's body.

LIVER

As the body's chemical processing center, the liver is the largest organ inside the body. About the size of a football and located behind the ribs in the upper right-hand portion of the abdomen, this meaty, rubbery glandular organ is vital to our existence. From its storage of vitamins, sugar and iron, through its production of critical proteins, to its proficiency in clearing blood of waste products, drugs and other poisonous substances, the liver supports the performance of every other organ in the body. We need the liver to live. Fortunately, up to 75% of the liver can be diseased or removed before it stops functioning. If the liver fails or shuts down, the person will die within 2 to 3 days. Liver dialysis, where a machine performs the detoxification functions of the liver, cannot support a person longer than a few days. This technology is used as a bridge between liver failure and liver transplant surgery.

LIVER'S FIRST-PASS EFFECT

Any medication that is swallowed has to be processed by the liver first. This "first-pass effect" influences how oral drugs are metabolized. The liver can modify the medication to its biologically active form to achieve therapeutic goals, or it can alter the medication to a less biologically active form, so higher doses are needed. The drugs themselves can stimulate the liver to produce proteins and other substances that impact the rest of the body. On the other hand, medications that are administered through the skin, such as transdermal preparations using skin patches, topical gels or sprays, or drugs that are delivered intravaginally or by injections, intravenously (IV), skin pellets or implants, avoid the liver's first-pass effect. Transdermal hormone preparations, such as estrogen patches, enter the blood stream directly, so they do not influence the liver. These transdermal hormone preparations by-pass the liver, and there is no "first-pass effect," so lower doses of estrogen can be used to achieve therapeutic goals.

Oral estrogen pills influence the liver's management of cholesterol and increase its production of clotting factors. Because transdermal estrogens do not affect the liver's handling of clotting factors or fatty triglycerides, transdermal estrogens can be prescribed to women who are not candidates for oral estrogens, e.g.- women with a history of blood clots or women who have elevated fatty triglyceride levels. Diabetics tend to have higher blood serum triglyceride levels, so estrogen patches are a good choice for their estrogen replacement therapy. Estrogen skin patches do not increase a menopausal woman's risk of strokes or blood clots, no matter how old she is.

LIVER & CHOLESTEROL

The liver controls the production and removal of cholesterol. Within the body, cholesterol is an essential component of every cell's membrane. Life-sustaining steroids, such as glucocorticoids and mineralocorticoids, as well as sex steroids involved in reproduction and perpetuation of the human species, are derived from cholesterol, as well. Because cholesterol is so vital to survival, Nature did not leave cholesterol acquisition to chance or diet. The liver manufactures 85% of the body's cholesterol, so cholesterol consumed in food plays a relatively insignificant role in determining blood levels of cholesterol. In February 2015, the Dietary Guidelines Advisory Committee, which is an advisory group appointed by the U.S. Department of Health and Human Services and the U.S. Department of Agriculture, has recommended that limitations on dietary cholesterol be removed from the 2015 edition of Dietary Guidelines for Americans.

Estrogen stimulates the liver to produce more of the "good" high-density lipoprotein cholesterol, known as HDL-cholesterol, "H" for Hurray, good cholesterol. HDL-cholesterol clears excess cholesterol from the bloodstream and prevents plaque build up in the arteries supplying our heart and brain. Estrogen directs the liver to decrease its production of the "bad" low-density lipoprotein cholesterol, known as LDL-cholesterol, "L" for Lousy, bad cholesterol. LDL-cholesterol delivers cholesterol to the arteries, and this increases plaque formation. These cholesterol plaques calcify, harden and narrow the arteries that deliver oxygen and nutrients to our organs. This artery-damaging disease process is known as atherosclerosis. Atherosclerosis causes heart attacks and strokes, and compromises blood flow to the genitals. Necrotic, unstable cholesterol plaques within damaged atherosclerotic blood vessels can break open, triggering the formation of a blood clot at the plaque site. If the clot blocks blood flow in an artery supplying the heart muscle, a heart attack occurs. If this blockage is in an artery supplying part of the brain, the person has a "brain attack" or stroke. Estrogen's influence on the liver's production of heart healthy ratios of HDL-cholesterol to LDL-cholesterol is one of the reasons that cardiovascular disease is so rare among premenopausal women. Appropriately timed and properly managed estrogen replacement therapy provides similar heart protection to menopausal women, as well.

LIVER & BLOOD CLOTS

If a person's blood does not clot properly, they can bleed to death. The liver manufactures clotting factors to stop excessive bleeding after cuts or injuries. Clotting factors are proteins that allow blood to clot properly. Because women bleed every month with their menstrual periods, and because they lose a lot of blood when they deliver a baby, Nature improved a woman's chance of surviving these recurrent bleeding episodes with the help of estrogen. Estrogen stimulates the liver to produce more clotting factors.

By powering up the liver's production of these clotting factors, estrogen causes blood to clot very efficiently, sometimes too efficiently, so blood clots can occur in the wrong places. Women of reproductive age are at greater risk of developing unwanted blood clots within deep veins located in their legs, pelvis, arms and shoulders, known as deep vein thrombosis (DVTs), than men. After age 50, however, men are at higher risk of DVTs than women. The estrogen drop associated with menopause decreases a woman's liver production of clotting factors. Low-dose oral estrogen replacement therapy, using FDA-approved, pharmaceutical grade, bioidentical estradiol, impacts the liver far less than conjugated equine estrogen (Premarin) pills or other synthetic oral estrogens. Of course, transdermal estrogen preparations, the estrogen skin patches, topical gels or skin sprays, do not influence the liver, so they do not increase a woman's risk of blood clots or strokes.

LIVER & HORMONE SHUTTLES

Oil and water don't mix; so fat-soluble molecules do not travel well in the salty waters of the bloodstream. Fat-soluble cholesterol needs to hook up either with high-density lipoprotein (HDL) or low-density lipoprotein (LDL) to be transported within the blood vessels. The cholesterol-derived sex hormones, estrogen, testosterone, and progesterone, along with thyroid hormones, are also fat-soluble, so on their own, they cannot travel within the bloodstream either. The liver produces sex hormone binding globulins (SHBG) and thyroid-binding globulins (TBG), which are the proteins that bind with fat-soluble hormones and deliver them to their target organs.

Estrogen increases the liver's production of these binding globulins. This can result in too much of the hormones being bound, and less of them free to achieve their hormonal missions. For example, if a woman is taking thyroid hormones when she gets pregnant, the escalating levels of estrogen stimulate her liver to produce more thyroid-binding hormone (TBG), so she may require higher doses of thyroid medication during pregnancy. On the other hand, menopausal ovaries no longer produce estrogen to encourage the liver's production of sex hormone binding globulin (SHBG). No longer bound by SHBG, emancipated testosterone is free to cause scalp hair loss, facial hair growth, and shape-shifting, from a woman's hourglass or pear silhouette to an apple-shape. Transdermal hormone preparations, such as estrogen skin patches, topical gels or sprays, do not influence the liver's production of sex hormone binding globulin (SHBG). Oral estrogen pills, however, do increase the liver's production of SHBGs that bind testosterone, which decreases the effects of freewheeling testosterone. When testosterone is bound, it's not free to fool around.

GALLBLADDER

The liver produces bile, a fluid that helps the body digest fats and helps the body absorb the fat-soluble vitamins A, D, E, and K. Bile consists of cholesterol, bile salts, and bilirubin. Bilirubin is a substance that forms when hemoglobin from red cells breaks down, releasing its iron, and giving stool its usual brown color. Bile is stored and released by the gallbladder. Located along the undersurface of the liver, the gallbladder is about 3 inches long and shaped like a hollow balloon. Bile helps digest fatty foods. The bile travels through the cystic duct and into the duodenum (the beginning of the small intestine). The pancreas releases digestive enzymes into the duodenum, as well. Together, bile and pancreatic enzymes help break down fatty food for intestinal absorption

Imbalances in the substances that make up bile cause gallstones. More than 80% of gallstones consist of hardened cholesterol, so they tend to be yellow-green in color. Pigment stones are made of bilirubin, which comes from the iron released from hemoglobin breakdown, so pigment stones are dark in color. 90% of people with gallstones have no symptoms, and the gallstones may be detected incidentally on imaging studies done for other purposes, or during abdominal or gynecological surgery. Obesity increases the amount of cholesterol in bile, which causes gallstone formation. Diets high in calories and refined carbohydrates, but low in fiber, increase the risk of gallstones. People with diabetes generally have high levels of triglyceride fatty acids in their system, and these fatty acids increase the risk of gallstones. As the body breaks down fat during prolonged fasting or rapid weight loss, the liver secretes extra cholesterol into bile, leading to gallstone formation. Medications that lower blood cholesterol levels, such as statins, increase the amount of cholesterol secreted into the bile, so they increase the risk for gallbladder problems, as well.

If bile thickens or a gallstone or scar tissue blocks bile flow from the gallbladder, symptoms will occur. After eating a fatty meal, milder symptoms of gallbladder dysfunction include indigestion, abdominal gas or bloating. If a gallstone lodges in a duct and causes blockage, the gallbladder contracts vigorously to try to dislodge the obstruction. This can cause sudden and rapidly intensifying pain in the middle and upper right area of the abdomen (biliary colic). The pain may radiate around to the back between the shoulder blades and up to the right shoulder area. To get the digestive tract running smoothly again, gallbladder trouble usually requires surgical removal of the diseased gallbladder.

Medical students are taught that the usual type of patient who has gall-bladder disease can be identified by the 5 F's: Female, Fat, Forty years or older, Fertile, with a Family history of gallstones. Women are more likely than men to develop gallstones. Estrogen increases cholesterol levels in bile and decreases gallbladder contractions, which causes gallstones to form. Pregnancy, estrogen-containing oral contraceptive pills (OCPs) or oral estrogen replacement therapy can exacerbate gallbladder issues. Unlike estrogen pills, transdermal estrogens, such as estrogen patches, topical gels or sprays, are absorbed directly into the bloodstream, so they do not influence liver metabolism or impact the gallbladder.

GAS & CONSTIPATION

To derive nourishment from what we eat, food needs to be processed through the entire length of the digestive tract. From the moment we swallow, synchronized peristalsis, the alternating contraction and relaxation of the muscles lining the digestive canal, moves food and water down the esophagus, through the intestines and colon, past the rectum and out the anus. We need muscles to digest food. For some women, fluctuating levels of female hormones during their menstrual cycle causes variable peristalsis action. For most women, stools are looser and more frequent at the time of menses, but firmer during the post-ovulation luteal phase of the cycle. After ovulation, the ovary secretes progesterone, which slows down peristalsis and evacuation. High progesterone levels during pregnancy also slow down intestinal transit time, causing problems with constipation, as well.

Irritable bowel syndrome (IBS) is a chronic disorder that affects the large intestine (colon) and causes intermittent episodes of cramping, abdominal pain, bloating, gas, diarrhea, and constipation. More women than men suffer from irritable bowels, and premenopausal female patients report exacerbation of their symptoms at the time of menses, when their estrogen is at an all time low.

Estrogen helps maintain muscle strength and action, so when menopausal women lose their estrogen, peristalsis function diminishes and becomes less synchronized. With menopause, the temperamental or irritable bowel produces more painful pockets of gas, bloating and flatulence, along with more issues with irregularity and constipation. After menopause, women taking estrogen replacement experience less bloating than women not taking hormone therapy. Steady levels of estrogen help keep the intestinal action moving along smoothly.

COLON CANCER

A woman's lifetime risk of developing colon cancer is 1 in 20, and colon cancer is the 2nd leading cause of cancer deaths in the United States. Since we've broached the topic of death, some pertinent numbers to be aware of are:

- The leading cause of death in the U.S. is cardiovascular disease - 1 in 3 deaths is due to heart attacks and strokes.
- The 2nd leading cause of death is cancer - 1 in 4 deaths is brought on by cancer.
  o Lung cancer is the leading cause of cancer deaths
  o Colon cancer is the 2nd leading cause of cancer deaths
  o Breast cancer is the 3rd leading cause of cancer deaths among women, and prostate cancer is the 3rd leading cause of cancer deaths among men
- The 3rd leading cause of death in the U.S. is preventable medical errors that occur in the hospital - 1 in 6 deaths is due to hospital-acquired infections, preventable blood clots, adverse drug events, falls, or diagnostic errors.

A person with colon cancer may have normal bowel movements and show no signs or symptoms of the disease. Or, they may notice a persistent change in bowel habits, such as repeated episodes of diarrhea, constipation, narrowing of the stool caliber, a sensation of needing to have a bowel movement that is not relieved by doing so (tenesmus), rectal bleeding, dark stools, blood in the stool, cramping or abdominal pain, weakness and fatigue, or unintended weight loss. Fortunately, regular screening finds colon cancer early, and screening can also prevent colon cancer altogether. When precancerous colon polyps and growths are detected, they can be removed before they have a chance to turn into cancer. From the time the first abnormal colon cell grows into a polyp, it usually takes 10 years for the polyp to develop into colon cancer.

Older age is one of the most important risk factors for colon cancer, with 90% of colon cancers occurring in people older than 50 years. People at average risk for colon cancer should start regular screening at age 50 and continue until age 75, as long as their results are negative. This may involve a colonoscopy every 10 years or testing stool samples annually for blood. Since stool contains cells that are shed daily from the lining of the colon, Cologuard screens for colon cancer by testing stool for DNA changes linked to any abnormal colon cell growths (cancerous or precancerous). Cologuard testing is usually done every 3 years. People at higher risk of developing colon cancer, such as individuals who suffer from an inflammatory bowel disease, have a family history of colon cancer or are part of a family with inherited cancer syndromes, or have colon polyps themselves, may need to start screening at a younger age. They may also need testing at more frequent intervals than others.

Other factors that are associated with increased risk of colon cancer are high red meat consumption, a low-fiber diet, history of chronic constipation (fewer than 3 bowel movements a week), being overweight or obese, smoking, or a personal history of having had breast, uterine or ovarian cancer in the past. The American Cancer Society recommends that adults engage in moderate exercise or physical activity, such as walking at a brisk clip for 30 minutes, 5 days a week, to decrease their risk of cancer. 10,000 steps a day walk cancer away. Taking low-dose (81 mg) baby aspirin regularly for 5 or more years decreases a postmenopausal woman's risk of colon cancer, as well decreases her risk of breast cancer, by 20%. Coincidentally, for a woman 65 years or older, the low-dose aspirin also helps decrease her risk of heart attacks or strokes by 20%. Inflammatory bowel disease, such as Crohn's or ulcerative colitis, occurs equally among men and women, but men have a greater cumulative risk of developing colon cancer than women.

For women suffering from these inflammatory bowel conditions, estrogen replacement therapy provides a protective effect for disease activity in their menopausal years. This is most likely due to the anti-inflammatory effects of estrogen.

Estrogen is beneficial to a woman's colon. The incidence of colon cancer is greater in men than in same aged premenopausal women, and men develop colon cancer at a younger age than women do. Women who have used estrogen-containing oral contraceptive pills (OCPs) reduce their overall risk of colon cancer. Premenopausal women with metastatic colon cancer live longer than their equally aged male counterparts. In contrast, estrogen deprived postmenopausal older women with colon cancer fare significantly worse than older men do. It is thought that estrogen-beta receptors (ER-beta) on the cells lining the intestine are involved in inhibiting the growth of abnormal colon cancer cells. When a woman loses her estrogen, she loses the cancer-preventing action of estrogen-beta (ER-beta) receptors.

A nutritious diet coupled with a healthy lifestyle works wonders at maintaining everlasting digestion. Following through on simple habits like, "an apple a day keeps the colostomy away," and "walk away from cancer," go a long way to avoiding digestive problems. For a woman, menopause hormone therapy reduces her risk of colon cancer, and this risk is further reduced with increased duration of female hormone replacement. 5 years of menopause hormone therapy results in a 40% risk reduction in colon cancer, 10 years yields a 50% reduction, and 15 or more years of menopause hormone therapy delivers a 66% reduction in a woman's risk of developing colon cancer. The protective effect of hormones is more marked in current users and long-term users of estrogen replacement therapy. 5 years after stopping her female hormones, a woman loses the colon cancer prevention benefits of estrogen. For a menopausal woman, estrogen replacement therapy helps keep her intestinal tract functioning as a trouble-free, cancer-free, digestive machine.

BREAST MATTERS

Of all the possible medical issues that can burden a woman, breast problems, particularly fear of breast cancer, tops her list of health concerns. Because cultures attach such great significance to the female breast, a woman's sexuality, maternity, and feminine identity are tied to her mammary glands. A palpable breast lump or a suspicious mammogram report is one of the most distressing clinical findings a woman will ever encounter. Fortunately, over 75% of all breast biopsies are benign. Due to breast cancer awareness campaigns, strides have been made in early detection and treatment of breast diseases. When breast cancer is found while it is still limited to breast tissue, a woman's chance for 10-year disease-free survival is over 90%.

BREAST ANATOMY

The breasts are specialized sebaceous glands contained within the fascia of the anterior chest wall. Sitting on top of the pectoralis major muscle, a mature breast is composed of 20% milk-producing glandular tissue and 80% fatty tissue laced with fibrous connective strands. There are no muscles in breast tissue, and the amount of fat determines the size of the breast. Fibrous bands, known as Cooper's ligaments, extend from the skin to the underlying pectoralis muscle's fascia and these bands provide some support to the breast.

Resembling triangular-shaped spokes of a wheel, the milk-producing glandular portions of the breast are composed of 15 to 20 lobes arranged in a radial fashion, extending out from the areolar-nipple complex. Milk is produced by the breast's lobules and transported through ducts to reach openings in the breasts' nipple. 2% to 5% of women have accessory breasts or nipples, which occur along the breast or milk lines, which run from the axilla (armpit) to the groin. The lymphatic distribution of the breast is complex. Although 75% of the lymphatic drainage goes to regional lymph nodes in the axilla (armpit), lymph can stream through channels along the sternum (breast bone), up above and below the collarbone, and along the side of the chest wall.

Breast tissue is sensitive to hormonal changes, such as shifts in estrogen and progesterone levels during the menstrual cycle. Under the influence of estrogen, the cells lining the milk ducts multiply and proliferate. After ovulation, progesterone production by the ovaries causes dilatation of the ductal system and differentiation of its alveolar cells into milk-producing secretory cells. Increased blood flow, capillary engorgement and water retention brought on by progesterone prepping the breasts for potential pregnancy, may cause women to experience breast tenderness and fullness after ovulation. If pregnancy occurs, estrogen and progesterone levels remain elevated after ovulation, so the woman may have breast and nipple tenderness during the first trimester of pregnancy. If pregnancy does not occur, progesterone levels plummet and estrogen levels decrease. As a result of plunging hormone levels, the endometrial lining of the uterus is shed as menstrual bleeding. At the same time, regression of the breast's alveolar milk producing cells occurs, the breast's ducts narrow back down, and fluid within the breast tissue is resorbed. Any premenstrual breast discomfort usually resolves with the onset of a woman's menstrual period.

With each menstrual cycle, the fibrous tissue surrounding the breast's lobules increases in density and amount, and the milk-producing glands expand. These heterogeneous tissue changes provide reproductive-aged, premenopausal women's breasts with lactation capabilities. However, heterogeneous, dense breast tissue obscures mammogram results, so mammograms are rarely indicated in women younger than 35 years old. Instead, breast ultrasound and magnetic resonance imaging (MRIs) are the preferred imaging modalities in younger women. The menopausal woman no longer needs breast-feeding capability, so milk-producing lobules and ducts in the breast recede and atrophy. The glandular components of the breast become replaced with varying degrees of adipose (fatty) tissue. The less dense, more fatty breast tissue in a menopausal woman renders her mammograms more accurate. On the other hand, heterogeneous, dense breast tissue visualized on a postmenopausal woman's mammogram is linked to increased risk of developing breast cancer.

PERSISTENT BREASTS

The persistently plump bosom of adult human females, whether the woman is breastfeeding or not, is a unique feature among primates. In all other breastfeeding mammals, a full breast is a clear indication that the female is suckling young. Not so in humans, since breasts do no recede in non-pregnant younger women or older postmenopausal women. Fertile women tend to store fat in their hips and thighs, so the waist of a fertile adult human female is slimmer than her hips. Other female primates do not deposit fat on their rumps, so they tend to have skinny posteriors and store fat in the abdomen, as do human males. Permanently conspicuous breasts, along with rounded buttocks, result in an hourglass figure. Seen from a distance, a woman's silhouette is plainly recognizable as distinct from the male of the species. Easily identifiable fertile females attracted ancestral males looking for a mating opportunity and ensured the perpetuation of the human species.

There are no lab animals whose mammary glands are similar to human breast tissue, so this creates a challenge in researching treatment and cures for breast diseases. Breast cancer in humans, for example, usually spreads via the lymphatics, mainly to the axillary (armpit) lymph nodes, followed by distant metastasis to the bone and brain. In contrast, rodent cancers metastasize almost exclusively to the lung via the bloodstream. The development of breast cancer cell lines and genetically engineered mice have helped our understanding of breast's molecular tumor biology.

FIBROCYSTIC BREASTS

The most common benign breast condition that occurs in women is fibrocystic breast changes, which usually happens between the ages of 30 and 50. More than half of all reproductive-aged women have fibrocystic breasts at some point. Fibrocystic changes are believed to be an exaggeration of the normal physiologic response of breast tissue to hormone fluctuations associated with the menstrual cycle. Fibrocystic breast issues are unusual after menopause. As the word, "fibrocystic" implies, fibrous tissue in the breasts thickens and affected regions of the breast have fluid-congested, cystic, lumpy-bumpy areas. This cystic nodularity and tenderness can occur in one or both breasts, and these changes are most often found in the upper, outer section of the breast, near the axilla (armpit). The classic symptoms of fibrocystic changes include premenstrual breast pain, rapid change and fluctuation in the size of the cystic areas, and occasionally spontaneous nipple discharge. Severe, localized pain may occur when a simple cyst undergoes rapid expansion. These symptoms resolve with the onset of the woman's menstrual period.

The treatment of fibrocystic breasts depends on the severity of symptoms and varies from mechanical support of the breasts, dietary changes, hormonal modulation, and in extremely rare instances, surgical therapy for intractable pain. Initial therapy consists of patients wearing a support bra, both day, and night. Some patients find reducing or eliminating their consumption of tobacco and methylxanthines helps decrease fibrocystic breast pain. Methylxanthines are found in coffee, tea, cola drinks, and chocolate. Vitamin E 400 IU taken daily helps some women with their breast symptoms, and others find that dietary supplementation of the essential fatty acid, gamma-linoleic acid, using 3 grams of evening primrose oil daily, decreases breast discomfort. Another dietary supplement, molecular iodine, (Violet), taken daily may help decrease premenstrual breast tenderness.

Since fluctuating hormones exacerbate fibrocystic breast symptoms, hormonal modulation involves eliminating menstrual hormonal fluctuations or creating stable levels of estrogen and progesterone in a woman's body. By eliminating estrogen and progesterone production by the ovaries, gonadotropin-releasing hormone (GnRH) agonists induce a chemical menopause, bringing estrogen and progesterone down to negligible levels. Danazol (Danocrine), a synthetic form of testosterone, inhibits ovulation and also induces a menopausal state, which depresses estrogen and progesterone levels. Because it is a form of testosterone, danazol has androgenic side effects, such as acne, unwanted facial hair, weight gain, and cholesterol elevations. Medicines that induce chemical menopause can cause hot flashes, sleep disturbances, vaginal dryness and bone thinning, so GnRH agonists or danazol are not used for more than 6 to 9 months.

Consistent and steady levels of estrogen and progesterone can easily be accomplished using monophasic low-dose oral contraceptive pills (OCPs). Monophasic means that the same dose of estrogen and progesterone hormones is found in all the hormonally active pills, so this provides stable levels of estrogen and progesterone throughout the month. Monophasic low-dose oral contraceptive pills (OCPs) can safely be used in a non-smoking woman until she is 56 years old. Since smoking increases a woman's risk of stroke, smokers should not use oral contraceptive pills (OCPs) beyond age 35. The selective estrogen receptor modulator (SERM), tamoxifen (Nolvadex) competes with estradiol for estrogen receptors in the breast, so it acts as an anti-estrogen on breast tissue. Tamoxifen is used in the treatment of breast cancer and to help decrease the chance of developing breast cancer in high-risk women. Some women with fibrocystic changes find that tamoxifen (Nolvadex) also helps decrease their breast pain.

Whether taking a dietary supplement or a prescription medication, it takes 2 to 3 months of therapy for any of these medical interventions to alleviate fibrocystic breast discomfort. For intractable fibrocystic breast symptoms not relieved by medical therapy, surgical removal of breast tissue may be considered. Total mastectomy, where all the breast tissue is removed, is an option; however, a subcutaneous mastectomy, where some breast tissue is left behind, produces a better cosmetic result, while still easing breast symptoms. Having fibrocystic breasts changes is not associated with an increased risk of breast cancer. Only women whose fibrocystic breast changes show epithelial hyperplasia harboring atypical cells on breast biopsy have increased risk of breast cancer.

FIBROADENOMA

Fibroadenomas, the second most common benign breast condition in women, do not change in size with the menstrual cycle, nor do they usually produce pain or tenderness. A fibroadenoma is a solitary, painless, firm and rubbery, solid (not cystic or fluid-filled) breast mass, which occurs in adolescents or young women in their 20s. Typically, the young woman discovers the painless breast mass accidentally while bathing. The average fibroadenoma is about 1 inch in diameter, the size of a chestnut. Fibroadenomas are distinguished from fluid-filled breast cysts using breast ultrasound. One third of breast fibroadenomas regress spontaneously. Multiple fibroadenomas are discovered in 20% of women who have a palpable fibroadenoma, and after surgical removal, fibroadenomas recur in 20% of patients. Fibroadenomas are considered an abnormality of normal breast development, rather than a newly growing breast tumor, and the long-term risk of going on to develop breast cancer later on is twice that for women with fibrocystic breasts.

NIPPLE DISCHARGE

Nipple discharge can occur with either benign or malignant conditions of the breast. 15% of women with benign breast disease may experience nipple discharge, whereas nipple discharge is present in less than 5% of women with breast cancer. Whether clear, yellow or bloody, the color of the nipple discharge does not distinguish between a benign or malignant process. Many women without any breast problems can manually express a few drops of sticky gray, green or black viscous fluid from their nipple. To be medically significant, discharge from the breast should be spontaneous and persistent in a non-lactating woman. Spontaneous nipple discharge is free flowing and can stain a woman's bra. Women taking antidepressant medications may also experience nipple discharge (galactorrhea), as well. Fibrocystic breast changes and benign intraductal papillomas are the two most common reasons for spontaneous, non-milky nipple discharge. Although there is over a 90% chance that nipple discharge is associated with a benign breast condition, it still needs to be thoroughly evaluated to rule out that very small chance it is breast cancer.

FAT NECROSIS

Fat necrosis happens when an area of fatty breast tissue is damaged, usually as a result of injury to the breast. Although this can happen after breast surgery or radiation, the majority of women do not remember the event that caused the injury. As the body repairs the damaged tissue, it is replaced by scar tissue that is firm with ill-defined borders. Sometimes the area of fat necrosis liquefies and becomes an oil cyst. Occasionally, there is skin retraction from the scarring process, as well. A fat necrosis breast lump can be hard to differentiate from cancer by breast exam or even a mammogram, so removal of the breast mass is usually recommended. Fat necrosis is more common in women with very large breasts, and there is no relationship between fat necrosis and subsequent risk of breast cancer.

BREAST CANCER

The cause of breast cancer is poorly understood, but epidemiologists (scientists who study the patterns of health and disease in populations) have documented some risk factors that increase a woman's chance of developing breast cancer. Except for being female and getting older, over 75% of women diagnosed with breast cancer have no family history of breast cancer nor do they have any known risk factors. Only 10% of breast cancers have a familial or genetic link. Other risk factors help identify about 15% of women who will eventually develop breast cancer. Fortunately, mammogram screening and improved treatment protocols have significantly decreased mortality associated with breast cancer.

BEING WOMAN

Women have breast cancer 100 times more frequently than men, so only 1% of breast cancer cases occur in men. Breast cancer is the second most commonly occurring cancer, and the 3rd most common cause of cancer deaths in women. Lung cancer is the #1 cause of cancer deaths among women, followed by colon cancer, and then breast cancer. Skin cancer is the most commonly occurring cancer among both men and women.

Even though a woman's lifetime risk of developing breast cancer is 1 in 8, her risk of dying from breast cancer is only 1 in 36. Nearly 50% of all women will die from cardiovascular disease; whereas, only 3% of women will die from breast cancer. In comparison to the number of women who die as a result of cardiovascular disease, hip fractures or dementia, the number of women who succumb to breast cancer is very small. We have definitely come a long way in screening and treatment of breast cancer.

AGE

A woman's greatest risk for developing breast cancer is age. The older she gets, the greater her risk. 80% of breast cancers are found in women over the age of 50. Fewer than 5% of all breast cancers are diagnosed in women under 40 years old, but disease prognosis is usually worse for younger women. Breast cancers that are diagnosed in younger women tend to be a fast growing, higher-grade tissue type and hormone-receptor negative (HR-). These ominous tumor characteristics make the breast cancer more aggressive and more likely to require chemotherapy.

Fortunately, breast cancer is relatively rare in young women.

- A 25 years old woman has a 1 in 20,000 chance of developing breast cancer.
- When she turns 30, that risk climbs to 1 in 2500.
- When she's 40, her risk increases to 1 in 200.
- When she turns 51, the average age for menopause, her risk for breast cancer is 1 in 50.
- By the time she reaches 65 years old, her risk for breast cancer is 1 in 16.
- If a woman lives to her mid-80s or beyond, her risk of being diagnosed with breast cancer is 1 in 8.

AGE vs. ESTROGEN

Although estrogen does not cause breast cancer, it can stimulate pre-existing malignant breast cells to grow faster. As a postmenopausal woman grows older, she has negligible levels of estrogen in her system. Yet, despite dwindling amounts of estrogen circulating in her body, breast cancer is more frequently diagnosed in older, estrogen-deprived, postmenopausal women. Why does a woman's risk of breast cancer increase as she grows older? How come estrogen-rich younger women are not plagued by breast cancer?

Breast cancer, like most cancers, is a disease of aging. As time goes by, not only is a woman's body subjected to the normal wear and tear of living, but her organs also sustain cumulative damage associated with unhealthy lifestyle choices. As breast cells age, they become more vulnerable to DNA glitches. Because of these aging DNA mishaps, when older cells divide, they make more genetic mistakes. These genetic flaws cause cells to create more abnormal versions of themselves. Breast cancer cells are breast tissue cells with DNA damage, and damaged DNA causes cancer cells to behave badly. Also, as a woman gets older, her immune system ages, becoming weaker and less able to ward off cancer cells. Unchecked, cancer cells continue to multiply and grow into a malignant tumor. Thus, merely by aging, a woman increases her risk of breast cancer substantially. At this late juncture in a woman's life, estrogen has very little to do with her chance of being diagnosed with breast cancer.

FAMILY HISTORY

Only 10% of breast cancers have a familial or genetic link. When it comes to family history and inheritance, a woman who has a 1st degree relative (a family member who is directly connected to the woman, such as a parent, sibling or offspring) with breast cancer, has a greater risk of developing the disease than a woman with a more distant relative (a grandparent, aunt or cousin) who has the disease. When strong genetic predispositions exist, breast cancer tends to occur at a younger age, and there is a higher prevalence for disease in both breasts.

A woman whose mother was diagnosed with breast cancer before the age of 60 has double the risk of going on to the develop breast cancer herself. If her mother was elderly (over the age of 60) when she had breast cancer, then the daughter's chance of developing breast cancer is less than having a younger mom with breast cancer. If an older/elderly woman over the age of 60 is diagnosed with breast cancer, then her daughter has a 40% increased risk of developing the disease. If a woman has two 1st degree relatives with breast cancer, then her risk increases 5 times.

85% of women with a 1st degree relative with breast cancer will never develop breast cancer themselves, and 85% of women diagnosed with breast cancer do not have any relatives with the disease. For the overwhelming majority of women diagnosed with this condition, breast cancer is fundamentally a stealth disease of older, estrogen-deprived, postmenopausal women.

BRCAs

Mutations in the BRCA (BReast CAncer) family of genes confer a lifetime risk of breast cancer that approaches 85%. This is in comparison to a lifetime risk of 12% (1 in 8 chance) of breast cancer for women without these genetic mutations. BRCA1 and BRCA2 genes function as tumor suppressor genes, and when there is a BRCA gene mutation, the body cannot suppress breast cancer cells or ovarian cancer cells. BRCA1 and BRCA2 gene mutations account for 90% of inherited breast cancers. These are autosomal dominant genetic changes, meaning that they get passed on to each subsequent generation, and each subsequent generation may be vulnerable to breast and ovarian cancer. BRCA status can be determined by genetic blood tests. Management recommendations include screening BRCA carriers with earlier mammograms and breast MRIs, as well as cancer prevention measures, such as chemoprevention with tamoxifen (Nolvadex) or surgical intervention with bilateral total mastectomy.

OVARIAN CANCER

About 10% to 15% of ovarian cancers occur because a genetic mutation, such as BRCA1 or BRCA2, has been passed down within a family. Although monophasic low-dose oral contraceptive pills (OCPs) decrease the risk of ovarian cancer by 50%, they may not be effective in overcoming a woman's inherited genetic mutation. In these cases, surgical removal of both fallopian tubes and both ovaries is usually recommended.

In the general population, 1 in 70 women will be diagnosed with ovarian cancer, and the average age at diagnosis is 65. The incidence of breast cancer is 10 times greater than ovarian cancer. Since there is no effective screening test for ovarian cancer, over 70% of women have advanced disease by the time they are diagnosed. Once symptoms such as increased girth, pelvic or abdominal pain, early satiety with eating, and frequent urination occur, ovarian cancer has reached an advanced, and usually incurable, stage.

A recent meta-analysis of 52 studies involving variable clinical scenarios, variable diagnostic techniques and variable follow-up, found a very slight 0.1% increased risk of developing ovarian cancer in menopausal women taking hormones. In contrast, neither the Women's Health Initiative (WHI) hormone intervention trial or WHI's extended post intervention follow-up study showed any real increase in ovarian cancer with menopause hormone therapy.

RADIATION

Excessive ionizing radiation to the chest, especially prior to age 30, increases a woman's risk of breast cancer. Women who received radiation treatment for postpartum mastitis, prolonged fluoroscopic X-rays for tuberculosis, radiation treatment for lymphomas, or have been exposed to radiation fallout from atomic bombs or nuclear power plants, are at increased risk of breast cancer.

CHILDBEARING & BREASTFEEDING

Women who deliver their first child prior to age 30 have a 30% less risk of developing estrogen receptor positive/progesterone receptor positive (ER+/PR+) breast cancer. Conversely, women who delay childbearing until after age 30 decrease their risk of hormone receptor negative (HR-neg) breast cancer by 60%.

Breast implants may interfere with a woman's ability to breastfeed, preventing her from receiving the cancer-protective benefits of breastfeeding. Over a woman's lifetime, breastfeeding for just 6 months decreases her risk of breast cancer by 20%. Having an abortion or miscarriage does not affect a woman's risk of breast cancer. Wearing underwire bras or using antiperspirants does not affect a woman's risk of breast cancer, either.

ALCOHOL

Consuming more than one alcohol drink a day not only increases a woman's risk of breast cancer by 50%, but it also increases her risk of strokes, as well.

SMOKING

16% of women smoke. Smoking cigarettes exposes the smoker and those immediately around her to thousands of unsavory chemicals. Hundreds of them are known toxins, such as carbon monoxide, hydrogen cyanide and ammonia, and 70 of these toxic chemicals cause cancer. There is no safe level of exposure to secondhand smoke, which is a combination of the smoke exhaled by a smoker and the smoke given off by a burning tobacco product.

Chemicals in tobacco smoke reach breast tissue and are found in breast milk. Smoking or a past history of smoking is associated with increased risk for developing breast cancer.

BODY WEIGHT

Postmenopausal women who weigh more than 40 pounds above their healthy body weight double their risk of breast cancer. Body weight is the most significant modifiable risk factor for postmenopausal breast cancer. Women carrying extra weight expose their breast tissue to excess estrogen.

During her reproductive years, the main type of estrogen circulating in a woman's body is estradiol (E2), which is produced by her premenopausal ovaries. Once a woman is menopausal, her depleted ovaries no longer produce estradiol (E2) estrogen. Her adrenal glands, however, continue to release testosterone and androstenedione androgens into her system.

Aromatase enzymes found in adipose (fatty) tissue convert these androgens into estrone (E1) estrogen, and estrone is then modified into estradiol (E2) estrogen. The main type of estrogen in a postmenopausal woman is estrone (E1). The heavier a woman is, the more her breasts are exposed to excess estrogen, particularly estrone (E1). After menopause, breasts concentrate estrogen into their tissues. Even though blood serum levels of estrogen are low in a menopausal woman, estrogen levels become higher in her breast tissue.

In the fatty tissue surrounding a breast cancer tumor, the modification of estrone (E1) to estradiol (E2) is decreased, so breast cancer tissue is exposed to more estrone (E1) relative to estradiol (E2). Estrone (E1) appears to attach preferentially to the alpha estrogen receptors (ER-alpha) on breast cells. Once estrogen hooks up with an ER-alpha receptor on the breast cell, it stimulates the breast cell to multiply. Breast cell's ER-beta receptor subtype, on the other hand, has anti-proliferative effects and is a tumor suppressor.

Estrone (E1), the main estrogen generated by adipose (fatty) tissue and the main estrogen found in menopausal women, preferentially binds to the breast cell's growth stimulating ER-alpha receptors over the ER-beta receptors. Estradiol (E2), the estrogen produced by premenopausal ovaries, the main estrogen found in reproductive-aged women and the preferred bioidentical estrogen used in menopause hormone replacement therapy, binds to both ER-alpha and ER-beta receptors with equal affinity. This creates a healthy balance between breast cell proliferation and tumor suppression.

Too much of anything is toxic. Carrying excess weight is toxic to breast tissue, and obesity (BMI > 30) increases a woman's risk of breast cancer far more than any menopause hormone therapy.

PHYSICAL ACTIVITY

Moderate physical activity decreases a woman's risk of breast cancer by 30%. A 30-minute walk, 5 times a week, will do the trick. Walk cancer away. 10,000 steps a day keeps disease and disability away.

The MELATONIN HYPOTHESIS

Melatonin is a hormone produced primarily by the brain's pineal gland at night. Its production is suppressed by exposure to light. Blind individuals are not optically receptive to light, so melatonin production is maintained at steady levels 24 hours a day. Blind women have a 50% lower risk of developing breast cancer compared to sighted women, and night shift workers have increased risk of breast cancer. Staying awake at night decreases melatonin production.

Melatonin blocks the alpha estrogen receptor (ER-alpha) on breast cells. This is the same estrogen receptor blocked by the selective estrogen receptor modulators (SERMs), tamoxifen (Nolvadex) and raloxifene (Evista), used to treat and prevent breast cancer.

Melatonin also inhibits the aromatase enzyme that converts testosterone to estrone (E1), which is then modified into estradiol (E2). This is the same enzyme that aromatase inhibitor (AI) medications used to treat breast cancer work to suppress. Essentially, melatonin acts both as a SERM and an AI to help decrease a woman's risk of breast cancer. Getting adequate sleep optimizes the pineal gland's production of cancer-suppressing melatonin.

STATINS

25% of Americans over the age of 50 are currently taking a cholesterol-lowering statin drug to prevent heart disease. Since 50% of patients admitted to the hospital with a heart attack have desirable cholesterol lipid levels, there's obviously more to heart disease than cholesterol. Statins may or may not be associated with breast cancer risk, but postmenopausal women and the elderly are at particular risk for statin-induced diabetes. The Women's Health Initiative study found that women who took a statin medication increase their risk of developing diabetes by 50%. Long-term data indicate that diabetes increases a woman's risk of dying from breast cancer.

ASPIRIN

Taking a low-dose (81mg) baby aspirin regularly for 5 or more years decreases a postmenopausal woman's risk of breast cancer, as well as her risk of colon cancer, by 20%. Inflammation markers, such as elevated prostaglandin E2 (PGE2) levels, are associated with a poorer breast cancer prognosis. As a nonsteroidal anti-inflammatory drug (NSAID), low-dose aspirin may help reduce breast cancer risk recurrence and improve survival. Coincidentally, for a woman 65 years or older, low-dose aspirin also helps decrease her risk of strokes and heart attacks by 20%.

VITAMIN D

In addition to its role in calcium metabolism and bone health, vitamin D has also been reported to have anticancer activities. It has been shown to inhibit cancer cell growth, induce apoptosis (cancer cell death) and decrease angiogenesis (new blood vessel growth that feeds the tumor). Studies suggest that living at higher geographical latitudes with lower sun exposures increases the risk of developing and dying of breast cancer, colon, and prostate cancers. Vitamin D levels are lower in ovarian cancer patients, as well. Vitamin D deficiency among breast cancer patients has been associated with poorer clinical outcomes and increased mortality.

ORAL CONTRACEPTIVE PILLS (OCPs)

Earlier medical studies evaluating women who took high-dose formulations of oral contraceptive pills (OCPs), also known as birth control pills (BCPs), prescribed back in the 1960s to the 1980s, showed a modest increased risk of breast cancer associated with their use. Hormone variations found in triphasic birth control pills, where each week of hormone pills in the birth control packet contains a different dose of estrogen or progesterone, is also associated with an increased risk of breast cancer. Recent clinical trials show that low-dose, monophasic oral contraceptive pills (OCPs) containing a stable low dose of estrogen and progesterone throughout the cycle do not increase a woman's risk of breast cancer. Contemporary low-dose monophasic oral contraceptive pills (OCPs) containing 35mcg or less of ethinyl estradiol estrogen not only reduce fibrocystic breast discomfort, but they also decrease a woman's risk of ovarian cancer by 50%.

BREAST CANCER DETECTION

Postmortem studies show that, over the age of 40, 10% of women who have succumbed to other causes of death harbor an occult, tiny cancerous breast growth detected at autopsy. Breast cancer grows very slowly, and it tends to be asymptomatic until the development of advanced disease. Breast pain is experienced by only 10% of women with breast cancer. Bilateral breast cancer, which is disease in both breasts, occurs in 1% of women newly diagnosed with breast cancer.

The classic sign of breast cancer is a solitary solid breast mass, which is fixed in its location and has indistinct borders, making it difficult to define precisely the size of the mass. Breast cysts or benign breast lumps tend to have smooth borders and are freely mobile within the breast. Advanced local breast disease puts traction on Cooper ligaments resulting in skin dimpling and nipple retraction. Interference of lymphatic and capillary drainage by tumor cells causes changes in the breast's skin texture with induration, edema (peau d'orange), inflammation and eventually ulceration.

If there is a persistent dominant breast mass that does not resolve with aspiration or needle drainage of the cyst fluid, or there is any uncertainty in the clinical examination or breast imaging studies, a biopsy of the area should be performed to rule out a malignancy. Fortunately, 75% of breast biopsies are benign.

BREAST SELF-EXAMINATION (BSE)

The best time for a woman to detect changes in her breast tissue is during her menstrual period when her hormone levels are at their lowest. Many women find that their ability to detect breast lumps improves by using the "wet" technique and feeling for breast masses while they are showering or bathing.

Breast cancer has been growing for about 10 years before reaching a diameter of 1 cm ("pea"-size). The average diameter of a breast mass discovered by women who routinely perform breast self-exams is 2 cm ("hazelnut"-size). Mammograms can detect breast cancer years before a breast mass can be felt, so non-palpable breast lesions requiring breast biopsy are most commonly discovered during mammograms. By facilitating early detection and diagnosis of breast cancer, screening mammograms reduce cancer-associated mortality rates.

SCREENING MAMMOGRAMS

Since the 1980s, women were being told that they should have annual mammograms starting at age 40. Then in November 2009, the United States Preventive Services Task Force (USPSTF) shifted these mammogram recommendations. The USPSTF is a congressionally mandated panel of independent experts who systematically review research and clinical practices in the areas of disease prevention and primary care. They then render evidence-based recommendations regarding screening tests and treatment modalities.

The USPSTF now recommends that routine screening mammograms should not start until a woman is 50 years old and that mammograms should not be performed annually, but every other year, between ages 50 to 75. USPSTF concludes that the current evidence is insufficient to assess the additional benefits and harms of screening mammography in women over the age of 75. Starting regular screening mammograms before the age of 50 should be based on the woman's potentially increased risk of breast cancer. Because of worrisome-appearing or false-positive mammogram reports, having more mammograms over the years may lead to more unnecessary breast biopsies, and perhaps increased damage to premenopausal breast tissue from radiation. Exceptions to the every-two-years mammogram rule include women with increased risk of developing breast cancer, such as women with a strong family history of breast cancer, women who bear the BRCA1 or BRCA2 gene mutations or postmenopausal women with dense, heterogeneous breast tissue visualized on their mammogram. These women may need more frequent mammograms.

Digital technology continues to improve mammogram screening for breast cancer. Computer-aided detection (CAD) allows for image manipulation through adjustments in contrast, brightness, and electronic magnification of selected regions of the breast image. This results in better visualization and interpretation of mammogram films. Despite improvements in digital mammography, no screening test is perfect, and this holds true for mammograms, as well. 15% of women with palpable breast cancer will have a normal mammogram result, so a persistent breast mass should be biopsied to determine tissue diagnosis.

BREAST MAGNETIC RESONANCE IMAGING (Breast MRI)

Unlike mammograms that use radiation to detect breast tissue changes, magnetic resonance imaging (MRI) scans use a strong magnetic field and radio waves to generate detailed images of anatomical structures. Breast MRI is an excellent imaging modality for women with a current diagnosis of breast cancer, a strong family history of breast cancer, or a known BRCA gene mutation. Breast MRI can detect multi-focal disease in the breast affected by breast cancer, detect disease in the opposite breast, and helps detect abnormalities in heterogeneous, dense breasts, which are difficult to interpret on mammograms. The ability of MRI to differentiate benign from the malignant tissue may help reduce the frequency of breast biopsies. Since breast MRIs cost 10 times more than mammograms and breast ultrasounds, MRIs are not utilized as routine breast cancer screening tools.

BREAST CANCER TREATMENT

The treatment of breast cancer is complex, with many variables to consider, such as tumor size, the tumor's tissue type, the hormone receptor status of the tumor, and the presence of tumor cells in the axillary (armpit) or sentinel lymph nodes. 75% of breast cancers are ductal carcinomas, originating from cells lining milk ducts within the breast, and 25% are lobular cancers, originating from breast cells that produce milk. Because of the constellation of clinical issues involved, breast cancer treatment varies from woman to woman. Until 30 years ago, radical mastectomy, with removal of the breast and underlying pectoralis major and pectoralis minor muscles, along with complete removal of the 30 to 60 axillary (armpit) lymph nodes, was the standard surgery for breast cancer. This is a cosmetically disfiguring operation, leaving a major deformity of the chest wall, and chronic lymph-edema and swelling of the arm after axillary lymph node dissection.

Major changes in the management of breast cancer over the past few decades have resulted from improved understanding of the biology of the disease. We now realize that a woman's breast cancer has existed in her body for years prior to being diagnosed. By the time the diagnosis of breast cancer is established, many women have systemic disease, meaning that tumor cells have already spread by lymphatics or the bloodstream throughout their body's system. Treatment of breast cancer now involves using "system-wide" treatments, such as hormone modulation or intravenous chemotherapy, to reach all parts of a woman's body. With the realization that breast cancer is a systemic disease and not just a localized cancerous growth in the breast, therapeutic emphasis has evolved to less radical surgery.

Treatment of breast cancer involves surgical excision of the cancerous tumor or removal of breast tissue, along with lymph node sampling or re-moval, radiation therapy, as well as systemic therapy, using adjuvant che-motherapy and/or hormone therapy. The major therapeutic objectives of treating breast cancer are control of local tumor growth, treatment of dis-tant metastasis, and improved qualify of life for women diagnosed with the disease.

Tumor grade and hormone receptor status help characterize cancerous breast tissue. Tumor grade describes how closely cancer cells look like nor-mal cells:

- Low-grade (grade 1) tumors are slow growing and have cells that resemble normal cells.
- High-grade (grade 3) tumors have cells that look very abnormal and are fast growing.
- Medium-grade (grade 2) tumors fall in between. The higher the tumor grade, the more abnormal the cancer cell's DNA.

The presence or absence of estrogen receptors, progesterone receptors and the human epidermal growth factor receptor 2 (HER2) in breast cancer is determined by tissue analysis of the tumor specimen removed from the patient's breast:

- A triple-negative breast cancer is estrogen receptor negative, progesterone receptor negative, and human epidermal growth factor receptor 2 (ER-/PR-/HER2), so it does not respond to hormone-blocking drugs such as tamoxifen (Nolvadex) or aromatase inhibitors (AIs). Non-hormonal chemotherapy is required for hormone receptor negative (HR-) tumors. 20% of breast cancers are the more aggressive hormone receptor negative (HR-) type, and this type of breast cancer tends to be more common in young, premenopausal women.

- 80% of breast cancers are hormone receptor positive (HR+), which means the breast cancer tissue has estrogen receptors (ER+), progesterone receptor positive (PR+) or human epidermal growth factor receptor 2 positive (HER2+), so this cancer type responds better to hormone therapies. Hormone receptor-positive (HR+) breast cancers are more common in older women, and these breast cancers tend to grow more slowly, respond better to hormone therapy, and have a better prognosis (outlook), compared to hormone receptor negative (HR-) breast cancer.

For hormone receptor positive (HR+) breast cancer, adjuvant hormone therapy includes oral medications that block the action of estrogen on breast cells, such as selective estrogen receptor modulators (SERMs), or work by lowering the amount of estrogen in a woman's body, such as aromatase inhibitors (AIs).

The selective estrogen receptor modulator (SERM), tamoxifen (Nolvadex), binds to estrogen receptors-alpha (ER-alpha) on breast cells, blocking estrogen from hooking up with these cells, thus preventing cells from multiplying. Tamoxifen can be used to treat both premenopausal and postmenopausal women with ER+ breast cancer. Tamoxifen can cause hot flashes, cataracts, and uterine cancer, and like any other oral estrogenic-type hormone, tamoxifen increases the risk of blood clots and strokes in women.

Aromatase inhibitors (AIs), such as anastrozole (Arimidex), letrozole (Femara) or exemestane (Aromasin), virtually eliminate any production of estrogen in postmenopausal women. AIs cannot stop the ovaries from making estrogen, so AIs are used only in postmenopausal women. AIs are now considered first-line adjuvant hormone therapy for postmenopausal women diagnosed with hormone receptive positive (ER+) breast cancer, since AIs work better than tamoxifen (Nolvadex). AIs inhibit or block the enzyme aromatase, which converts testosterone and androstenedione androgens secreted by a postmenopausal woman's adrenal glands, into estrone (E1) estrogen, which is then modified into estradiol (E2) estrogen. Since aromatase inhibitors (AIs) eradicate estrogen's existence in a postmenopausal woman's body, AIs cause hot flashes, muscle and joint aches, carpal tunnel syndrome, vaginal dryness, fatigue, insomnia, mental fuzziness, depression, cholesterol elevations and bone thinning. Because of these side-effects, AIs are difficult drugs to take.

The initial size of the breast tumor is the single best predictor of the likelihood of positive axillary (armpit) lymph nodes. The number of positive axillary lymph nodes harboring metastatic tumor cells is the single best predictor of breast cancer survival. With current modalities available for the treatment of breast cancer, women whose initial tumor is less than 1 cm in diameter, and who have negative axillary lymph nodes, have excellent disease-free survival, with a 10-year relapse rate of less than 10%.

Because microscopic spread of tumor cells via lymphatics or through the bloodstream has probably already occurred prior to breast cancer ever being diagnosed, 66% of all women with breast cancer eventually develop distant metastatic disease, regardless of the type of initial therapy. Although the disease may recur many years later, sometimes decades, after initial diagnosis, only 3% of women will die from breast cancer. The majority of postmenopausal women diagnosed and treated for breast cancer will succumb to something else, such as cardiovascular disease, dementia or osteoporosis-related hip fracture, long before their breast cancer recurs.

ESTROGEN RECEPTORS

There are two types of receptors for estrogen: estrogen receptor-alpha (ER-alpha) and estrogen receptor-beta (ER-beta). In breast tissue, the ER-alpha causes growth and proliferation of mammary breast cells. ER-beta, on the other hand, not only inhibits multiplication of breast cells, ER-beta hampers or down-regulates ER-alpha's tendency to stimulate breast cell proliferation. Postmenopausal women's breast tissue is ER-alpha dominant, whereas younger women's is ER-beta dominant. In addition to younger women's breast cells having fewer DNA glitches, estrogen-receptor dichotomy helps explain why estrogen-rich, younger women are not plagued by breast cancer. Although young women are swimming in estrogen, they do not experience the increased risk of breast cancer postmenopausal estrogen-deprived women suffer. Younger women have greater numbers of ER-beta's on their breast cells. This inhibits multiplication and proliferation of breast cells. Postmenopausal women's breasts are populated with breast stimulating ER-alpha's and depleted of ER-beta's.

The selective estrogen receptor modulators (SERMs), tamoxifen (Nolvadex) and raloxifene (Evista) medications used to prevent the recurrence and decrease the occurrence of breast cancer, work by blocking estrogen's coupling with ER-alpha's and up-regulating ER-beta's. Blocking ER-alpha activity prevents cells from multiplying, and increasing ER-beta activity inhibits the proliferation of breast cells even further. It has been hypothesized that enhancing the ER-beta's could be a useful way to protect against breast cancer. Through the manipulation of estrogens and estrogen receptors, cancer cells can be killed from within the cancer cell, thereby minimizing adverse effects on healthy tissue. Since other types of chemotherapy can suppress the bone marrow and immune system, and radiation therapy can damage surrounding organs, these modalities cannot be used long-term to prevent breast cancer recurrence. On the other hand, many women can safely stay on SERM hormone therapy, e.g.- tamoxifen (Nolvadex) or raloxifene (Evista), for years.

Unfortunately, chemotherapy and radiation do not kill the stem cells that give birth to breast cancer cells. Cancer stem cells do not have either

ER-alpha or ER-beta receptor sites, so the SERMs cannot perform their tumor-suppressing magic on breast cancer stem cells. Less than 1% of the cells in a tumor are the cancer's root stem cells, but as long as they exist in the body, the breast cancer may recur, despite chemotherapy, despite radiation therapy and despite SERM therapy. Until there are safe and effective strategies for eliminating breast cancer stem cells, the war on cancer goes on.

The GAIL MODEL

The Breast Cancer Risk Assessment Tool (the Gail Model) was designed by researchers at the National Cancer Institute and the National Surgical Adjuvant Breast and Bowel Project to help quantify a woman's risk of developing breast cancer. It takes into account risk factors for breast cancer, such as being an older woman, having two or more first-degree relatives (mother, sister, or daughter) diagnosed with breast cancer, starting menstrual periods at a younger age, being over 30 years old when she delivered her first baby, never having a baby, having breast biopsies in the past, having breast biopsies showing atypical hyperplasia, or being African-American.

Using the Gail model, a woman with a 5-year risk score of 1.66% or higher is classified as "high-risk " for developing breast cancer. Although the tool helps estimate a woman's risk of developing breast cancer within the next 5 years and over her lifetime, it cannot predict whether or not a particular woman will get breast cancer.

BREAST CANCER CHEMOPREVENTION

For women over the age of 35 who are at increased risk of breast cancer, taking medications normally used in breast cancer treatment, such as a selective estrogen receptor modulator (SERM) or an aromatase inhibitor (AI) can improve their odds of staying cancer-free. Clinically referred to as chemoprevention, taking either of the SERMs, tamoxifen (Nolvadex) or raloxifene (Evista) or any of the AIs for 5 years can reduce a woman's risk of estrogen receptor-positive (ER+) breast cancer by 50%.

Since 80% of breast cancers are estrogen receptor positive (ER+) tumors, chemoprevention of invasive breast cancer is a strategy worth considering in high-risk women. Women with a strong family history of breast cancer, women with a breast biopsy showing atypical hyperplasia or lobular carcinoma in situ (LCIS) or women with a 5-year risk of developing breast cancer of 1.66% or higher according to the Gail model, are potential candidates for chemoprevention.

For premenopausal women who pursue breast cancer chemoprevention, tamoxifen is their only option currently. Raloxifene has been tested only in postmenopausal women, so its benefit in premenopausal women is unknown. Aromatase inhibitors (AIs) do not inhibit estrogen production by the ovaries, so they are not effective in reducing estrogen levels premenopausal women. Raloxifene and AIs are used only in postmenopausal women; whereas, tamoxifen can be used in both premenopausal and postmenopausal women. Premenopausal women taking tamoxifen should also consider non-hormonal methods of birth control, since hormonal methods of contraception, such as oral contraceptive pills (OCPs), may alter the breast-protection effectiveness of tamoxifen. Tamoxifen can induce ovulation in women with polycystic ovary syndrome (PCOS), as well. Women who are pregnant or are trying to get pregnant should not take a SERM since they may cause birth defects. SERMs also get into breast milk, so a woman should avoid SERMs while breastfeeding.

Both tamoxifen and raloxifene (Evista) help maintain a woman's bone density, so they can pull double duty by preventing invasive breast cancer in postmenopausal women with osteoporosis. Women taking tamoxifen are more likely to experience troublesome side effects as compared to raloxifene users. Endometrial uterine cancer, cataracts and decreased breast protection while taking a selective serotonin reuptake inhibitor (SSRI) antidepressant, are complications related to tamoxifen, but not raloxifene. Similar to other oral estrogen medications, both tamoxifen and raloxifene increase a woman's risk of blood clots and strokes.

Tamoxifen is a prodrug that is activated by the liver's cytochrome P450 isoenzyme 2D6 (CYP2D6) into tumor-fighting endoxifen. Endoxifen binds to the breast cells' estrogen receptors and suppresses breast cancer growth. SSRI antidepressants inhibit the CYP2D6 enzyme and prevent tamoxifen from morphing into its biologically active, tumor-fighting form, so this decreases tamoxifen's anti-cancer effectiveness. SSRIs are prescribed not only to treat depression but are used to help relieve hot flashes that can be caused by tamoxifen. The SSRIs paroxetine (Paxil, Briselle), fluoxetine (Prozac), and sertraline (Zoloft) block the CY2D6 enzyme and cripple tamoxifen's effectiveness. Of all the SSRIs, venlafaxine (Effexor) has the least impact on inhibiting the CYP2D6 enzyme and is the safest choice when used with tamoxifen. For those women who cannot take venlafaxine (Effexor), citalopram (Celexa) would be the second choice. Any SSRI can be used while a patient is on raloxifene. Relizen, also known as Femal or Serelys, is a non-hormonal herbal supplement made from pollen extract harvested in southern Sweden. Relizen reduces menopausal hot flashes without interfering with the CYP2D6 enzyme action needed for effective tamoxifen therapy.

Around 30% of breast cancers are linked to poor lifestyle habits, so the risks and benefits of using medications to try to prevent breast cancer need to be considered in the context of the woman's clinical history and personal outlook. The presence of breast cancer risk factors does not mean that cancer is inevitable, since many women with risk factors never develop breast cancer.

MENOPAUSE HORMONE THERAPY & BREAST CANCER

Breast cancer is the result of a 10-year evolution of a group of cells that were becoming increasingly abnormal and malignant. Long-term clinical trials involving 1.5 million women confirm that menopause hormone therapy does not initiate or cause breast cancer. However, by promoting the growth of pre-existing breast cancer cells, hormone therapy allows a woman's breast cancer to be diagnosed earlier. Since estrogen is a known stimulus for breast cancer growth, anti-estrogenic therapies are now standard therapy for estrogen-receptor positive (ER+) tumors.

For a menopausal woman, estrogen replacement therapy does not increase her risk of developing breast cancer. The Women's Health Initiative (WHI) study showed that postmenopausal women who took estrogen replacement for 6.8 years reduced their risk of developing breast cancer by

25% compared to women on placebo. Among 57,000 menopausal women in the California Teachers Study, it took almost a decade of estrogen therapy to detect a statistically significant increase risk of breast cancer. In the Nurses' Health Study involving 29,000 postmenopausal women, there was no increased risk of breast cancer in women taking estrogen for 20 years. When progesterone is added to estrogen replacement therapy, the risk of breast cancer increases slightly.

Progesterone, specifically synthetic progestin, is the bad boy of menopause hormone therapy. In the E3N-EPIC Study involving 80,000 French postmenopausal women followed for 8 years, estrogen with natural micronized progesterone was not associated with an increased risk of breast cancer, whereas women taking estrogen with a synthetic progestin increased their risk of breast cancer slightly. The WHI study showed that women who took estrogen with a synthetic progestin for 5.2 years increased their risk of breast cancer by 25%.

This increased relative risk of 25% means that, since 4 out of 100 women between the ages of 50 to 79 are naturally destined to develop breast cancer over the next decade, if all 100 of these women took estrogen with a synthetic progestin, then 5 of them would go on to develop breast cancer. So, an increased relative risk of 25% is an absolute increased risk of one person out of 100. One is a lonely number, but a menopausal woman's chance that she is specifically at particular risk of developing breast cancer while taking estrogen with a synthetic progestin is less than 1% (0.8% to be exact). Although the use of combined estrogen-plus-synthetic progestin slightly increases breast cancer risk, use of these hormones before breast cancer diagnosis reduces a woman's risk of death after a breast cancer diagnosis.

Not only does menopause hormone therapy decrease all-cause mortality, that is, it decreases a woman's chance of dying from cardiovascular disease, diabetes, dementia, osteoporosis, wound infections, etc., but it also decreases her chance of dying from breast cancer, as well. Several years after discontinuing combination estrogen-plus-progesterone menopause hormone therapy, any slightly increased risk of breast cancer dissipates.

1 out of 3 women will undergo a hysterectomy by age 65. For menopausal women who no longer have a uterus, they can enjoy all the benefits of estrogen without worrying about progesterone in any shape or form. Estrogen stimulates the endometrial lining of the uterus to proliferate and grow and grow. Endometrial tissue overgrowth can lead to abnormal uterine bleeding, uterine polyps and uterine cancer. Progesterone prevents this uncontrolled endometrial tissue growth and protects the woman from uterine cancer.

Progesterone does not necessarily protect the woman's breasts. Instead, progesterone, the "pro-gestation or pro-pregnancy" hormone, prepares the breasts for lactation and breastfeeding. This boost in milk-producing fibroglandular tissue in non-ovulating menopausal women augments breast tissue's heterogeneity, which increases breast density on mammograms. Increased breast density on a mammogram is associated with increased breast cancer. In the Women's Health Initiative (WHI) study, use of estrogen-only, conjugated equine estrogen (Premarin) 0.625mg augmented mammographic breast density by only 1.6%, as compared to the 6% increase caused by the combination of conjugated equine estrogen (Premarin) 0.625mg with synthetic medroxyprogesterone (Provera) 2.5mg. Bioidentical or "body"-identical progesterone, a hormone that is chemically identical to the progesterone found in a woman's body, seems to be less problematic for breasts than synthetic progestins. Oral micronized progesterone (Prometrium) pills or micronized progesterone vaginal gels (Crinone or Prochieve) are FDA-approved, pharmaceutical-grade, bioidentical natural progesterone preparations that will prevent endometrial tissue overgrowth and protect the uterus.

A novel pharmaceutical approach to protecting the uterus from estrogen stimulation is a tissue-selective estrogen complex (TSEC), which combines estrogen with a selective estrogen receptor modulator (SERM). An oral pill that couples conjugated equine estrogen 0.45mg (Premarin) with the SERM, bazedoxifene 20mg (Duavee), is used to treat menopausal hot flashes and prevent osteoporosis. Because of its anti-estrogen action on the endometrial lining of the uterus, the bazedoxifene SERM component acts like progesterone in protecting the uterus. By inhibiting breast cancer cell growth, bazedoxifene also acts as an antiestrogen on the breast, as well.

When SERMs are solo performers, such as tamoxifen (Nolvadex) prescribed for breast cancer treatment and prevention, raloxifene (Evista) prescribed for breast cancer prevention and treatment/prevention of post-menopausal osteoporosis, or ospemifene (Osphena) prescribed for menopausal vaginal dryness and painful intercourse, SERMs cause hot flashes. With a TSEC, such as Duavee, a SERM is coupled to estrogen, so the estrogen component provides estrogen-related health benefits, such as treatment for hot flashes.

For a menopausal woman who wants to emancipate herself from the risks of progesterone or progestin, but does not want to add another type of chemical into her body, then a progestin-containing intrauterine device (IUD) is a suitable option. The IUD acts as a vehicle for delivering progesterone to the only target organ that needs it- the uterus, so a menopausal woman's breasts are not exposed to progesterone. By releasing a tiny amount of levonorgestrel progestin into the uterine cavity, the Mirena/Liletta IUD protects the lining of the uterus from estrogen's stimulation, without exposing the rest of the woman's body to unnecessary progesterone. Insertion of the IUD is a simple 10-minute procedure completed in the gynecologist's office. The procedure is comfortable when the prostaglandin, misoprostol (Cytotec), is used to help soften and dilate the cervix. The Mirena/Liletta IUD lasts 5 to 7 years, and it can be replaced during the same time the old one is removed. With a progestin IUD in place, a menopausal woman with a uterus safely enjoys all the benefits of estrogen replacement therapy without subjecting her breasts, or the rest of her body, to progesterone. This truly is easy, breezy, estrogen replacement therapy.

For a woman who needs a touch of testosterone added to her menopause hormone therapy, testosterone will not increase her chance of breast cancer. In the WHI observational study involving 72,000 postmenopausal women followed for 10 years, hormone therapy using the oral pill containing conjugated esterified estrogen with methyltestosterone was not associated with a significantly increased risk of breast cancer.

When it comes to breast cancer, a woman cannot change her age or her family history. She can help minimize the impact of certain risk factors through improved lifestyle choices and avoiding tissue-damaging toxins. When she reaches menopause, she arrives at another fork in the road on her path to health maintenance. With all the holistic health benefits that appropriate estrogen replacement therapy has to offer in naturally alleviating bothersome menopausal symptoms of hot flashes, night sweats, vaginal dryness, insomnia, fatigue, memory slips and irritability, as well as estrogen's natural flair for preventing cardiovascular disease, dementia, osteoporosis, urinary incontinence, vaginal atrophy, and other tissue or organ deterioration exacerbated by hormone deficiency, nothing compares to Nature's estrogen power for keeping a woman happy and healthy. Estrogen does not cause breast cancer and progesterone-free breast protecting hormone options are now available for menopausal women.

Menopausal women whose hormone deficiency is replaced appropriately enjoy a better quality of life than their estrogen-deprived counterparts. For those who want to remain sovereign and self-propelled throughout their golden years, menopause hormone therapy should not be sidetracked by looming thoughts of breast cancer. We have a clearer understanding of the timing, type and dose of menopause hormone therapy needed to maximize the health benefits of estrogen while simultaneously eliminating the risks associated with old-fashioned hormone regimens.

BONES, BABY, BONES

To be able to move or not to move, that's the real issue. For a menopausal woman, "whether 'tis nobler in the mind to suffer the misfortunes of a stationary dependent existence, or take arms against musculoskeletal disability," involves the prevention of osteoporosis. Participating in activities of daily living and tending to one's sustenance and maintenance require rudimentary kinetics and locomotion. To remain in motion, a woman needs to have working muscles, moving joints, and resilient bones. Estrogen helps make it all happen, every step of the way.

BONING UP on BONES

The human skeleton dangling from a hook looks creepy, but in a live human being, the skeleton gives the body its structural framework, provides protection to vital organs, and allows mobility. Bones of the skull protect the brain, ribs protect the heart, lungs, and liver, the vertebral backbone protects the spinal cord, and pelvic bones protect the uterus and bladder. A baby is born with 300 different bones. As the child matures, small bones fuse, so an adult walks around with 206 bones. Without skeletal bones' scaffolding, the body would collapse into a gelatinous blob.

In an archeological dig, bones are fossilized pieces of mineralized, inert structures. In the living body, bones are alive and well, existing with dedicated nerves and blood supply. That's why it hurts to break a bone, and the fracture site swells. When bones break, these cells deposit bone and remodel the fracture site, allowing the bone to function again. Bone has an outer layer of hard or compact bone. This "cortical bone" is very dense, tough and strong. Inside the cortical layer is a spongy bone, also known as "trabecular bone," which resembles a honeycomb and is a lighter bone and slightly flexible. In the middle of some bones is the jelly-like bone marrow, which produces red and white blood cells, as well as platelets. Bone's weight-bearing strength and resiliency are derived from calcium and phosphorous, along with magnesium, zinc and other trace minerals deposited onto a collagen protein matrix.

Like any other living tissue, bone is metabolically active. Simple day-to-day activity causes traction and stressors on bones, resulting in microfractures. These microfractures require repair and remodeling to maintain bone health, strength, and resiliency. "Osteoclasts" ("c" for crashers) are bone cells that remove old, damaged or diseased bone by resorption. This creates space so that new bone can be deposited by the bone building "osteoblasts" ("b" for builders). In a normal adult, 20% of the skeleton is remodeled every year. Calcium and phosphate crystals are incorporated into a collagen protein matrix to mineralize bone.

99% of the body's calcium is stored in the bony skeleton and teeth, so only 1% of the body's calcium is busy tending to crucial physiological activities keeping a person alive. Calcium is required for the heart to beat, for blood to clot, for nerves to transmit messages, for muscles to contract, and for the release of hormones and enzymes throughout the body. The brain works by fluxes of calcium in and out of nerve cells, so the brain demands calcium. For normal body functioning, blood serum calcium levels need to be maintained within a very narrow range. If calcium levels deviate from this tight and narrow, a person feels lousy. Their heart rate roams; they suffer from painful bones, psychic moans, abdominal groans and kidney stones. Depressed calcium levels can precipitate tetanus, a life-threatening condition where severe muscles spasms block air exchange to the lungs.

Calcium consumed through the diet or provided by oral supplements requires adequate vitamin D to be absorbed through the intestines. Without adequate vitamin D, calcium supplements are wasted. If there is not enough calcium circulating in a woman's system, her body will excavate needed calcium from its built-in quarry, the skeleton. By digging holes in the bone, osteoclasts release calcium into the bloodstream, so the body's vital processes can function. The balance of osteoclast and osteoblast cellular activity impacts bone remodeling, and this activity is controlled by the interplay of calcium, vitamin D, estrogen, testosterone and other hormones.

Hormones that impact bone include:

- The sex steroids, estrogen or testosterone, judiciously inhibit osteoclasts and stimulate osteoblasts, with a net gain in bone density, strength, and resilience.
- Excess thyroid hormone speeds up bone metabolism, causing bone thinning.
- Calcitonin, a hormone secreted by parafollicular cells within the thyroid gland, inhibits osteoclasts' excavation of bone and reduces blood calcium levels.
- Parathyroid hormone, a hormone secreted by the four tiny parathyroid glands (each the size of a grain of rice) located on the back of the thyroid gland, increases blood calcium levels by stimulating osteoclasts. An overactive parathyroid gland causes bone thinning.
- Excess cortisol hormone production from the adrenal glands inhibits osteoblasts, so bone building decreases and bone thins.

When nutrition, weight-bearing exercise, genetics, hormones and menstrual cycles are all working in harmony, a woman reaches her peak bone density around age 30 to 35. After age 35, bone mass starts to decrease, and with the precipitous drop in estrogen levels associated with menopause, bone density takes an accelerated downward spiral. Within 5 years of menopause, a woman has lost 20% of her bone mass. After this menopausal descent, age-related bone loss continues at a rate of 1% to 2% per year. Loss of estrogen disrupts calcium metabolism. Estrogen deficiency diminishes the intestines' ability to absorb calcium, weakens the kidneys' capacity to hold on to calcium, and impairs the body's knack for generating vitamin D. All in all, this spells trouble for a woman's bones.

A 30% loss of bone density needs to occur before "thin bones" can be visualized on routine plain-film x-rays, like a chest x-ray or an x-ray of a broken bone. That's why a menopausal woman who sustains a low-impact fracture, such as tripping and breaking her wrist, or slipping and breaking her hip, or even simply notices that she is getting shorter, should have a bone density scan to determine the status of her bones.

OSTEOPOROSIS

Osteoporosis literally means "bone porous," a condition in which bones become very weak and break easily. Osteopenia is the bone-thinning precursor to osteoporosis. If osteopenia is not addressed, it can progress to the severely thinned bones of osteoporosis. Under a microscope, bones look like a honeycomb. With osteoporosis, individual trabecular plates of bone are lost, so there are bigger and bigger holes in the honeycomb. These porous bones have significantly reduced bone mass, which results in an architecturally weakened structure that breaks easily. Areas of the skeleton housing more trabecular bone, such as the wrist, spine, and hip, are particularly vulnerable to this bone loss process. Osteoporosis is the most common bone disease that occurs in humans. 50% of postmenopausal women will sustain an osteoporosis-related fracture at some point in her lifetime. Half of these fractures involve the spinal column; a quarter involve the hip, and the remaining quarter involve the wrist. Osteoporosis affects the jawbone as well; oral alveolar bone loss can lead to tooth loss.

Osteoporotic bones can be so fragile that they break simply by bumping into furniture or sneezing. Sometimes, osteoporotic bones become so weak, they break spontaneously. Osteopenia and osteoporosis are silent diseases. They manifest themselves for the first time only after a woman has sustained a fracture involving minimal trauma. Osteoporosis is preventable and treatable, but because there are no warning signs prior to a fracture, many people are not diagnosed in time to receive therapy during the early phase of the disease.

66% of osteoporotic compression fractures of the vertebral spine are asymptomatic, so a woman may not even notice anything wrong early on. If a woman has lost more than 1½ inches of height since age 35, she is at risk for osteoporosis and hip fractures. As these compression fractures of the spine accumulate, she stoops over and becomes more and more uncomfortable. Not only is this dowager's hump disfiguring, but multiple thoracic spine fractures also result in restrictive lung disease, which compromises oxygen exchange and increases an older woman's susceptibility to pneumonia. Lower thoracic and lumbar vertebral spine compression fractures alter abdominal anatomy, leading to intestinal compression, digestive problems, pelvic organ prolapse (POP) and urinary incontinence.

As if osteoporotic compression fractures of the vertebral spine were not enough, an estrogen-deprived older woman faces disabling and deadly osteoporosis-related hip fractures. As a postmenopausal woman ages, she experiences dizziness, poor vision, gait instability, balance problems, urinary urge incontinence and medication side effects, which increase her vulnerability to falling and breaking a hip. During the prolonged period of recuperation that follows a hip fracture, many otherwise healthy women succumb to other diseases. 20% of women who sustain a hip fracture die within the first year of the fracture, usually due to a blood clot or pneumonia. More than 50% of the remaining survivors end up spending the rest their crippled lives in a nursing home.

OSTEOPOROSIS RISK FACTORS

For women, lack of estrogen is the strongest risk factor for weakening bones. Without estrogen, women develop osteopenia and osteoporosis. 50% of postmenopausal women will sustain an osteoporosis-related fracture. A woman's bones needs estrogen to do the things bones need to do, which is to stand tall, stay strong, and keep moving. Women who enter menopause with low bone density are more likely to develop osteoporosis than women who enter menopause with normal bone density. 80% of people suffering from osteoporosis are women. Menopause is unfriendly to a woman's skeletal system, so her bones, joints and muscles suffer without estrogen.

When a non-pregnant premenopausal woman loses her menstrual cycles for more than 6 consecutive months, she starts losing bone density and increases her risk for osteoporosis. Premenopausal hormonal hazards for bone thinning include:

- Anorexia nervosa, orthorexia nervosa, bulimia, or the female athlete triad (loss of menstrual periods linked to an eating disorder associated with excessive exercise), causes young women to stop menstruating, which means their ovaries are no longer producing estrogen, so they lose bone at a young age.
- Stress can turn off a woman's menstrual cycles as well, so when a woman goes for 6 or months without a period, she is at risk of losing bone.
- Elevated prolactin hormone levels, whether produced by a pituitary gland tumor in the brain or brought on as a side effect of psychiatric medications, such as antidepressants, antipsychotics, and narcotics, suppress ovulation and decrease the ovaries' production of estrogen, which leads to bone thinning.

Hormonal medications that prevent a woman's body from producing estrogen also increase her risk of osteoporosis, as well. Medications such as:

- Progestin-only contraceptives, such as medroxyprogesterone acetate (Depo-Provera) shots, levonorgestrel implants (Implanon, Nexplanon) and the minipill norethindrone (Nor-QD, Ortho Micronor), suppress ovulation and prevent pregnancy. Progestin-only contraceptives prevent pregnancy, but they also prevent the ovaries from producing bone-protecting estrogen. On the other hand, hormonal contraceptives containing a combination of estrogen plus progestin, such as low-dose oral contraceptive pills (OCPs), patches or vaginal rings, suppress ovulation and prevent pregnancy, while simultaneously providing a woman with bone-preserving estrogen.

- Progestin IUDs do not bother bones. Since less than 10% of the low dose levonorgestrel progestin found in the Mirena/Liletta IUD or Skyla IUD is absorbed into a woman's bloodstream, it does not inhibit the ovaries' production of estrogen. Progestin IUD's contraceptive power comes from its ability to thicken cervical mucus, thereby blocking sperms' entry into the uterus, as well as its capacity to prevent the uterine lining from becoming thick and juicy. Any sperm that may have made it through the cervical mucus plug faces this hostile, arid uterine environment, making it impossible for sperm to swim to the fallopian tube to meet up with the fertile oocyte/egg.
- Aromatase inhibitor (AI) medications, such as anastrozole (Arimidex), letrozole (Femara), exemestane (Aromasin), which are used to treat and prevent breast cancer, totally eliminate estrogen production in a postmenopausal woman's body, so they are associated with bone thinning, joint pains, and muscle aches.
- Gonadotropin releasing hormone (GnRH) medications, such as Lupron or Zoladex, are used to chemically induce a menopausal state to treat endometriosis or uterine fibroids. Being on these menopause-inducing drugs for more than 6 months can cause bone loss.

In addition to hormone medications that manipulate bone metabolism, other risk factors for osteoporosis include:

- Age older than 65 years
- Family history of osteoporosis
- Being thin (weighing less than 127 pounds) or having a small body frame
- Smoking
- Excess alcohol drinking (more than one drink a day)

Suffering from other health problems can cause bone thinning, and drugs used to treat these health problems can exacerbate bone loss. Health problems that increase the risk of developing osteoporosis include:

-   Rheumatoid arthritis, ankylosing spondylitis lupus, scoliosis
-   Diabetes
-   Gastrointestinal bypass procedures, inflammatory bowel disease (Crohn's, ulcerative colitis), celiac disease, lactose intolerance or other malabsorption syndromes
-   Cushing's syndrome
-   AIDS/HIV
-   Chronic liver or kidney disease
-   Multiple myeloma, multiple sclerosis, Parkinson's disease, stroke
-   Sickle cell disease or thalassemia
-   Older women with chronic hyponatremia (blood serum sodium levels persistently below 135mmol/L) are at increased risk for osteoporosis, as well. Chronic hyponatremia increases osteoclast activity.

Drugs that cause bone loss include:

-   Blood thinners such as heparin and warfarin (Coumadin) cause bone thinning. Heparin and warfarin have been used clinically since the 1940s and 1950s, so decades of use have elucidated their adverse effects on bone health. The newer blood thinners, such as rivaroxaban (Xarelto) have been on the market since 2008, so time will tell what their impact on the bone will be.
-   Anti-seizure medicines such as phenytoin (Dilantin) and phenobarbital stimulate the liver to deactivate vitamin D. Without vitamin D, the intestines do not absorb calcium.
-   Steroid (glucocorticoid) medicines, such as cortisone, prednisone or dexamethasone, used for 3 or more months, stimulate bone resorption and inhibit bone deposition.

- Psychiatric medicines such as lithium (Eskalith), selective serotonin reuptake inhibitors (SSRIs) such as fluoxetine (Prozac), paroxetine (Paxil), sertraline (Zoloft) or escitalopram (Lexapro), serotonin norepinephrine reuptake inhibitors (SNRIs) such as duloxetine (Cymbalta) or venlafaxine (Effexor) cause bone thinning. Serotonin transporters are found in bone, and by influencing bone metabolism SSRIs increase a woman's risk of osteoporosis-related fractures.
- Proton pump inhibitors (PPIs) such as omeprazole (Prilosec), lansoprazole (Prevacid) or esomeprazole (Nexium) decrease stomach's acid production, which interferes with calcium absorption.
- Drugs used to prevent organ transplants from being rejected and some chemotherapy agents used to treat cancers cause bone thinning.
- Loop diuretics, such as furosemide (Lasix) or bumetanide (Bumex) increase the kidneys' elimination of calcium. Thiazide diuretics, such as chlorothiazide (Diuril) or hydrochlorothiazide (Microzide), on the other hand, cause less calcium loss by the kidneys.

Lifestyle choices that promote bone health include:

- Eating a well-balanced, nutritious diet that provides adequate protein, vitamins, and minerals, is good for the bones. 7 fruits and vegetables a day keeps disease away.
- Not smoking.
- Limiting alcohol drinking to no more than 1 serving a day, either 5 ounces of wine or 12 ounces of beer or 1.5 ounces of whiskey a day
- Exercising. Exercise makes the bones stronger. People who are bedridden or sedentary are at high risk for osteoporosis. Weight-bearing exercises, such as walking, dancing, hiking and aerobics, along with muscle-strengthening exercises, such as carrying 2 ½ pound weights while walking, engaging in Pilates or yoga, improve bone strength, balance and coordination, as well as decrease muscle wasting. Balance training exercises and activities such as Tai Chi can

also help prevent falls. Although swimming and biking are good for overall health, they are not weight-bearing exercises. 10,000 steps a day keeps disease and disability away.

- Safety first. One should become familiar with her terrain and make her home safe from falls by removing clutter, eliminating loose throw rugs, placing assistive devices in bathrooms and improve lighting.

- Adequate vitamin D blood serum levels. The body needs vitamin D to absorb calcium, and calcium helps build and maintain strong bones. When it comes to how much calcium and vitamin D to take, it is handy to remember "a 1000 & 1000." The oral intake (diet plus supplement) of calcium should be 1000mg a day. Most menopausal women consume about 500mg of calcium through their diet daily, so a 500mg calcium supplement taken daily with food should be adequate. Dairy products are the best source of calcium due to their high elemental calcium content, high absorptive rate, and relatively low cost. A serving size of dairy equals one cup (8 ounces) of milk, one cup of yogurt or 1.5 ounces of cheese. Each one of these dairy servings provides 300mg of calcium.

- Calcium supplements. Calcium carbonate antacids (Tums) are inexpensive and contain the most amount of elemental calcium (40%). Aluminum-containing antacids such as Maalox or Mylanta inhibit gastrointestinal absorption of calcium. Calcium carbonate derived from "natural" or "refined" sources, such as bone meal or oyster shell, may contain lead, so they should be avoided. Calcium citrate contains 22% elemental calcium and does not require gastric acid for absorption, so it is a better choice for older women with reduced gastric acid production or women taking proton-pump inhibitor (PPIs) medications. Excess calcium supplements may cause calcium to be deposited in the wrong places, leading to kidney stones and heart disease due to calcified coronary arteries.

By obtaining any needed calcium through excavation from the skeleton's quarry, the body maintains a tight reign on calcium levels in the blood. Blood serum calcium levels do not reflect the woman's true calcium needs. Adequacy of calcium intake can be assessed with a 24-hour urine collection measuring calcium. Calcium intake (diet plus supplement) totaling 1000mg of calcium a day is satisfactory for most menopausal women.

Unlike calcium blood tests, serum vitamin D levels are helpful in monitoring vitamin D needs, as well as a woman's response to vitamin D therapy. The 400 IU of vitamin D3 found in a multivitamin is inadequate for most menopausal women. Unless otherwise indicated by low serum vitamin D levels, taking 1000 IU of vitamin D3 daily should cover a woman's vitamin D needs. Taking a vitamin D3 supplement of 1000 IU a day, along with the 400 IU of vitamin D3 found in a multivitamin, is fine.

DIAGNOSING OSTEOPOROSIS

Like hypertension, osteoporosis is a silent disease, and like untreated hypertension, osteoporosis can kill. Fortunately, bone thinning can be diagnosed early and easily, and treatment can prevent disabling and deadly osteoporotic fractures from occurring. The most common clinical tool used to diagnose osteoporosis is the dual-energy X-ray absorptiometry (DEXA) scan. DEXA measures bone mineral density by detecting the extent to which bones absorb photons that are generated by very low-level x-rays. The amount of radiation a DEXA scan generates is much less than the radiation associated with a plain chest x-ray. Bone mineral density is measured in the spine, hip and wrist, the areas most likely to be affected by osteoporosis, with the hipbone's density being the most reliable in determining fracture risk.

The DEXA bone density scan results, along with the patient's medical history, are useful in evaluating the probability of a fracture occurring, determining whether any preventative treatment is needed, and monitoring the efficacy of therapeutic interventions. Because of the physics of the test's methodology, to accurately detect bone density changes, repeat DEXA scans should be done no sooner than at 2-year intervals.

DEXA bone density screening is recommended for:

- All women age 65 or older.
- Menopausal women under age 65 years with one or more risk factors for osteoporosis.
- Women going through menopause with risk factors for osteoporosis. Bone density test results may help women make decisions regarding estrogen replacement therapy.
- Any woman over the age of 50 who suffers a low-impact fracture, such as a fracture due to falling, slipping or tripping.
- Postmenopausal women who have stopped taking hormone replacement therapy. This will help determine how much bone density is lost after discontinuing estrogen replacement.

DEXA Test Scores

When assessing bone density, DEXA scans report a T-score and a Z-score. The Z-score compares a woman's bone density to what is normal for other women in her age bracket. Among older adults, low bone density is common so Z-scores may be misleading. An older person may have a normal Z-score (Z-scores above -2.0 are normal), but still be at high risk for breaking a bone, so Z-scores are not used to guide therapy in menopausal or older women. Z-scores are relevant for children, teens and women having menstrual periods. The T-score shows how much a woman's bone density is above or below normal when compared to an average healthy 30-year-old woman's bone density. The T-score is not used in children and teens because their bones are still growing.

The T-score is used to diagnose osteoporosis and osteopenia in women going through menopause and in postmenopausal women over the age of 50. The T-score is used to direct therapeutic interventions used to maintain bone density and prevent future fractures. The lower a T-score, the lower the bone density. Sometimes the T-score can be normal in one area of bone, but show osteopenia or osteoporosis in a different bone. The lowest T-score is used to render a diagnosis.

Guide to T-scores:

A T-score of -1 or above … is Normal bone density, so

T-scores of -1.0, -0.5, 0, +0.5, or +1.0 … indicate Normal bone density

Normal T-scores carry a lifetime risk for a hip fracture of 15%.

A T-score between -1 and -2.5 … defines Osteopenia or low bone density, so

T-scores of -1.1, -1.5, -1.8, -2.0, or -2.4 … indicate Osteopenia

Osteopenia T-scores carry between 20% to 50% lifetime risk for fracture.

A T-score of -2.5 and below … defines Osteoporosis, so

T-scores of -2.5, -2.8, -3.0, -3.5, or -4.0 … indicate Osteoporosis

Osteoporosis T-scores carry over a 60% chance of having a hip fracture.

FRAX & ABSOLUTE FRACTURE RISK

If a woman has a T-score consistent with osteoporosis, then she should proceed with an osteoporosis medication to decrease her chance for sustaining a disabling or deadly, osteoporotic fracture.

The management of osteopenia (bone-thinning) T-scores in middle-aged women (late 40s to late 50s) is less straightforward and depends on other clinical factors. Except for estrogen replacement therapy, most of the other medications prescribed for osteoporosis prevention and treatment have been primarily used in elderly women. Many of these osteoporosis medications are cumbersome to take, and some have rare, but serious side effects. If a woman has a T-score consistent with osteopenia, she should ramp up the bone-protecting lifestyle habits described earlier. To determine if a woman with osteopenia would be a candidate for pharmaceutical intervention, her personal medical history, her current health, her risk factors for advancing into osteoporosis, and her likelihood of breaking a bone, all need to be considered.

FRAX Tool

To help guide the decision process for treating osteopenia, the World Health Organization (WHO) established a Web-based Fracture Risk Assessment Tool (FRAX), which estimates a woman's absolute risk for an osteoporotic fracture occurring over the next 10 years. It takes into account her hip T-score value, her age, body mass index (BMI), personal history of low-impact fracture, parental history of hip fracture, smoking status, alcohol consumption, and other medical conditions.

According to the U.S.-adapted FRAX algorithm, either a 10-year probability of a hip fracture of ≥3%, or an overall 10-year risk of any type of osteoporotic fracture of ≥20%, meet criteria for initiating pharmaceutical treatment to prevent fractures in osteopenic women. Osteopenia in the presence of one or more risk factors for osteoporosis, or progressive bone loss, as documented by serial DEXA scans, may also warrant pharmaceutical intervention to prevent fractures.

PHARMACOLOGICAL TREATMENT of OSTEOPOROSIS

When it comes to the prevention and treatment of postmenopausal osteoporosis, there are a number of pharmaceutical options to choose from. Although the medications may not cause large increments in T-scores, they all reduce the incidence of osteoporosis-related fractures by around 40% to 50%. They achieve this fracture reduction predominantly through their anti-resorptive action on the bone, meaning they maintain bone density by inhibiting the bone-resorbing osteoclasts.

BISPHOSPHONATES

Bisphosphonate medications are approved for the prevention and treatment of postmenopausal osteoporosis. They are considered the gold standard of therapy for the disease and are the most widely prescribed agents for the treatment of osteoporosis globally. Bisphosphonates prevent bone thinning by suppressing the bone-excavating osteoclast cells, and they are available as oral or intravenous (IV) medications. They include the drugs alendronate (Fosamax), risedronate (Actonel), ibandronate (Boniva oral and IV) and zoledronic acid (Reclast IV). In order to use bisphosphonates, normal kidney function must be documented with an estimated glomerular filtration rate (eGFR) of at least 60 mL/min or creatinine clearance around 100 mL/min.

Oral bisphosphonates are poorly absorbed through the gastrointestinal tract (less than 1% of the dose gets into the bloodstream), but once that little bit gets to the bone, it stays embedded in the skeleton for a long, long time. Specific and rigid guidelines must be followed for maximizing the stomach's absorption of oral bisphosphonates. Bisphosphonates must be taken first thing in the morning, on an empty stomach, with a full 8-ounce glass of water. No additional food or drink should be consumed for 30 to 60 minutes after swallowing the pill, and no lying down for 30 to 60 minutes after taking the pill.

About 30% of women taking oral bisphosphonates experience heartburn, stomach upset or intestinal problems, so they may need to switch to IV bisphosphonates or use another type of osteoporosis medication. In addition to gastrointestinal difficulties, other side effects of bisphosphonates include severe bone, joint and muscle pain. Clinical studies show that bisphosphonates increase the risk of new-onset atrial fibrillation, an abnormal heart rhythm requiring hospitalization. Although rare, osteonecrosis of the jaw or atypical femur fractures are complex and difficult complications linked to bisphosphonate use.

OSTEONECROSIS of the JAWBONE

Osteonecrosis literally means, "bone dead," of the jaw is a severe bone disease that is associated with bisphosphonate use. It usually happens after invasive dental surgical procedures, such as extractions or implants, not from teeth cleaning or cavity filling. It can also occur spontaneously, without any prior dental work.

Jawbones are areas of high bone turnover and remodeling, so when osteoclasts are suppressed by bisphosphonates, bone healing and remodeling are also suppressed. Extracting a tooth leaves a hole in the jawbone that needs to be remodeled to heal. When osteoclasts are suppressed by bisphosphonates, they cannot fill the pothole, so to speak, so the bone does not heal, and that area of the bone dies. Segments of dead jawbone become exposed through the gum line or oral soft tissue. The surrounding tissue becomes inflamed, and can become infected by bacteria within the oral cavity. Osteonecrosis of the jaw is a chronic, painful condition that requires repeated surgical debridement treatments and on-going wound management. Unfortunately, most of time, the affected bone never heals, so complex oral maxillofacial surgery involving bone grafts and jaw reconstruction are needed.

ATYPICAL FEMUR FRACTURE

Atypical femur (thigh bone) fractures are an unusual type of fracture that has been linked to bisphosphonate use. Less than 1% of all hip and thigh fractures are of this atypical variety, but over 90% of people who sustain these unusual femur fractures have taken bisphosphonates for more than 5 years.

These fractures are described as "atypical" because, unlike other femur fractures, they occur spontaneously, without any history of trauma. These bisphosphonate-related atypical femur fractures involve the strongest part of the strongest bone in the body. This area is the upper 1/3 segment of the shaft of the femur, technically known as the subtrochanteric and diaphysis region. In contrast, when an osteoporosis-related hip fracture happens from the impact of falling, the breakage occurs in the femoral neck or intertrochanteric region located at the top end of the femur adjacent to the pelvic bone.

For weeks or months prior to when an atypical femur fracture occurs, women may experience thigh pain or groin pain. The thigh pain worsens with standing or bearing weight. 33% of the time atypical femur fractures occur in both thighbones. These are complete transverse or oblique fractures, meaning the bone breaks straight across, like snapping a dry twig. Bisphosphonate over-suppression of osteoclasts' bone remodeling capabilities can render bones too weak and brittle to repair microfractures that occur from normal day-to-day living. The accumulation of bone microdamage and altered structural integrity at the femur's point of maximal, weight bearing stress makes it vulnerable to spontaneous breakage. If the potential for a break is detected, then discontinuing bisphosphonate therapy and preventive surgical nail fixation along the length of the femur is recommended.

Bisphosphonates have extended bone-staying power, so to minimize the possibility of these rare, but complicated bone healing problems, these medications should be stopped after 5 years of therapy. During this "drug holiday," lifestyle measures promoting bone health should be maintained. 2 to 3 years after stopping therapy, a woman's DEXA bone density can be repeated to determine if pharmaceutical intervention should be reinstated.

CALCITONIN

Calcitonin (Miacalcin, Fortical) is a synthetic hormone used for the treatment of osteoporosis in postmenopausal women who are at least 5 years beyond menopause. Normally, the parafollicular cells within the thyroid gland secrete calcitonin to tone down calcium levels in the bloodstream. Calcitonin suppresses osteoclasts' resorption of bones, so less calcium is released into the bloodstream. Administered as a daily nasal spray, calcitonin reduces the risk and pain of vertebral spine fractures, but it is not that effective in preventing hip fractures.

DENOSUMAB

Denosumab (Prolia) is used in postmenopausal women whose osteoporosis seems to be resistant to other therapeutic modalities. It is administered as a subcutaneous injection every 6 months. It is an immunological mediator that targets RANKL, a member of the tumor necrosis factor superfamily, and by inhibiting RANKL the development and activity of osteoclasts are stifled. Denosumab acts through immunological mechanisms, so it is a medicine that may affect the body's ability to fight infections. It can cause serious skin infections and endocarditis, which is an inflammation of the inner lining of the heart caused by infection. Because it suppresses osteoclasts' remodeling capabilities, denosumab is associated with osteonecrosis of the jaw and atypical femur fractures.

TERIPARATIDE

Teriparatide (Forteo, PTH 1-34) is the parathyroid hormone (PTH) that modulates calcium levels in the body. In response to low blood levels of calcium, the parathyroid gland releases parathyroid hormone, which stimulates osteoclasts to break down bone and release calcium into the bloodstream. Chronically elevated parathyroid hormone depletes bones; however, intermittent exposure to parathyroid hormone paradoxically activates bone building osteoblasts more than it will stimulate bone-excavating osteoclasts. The body registers the once a day teriparatide injection as an intermittent burst of parathyroid hormone, so the net effect is stimulation of new bone formation, leading to increased bone density.

Side effects of teriparatide include leg cramps, nausea, and dizziness. It carries a special warning in its drug packaging because it is linked to bone cancer in lab rats. The safety and efficacy of teriparatide use beyond 2 years has not been demonstrated, so it is common practice to follow 2 years of teriparatide therapy with an antiresorptive agent, usually a bisphosphonate, to maintain the teriparatide-accrued bone density. Women with bone cancer, or who are at increased risk of bone cancer, e.g.- Paget's disease of the bone, or women with bone metastasis from another cancer, should not take teriparatide therapy.

STRONTIUM

There are over 100 chemical elements on the periodic table, yet 96% of the mass of the human body is made up of just 4 of these elements: carbon, hydrogen, oxygen and nitrogen. More than 70% of the body is composed of water (H_2O), with the residual a sparse sampling of minerals. Calcium is the most common mineral in the body, composing 1.5% of the body's makeup, followed by phosphorous, which makes up 1% of the body's mass. Nearly all of the calcium and phosphorous in the body is found embedded in the collagen protein matrix that gives bone its strength and structure. Within the bone and connective tissue, the human body also contains 350mg of the element, strontium.

Strontium is chemically similar to calcium. Both are reactive alkaline earth metals with an oxidation number of +2. Unlike noble metals, such as silver, gold or platinum, which tend to exist as inert loners, strontium and calcium are the reactive marrying kind, so they are not found footloose and free in nature. They are bound to other chemicals, such as carbonates or citrates.

Although strontium is named after the Scotland town where it was discovered, when strontium is mentioned, many people think of the dangerous, radioactive component of nuclear fallout produced during atmospheric testing of nuclear weapons in the 1950s. These days ultra-pure radioactive strontium-90 is used medically in arterial stents to maintain blood flow, and strontium is used to treat excess capillary growth associated with wet-form, age-related macular degeneration (AMD) of the eye's retina. Bone cancer and metastatic bone pain are treated with radioactive strontium-89.

Naturally occurring strontium is neither radioactive nor toxic at levels normally found in the environment. In fact, strontium is one of the most abundant elements on earth. There is more strontium in the earth's crust than carbon, and strontium is the most abundant trace element found in the oceans' seawater. Because of its chemical similarity to calcium, strontium can replace calcium in some biochemical processes in the body. When strontium replaces a small proportion of the calcium found in teeth, it renders teeth resistant to cavities. Strontium is a helpful ingredient found in toothpaste used to strengthen sensitive teeth (Sensodyne).

Since the late 1950s, strontium has been found to prevent osteoporosis-related fractures. The largest and longest running clinical trials on strontium involve older women in their 70s. Since hip fractures occur more frequently in elderly women, recent studies show strontium to be particularly helpful in this older age group. In 1959, researchers at the Mayo Clinic investigated the effect of natural strontium lactate on individuals suffering from osteoporosis. 84% of the patients reported marked relief of bone pain while the remaining 16% experienced moderate improvement in bone pain. X-rays taken at the beginning and end of the 3-year study showed increased bone mass in 80% of the cases. Unfortunately, measurement of bone mineral density was crude in 1959, but the fact that any positive changes were visualized on plain film x-rays is impressive.

Because of the fallout from the "strontium scare" of the 1950s, little follow-up on these findings was conducted until 30 years later. Subsequent long-term clinical trials further confirmed natural strontium's bone strengthening power. Just a little bit of strontium incorporated into the bone structure strengthens bone, and since strontium (atomic number 38) is heavier than calcium (atomic number 20), it can over-dramatically increase DEXA scan T-scores. This variance needs to be considered when interpreting bone density reports.

Unlike other osteoporosis prevention and treatment medications that either inhibit osteoclasts bone resorption (bisphosphonates, calcitonin, denosumab), or deposit bone by stimulating osteoblasts (teriparatide), strontium is a dual action bone agent (DABA). It increases bone formation while simultaneously decreasing bone resorption, leading to a balance of bone turnover in favor of bone formation. By increasing bone mineral density and improving the architectural integrity of trabecular bone, natural strontium decreases the risk of osteoporosis-related fractures. Earlier studies confirming the positive effect of strontium on bone health involved various different natural strontium salts, so the bone-protecting therapeutic factor is the strontium itself.

Since substances found in nature cannot be patented, more recent pharmaceutical trials used a patent-protected synthetic version of strontium known as strontium ranelate (Protelos), which is a prescription medicine available in Europe and Australia. The synthetic strontium ranelate (Protelos) compound appears to be associated with an increased risk of developing blood clots, and there are concerns about its cardiac safety in women with risk factors for heart disease, such as obesity, smoking, or a prior history or cardiac issues or strokes. These problems have not been found with naturally occurring strontium salt supplements.

Because calcium and strontium are chemically similar, they can be coupled with similar compounds. Since calcium is available as calcium carbonate or calcium citrate supplements, natural strontium is available as strontium carbonate or strontium citrate supplements, as well. These naturally occurring strontium salts can be purchased as food supplements, and strontium citrate seems to be better absorbed than strontium carbonate. The dose of strontium needed to prevent osteoporosis is 227mg daily. To treat osteoporosis, 680mg of strontium a day is recommended. Naturally occurring strontium salts are a safe and useful therapeutic option for postmenopausal women who need protection from osteoporosis-related fractures.

THE ESTROGEN-BONE CONNECTION

When a menopausal woman loses her estrogen, bone metabolism shifts into bone resorption overdrive. No longer modulated by estrogen, bone-resorbing osteoclasts go wild, breaking down bone. The estrogen-deprived, bone-building osteoblasts simply cannot keep up with osteoclasts' destruction. Because estrogen supports the bone's collagen protein matrix upon which the calcium was deposited, once estrogen is lost, the bone's scaffolding deteriorates, as well. This bone thinning process is particularly evident in the trabecular (honeycomb-like) bone located at the wrist end of the forearm, the vertebral bones of the spine, and in the femoral neck (hip bone). Weakened by osteoporosis, these porous bones break easily with low-impact or minimal-impact trauma.

Since the principle cause of osteoporosis in women is the loss of estrogen, it stands to reason that the most natural and holistic remedy for preserving bones is estrogen replacement therapy. Indeed, nothing protects menopausal women from disabling and deadly osteoporosis-related fractures as effectively, safely and naturally as menopause hormone therapy. In addition to bone protection, hormone replacement helps with calcium and mineral absorption, vitamin D synthesis, maintaining skeletal muscle mass, strengthening the bones' collagen protein matrix, and sustaining the nerve pathways needed to effect movement and locomotion.

Estrogen replacement therapy decreases osteoporosis-related fractures throughout a postmenopausal woman's body (wrist, spine, and hip) by 50%. If a woman stops her estrogen replacement therapy, she will lose bone and bone's collagen matrix, so her bones deteriorate. Strong bones need adaptive bone-remodeling processes, with adequate raw materials and a suitable balance between osteoclast (bone-remodeling) and osteoblast (bone-building) cellular activity. Bone is living tissue, so when bone maintenance is withdrawn, bone deteriorates and weakens, rendering a postmenopausal woman vulnerable to devastating and deadly osteoporosis-related fractures.

Nothing beats estrogen for bone protection, but there are other synthetic hormones with estrogenic action, which can be used for the prevention of postmenopausal osteoporosis. These include the SERM, raloxifene (Evista), the TSEC, conjugated equine estrogen plus bazedoxifene (Duavee), and the synthetic steroid, tibolone (Livial).

RALOXIFENE

Raloxifene (Evista) is a selective estrogen receptor modulator (SERM) approved for the prevention and treatment of postmenopausal osteoporosis. A SERM is a non-steroidal estrogen agonist/antagonist, so it acts like estrogen on some tissues and acts as an anti-estrogen on other tissues in a woman's body. It is not a steroid, so it is not made from cholesterol, and its chemical structure does not resemble estrogen. Raloxifene acts as an anti-estrogen on the breasts and uterus but acts like estrogen in reducing the risk of vertebral spine fractures. Raloxifene is also prescribed as chemoprevention for breast cancer in postmenopausal women who have osteoporosis and also are at high risk for developing breast cancer. 33% of women on raloxifene experience hot flashes, sleep disturbances and depression, and raloxifene increases a woman's risk for blood clots and strokes. Estrogen protects all bones in a woman's body from osteoporosis-related fractures, whereas, raloxifene focuses mainly on her spine. Neither wrist fractures nor hip fractures are reduced with raloxifene.

TSEC

For women who have not had a hysterectomy, a new pharmaceutical option for the prevention of postmenopausal osteoporosis is a tissue selective estrogen complex (TSEC). By combining estrogen with a selective estrogen receptor modulator (SERM), these medications harness the health benefits of estrogen replacement therapy without subjecting a menopausal woman to the drawbacks of progesterone.

Menopausal women who have a uterus require progesterone to offset estrogen therapy's stimulation of uterine tissue overgrowth. Estrogen replacement therapy has not been associated with an increased risk for breast cancer. It is the combination of estrogen-plus-synthetic progestin that slightly increases a woman's risk of breast cancer, so the less a menopausal woman's breasts are exposed to progesterone, the better. Coupling estrogen to the uterine protection power of a SERM eliminates a woman's need for progesterone. Duavee is a daily oral pill that combines 0.45mg of conjugated estrogen, (the estrogen found in Premarin) with 20mg of bazedoxifene, a SERM that does not cause a change in breast density and offsets estrogen's stimulation of the uterus. On its own, bazedoxifene is a SERM with bone protection capabilities, as well.

A TSEC, like Duavee, is a progesterone-free alternative to traditional estrogen-plus-progestin therapy for relief of menopausal symptoms and prevention of osteoporosis, in women with a uterus. Because a TSEC is a combination of an oral estrogen with a SERM, this medication increases a woman's risk of blood clots and strokes. Menopausal women who have had a hysterectomy do not need uterine protection, so Duavee is not used in women without a uterus.

TIBOLONE

Tibolone (Livial) is a tissue-specific steroid that combines the effects of estrogen, progesterone and testosterone in a daily oral pill. It is not available in the United States, but since the 1990s it has been successfully used by millions of postmenopausal women in over 90 other countries for the prevention of osteoporosis-related fractures and treatment of bothersome menopausal symptoms.

Tibolone's estrogen metabolite prevents osteoporosis, relieves hot flashes and night sweats, and improves vaginal tissue health and lubrication. Its progesterone metabolite protects the endometrial lining of the uterus. Unlike oral estrogen, SERMs or TSECs, tibolone does not increase a woman's risk for blood clots. Tibolone's testosterone metabolite improves mood and memory and lifts libido. Tibolone helps maintain lean muscle mass, as well, so the number of falls in tibolone-treated women is 25% less than in their same-aged untreated counterparts.

Like estrogen replacement therapy, tibolone not only protects a menopausal woman's bones from osteoporosis-related fractrues, it provides her with other hormonal health benefits that maintain her quality of life.

WHAT about JOINTS?

If skeletons consisted of just one solid bone, movement would be impossible. So, the skeleton is divided into many bones that articulate or connect with each other at joints. When joints develop problems, a woman suffers from arthritis, meaning, "joint inflammation." Unlike osteoporosis, which is a silent bone disease, arthritis makes itself known. Degenerating joints moan and groan with pain.

Osteoarthritis, "the wear and tear damage" of bone joints, is the most common cause of long-term disability in women older than 65. Osteoarthritis results from the loss of cartilage in a joint, which causes bone to rub on bone and joints to swell and become deformed. This is a painful condition with marked loss of joint motion and mobility. When arthritic joint pain becomes unbearable, the involved joint is surgically fused or replaced with a metal prosthesis. Although it can involve any area of the body, the most common joints for osteoarthritis are in the hands, particularly the thumb, and in weight-bearing joints, such as the spine, hips, knees and feet.

Osteoarthritis strikes postmenopausal women more often than men, and older women have more joints involved with more severe degenerative changes than same-aged men. Estrogen replacement therapy counters osteoarthritic joint degeneration. Menopausal women taking estrogen replacement therapy experience fewer joint symptoms have less joint pain and need significantly fewer hip and knee joint replacements. By reducing inflammatory chemicals and cartilage turnover within joints, estrogen reduces joint destruction.

RHEUMATOID ARTHRITIS

Rheumatoid arthritis is an autoimmune condition that typically affects the joints in the hands and feet. The immune system misfires and mistakenly attacks normal joint tissues. This causes painful joint swelling, bone erosion, and joint deformity. Low levels of estrogen trigger inflammatory arthritic flares, whereas high levels of estrogen offer protection. For women, the risk of developing rheumatoid arthritis peaks at ages 50 to 54, the menopausal years. Women on estrogen replacement therapy are less likely to develop rheumatoid arthritis.

GOUT

Gout has long been associated with portly men, especially those who could afford to overindulge in rich foods and alcohol. Gout in premenopausal women is uncommon because estrogen helps the kidneys eliminate excess uric acid from their system. But, once a woman loses estrogen, her uric acid levels rise, and she becomes vulnerable to this painful "joint disease of kings." Once a woman is menopausal, it usually takes 8 to 10 years of uric acid accumulation to reach a point where needle-like uric acid crystals are deposited in joints, causing inflammatory gouty arthritis. This arthritic pain, which usually involves the big toe, but other joints can be involved as well, can be excruciating. By around age 60, the number of cases of gout in women and men is about equal. After age 80, more women than men have gout. Menopause hormone replacement therapy decreases gout attacks.

BARE BONES

A woman's lifetime risk of developing breast cancer is 1 in 8. Her chance of dying from breast cancer is 3%. The chance that breast cancer causes a woman to end up helpless in a nursing home is 0%. On the other hand, a woman's lifetime risk of developing a hip fracture is 1 in 6. Her chance of dying within a year of that hip fracture is 20%. The chance that the hip fracture will condemn her to a nursing home is 40%.

Statistically, osteoporosis is far more incapacitating and deadly for a woman than breast cancer. Every year, 50% of the older population takes a fall, either from losing their balance, tripping or slipping at home. Women are 3 times more like than men to break their hip from one of these falls. Women also spend more time in hospitals due to osteoporosis-related problems than they do for heart attacks, diabetes or breast cancer.

Menopausal hot flashes are a harbinger of low bone density, but they herald a lower risk of breast cancer. Women who suffer from menopausal hot flashes have an 80% increased risk of sustaining an osteoporosis-related hip fracture in the future, but they have a 50% reduced risk of breast cancer. Obviously, protecting a menopausal woman's thinning bones with appropriate estrogen hormone replacement therapy is not going to increase her risk of breast cancer. Menopausal women suffering from severe pelvic organ prolapse (POP) problems, such as a dropped bladder or descending uterus, tend to have lower bone density, with an increased risk for osteoporosis-related fractures. Estrogen-dependent collagen protein provides form and function throughout a woman's body. When she loses estrogen, collagen breaks down, so her skin wrinkles, pelvic organs dry out and prolapse, and bones break. Without estrogen-provided collagen support, tissues deteriorate and organs collapse.

Over 75% of bone loss that occurs in a woman during the first 15 years after menopause is due to estrogen deficiency, rather than aging. Getting shorter and hunched over with a dowager's hump may look like a natural consequence of aging, but it's actually a manifestation of estrogen deprivation. When it comes to protecting a woman from osteoporosis-related fractures, non-estrogenic medications are suboptimal. They are too difficult to take, unnatural or fraught with unusual and distressing complications.

Footing and balance decline in an estrogen-deprived, postmenopausal woman. The fact that menopause hormone therapy improves both postural stability, as well as bone density, helps explain why estrogen is superior to bone preserving raloxifene (Evista), or the bisphosphonates, in preventing wrist and hip fractures due to falling. The dynamics of appropriate menopause hormone therapy and fracture protection are too multifactorial to be explained solely by estrogen's effect on maintaining bone density. A menopausal woman's brain processing speed and her postural stability are maintained with estrogen therapy. Her sensory perception, comprehension, and coordination, stay the course, as well. Without estrogen, muscles weaken, joints creak, bones break, confusion surfaces, and frailty sets in.

On the basis of United States Life Tables, a woman aged 65 can expect to live an average of 20 more years. No longer is it an issue of how long a woman is going to live, but how she lives that matters. As a woman grows older, the ability to live independently and tend to her activities of daily living (ADLs) is golden. A pleasant quality of life with dignified aging comes to those who, not only talk the talk but whose bones allow them to walk the walk. Will she be a vibrant and active senior, pursuing personal interests, and participating with family and friends? Or, will she end up a frail, infirm and dependent spectator, languishing in a nursing home somewhere?

The bone protecting power of on-going estrogen replacement therapy has been demonstrated to take place in women over age 65, and even in women over age 75. It's never too late for estrogen's bone protection. As a woman gets older, however, the dosing of her medications need to be adjusted to accommodate her aging metabolism and declining liver and kidney function. This holds true of estrogen replacement therapy, as well. Lower doses of estrogen help maintain bone density in older women, and using transdermal hormone preparations, such as estrogen skin patches, gels or sprays, eliminate any increased risk of strokes or blood clots associated with oral estrogen pills. This allows a menopausal woman to continue safely taking estrogen well into her elderly years, so it's a win-win for an older woman. She derives all the health benefits of long-term estrogen replacement therapy with minimal risk.

Osteoporosis is a devastating disease that kills and cripples women, yet it is totally preventable. Steps a woman can take to prevent this menopausal tragedy include a healthy lifestyle, exercises, adequate calcium and vitamin

D intake, and, most importantly, well-orchestrated estrogen replacement therapy. The root cause of osteoporosis-related fractures in postmenopausal women is estrogen deficiency, so it's not surprising that nothing takes care of a woman's bones as naturally and effectively as estrogen. At any age, a woman needs estrogen to stay strong, estrogen strong.

LET'S GET CARDIOVASCULAR

What does menopause have to do with a woman's heart? Well, love makes the world go round, but estrogen keeps a woman's life-sustaining blood flowing. The human heart beats 100,000 times a day, pumping oxygen and nutrient carrying blood through a 100,000-mile network of arteries, veins, and capillaries. In a woman, all this pumping action over long distances circulates better and flows smoother with estrogen's support. Estrogen deprivation not only causes profound heartbreak, but it also leads to heart attacks, strokes and sudden death in postmenopausal women.

During the 40 years' span between puberty to menopause, estrogen's life force has been shielding a premenopausal woman from heart disease and strokes. Unfortunately, once she loses her estrogen protection, cholesterol streaks and inflammatory chemicals are free to oxidize and damage blood vessels, her heart loses its rhythm, and faulty blood flow curtails optimal brain function. This silent and progressive destruction of blood vessels supplying a menopausal woman's vital organs takes 10 to 15 years of estrogen deprivation to inflict permanent organ damage. No one dies from menopausal hot flashes. Instead, hot flashes and night sweats portend a future of crippling cardiovascular diseases associated with estrogen deficiency.

Cardiovascular disease (heart disease and strokes) is the #1 killer of women worldwide. It claims more lives each year than all breast cancers, Alzheimer's, HIV/AIDS, accidents, and malaria combined. Heart disease has been thought of as a "man's disease," yet heart disease has been the leading cause of death for women since 1908. Death rates from cardiovascular disease are higher in women than men, as well.

45% of women will die from heart disease and strokes. Only 3% of women will die from breast cancer. Although cardiovascular disease kills 10 times more women than breast cancer, most women are far more afraid of being diagnosed with breast cancer than they are from having a heart attack. In women, heart disease is too often a silent killer - 66% of women who suddenly die from a heart attack had no previous symptoms.

Each year, more women than men die from heart disease, and the gap between men and women's survival after a heart attack continues to widen. Women are twice as likely as men to die within the first few weeks of suffering a heart attack. 42% of women who have heart attacks die within a year, compared with 24% of men. Women are twice more likely than men to die following heart bypass surgery. Compared to 25% of men, 50% of women who survive a heart attack will be disabled with heart failure within six years of their adverse cardiac event. Surprisingly, despite women's increased risk of morbidity and mortality from cardiovascular diseases, women comprise only 24% of participants in heart-related studies.

ATHEROSCLEROSIS

The cardiovascular system involves cardio- (heart) plus vascular (blood vessels) within the body, so cardiovascular disease includes heart disease, heart failure, hypertension, and strokes. Atherosclerosis is a disease process where calcified, cholesterol plaques (atheromas) accumulate in arteries, causing hardening and narrowing (sclerosing) of the blood vessel. This compromises blood flow to the organs dependent on these channels for oxygen and nutrients. Unstable or necrotic cholesterol plaques within atherosclerotic vessels can break open, causing a blood clot to form at the cholesterol crater and occlude the artery. Depending on which artery is blocked, the clot can cause either a heart attack or a stroke. A heart attack (myocardial infarction, MI) occurs when blood flow through a coronary artery supplying the heart is blocked, causing that part of the heart muscle to die. Similarly, a stroke is a "brain attack," because blood flow to a part of the brain is blocked, causing that part of the brain to die. Strokes (cerebrovascular accident, CVA) are due to problems with cerebral arteries supplying blood to the brain.

MAN's HEART vs. WOMAN's HEART

Since it takes 10 to 15 years of estrogen-deprivation for atherosclerosis to progress enough to cause a heart attack or stroke in a postmenopausal woman, women present with heart disease 10 years later than men. Men are hit with heart attacks in their late 50s to early 60s. Women, on the other hand, are retired, "little old ladies" in their late 60s to early 70s when they suffer a heart attack. Not only is there an age difference between when men and women show up with cardiovascular disease, but they also have differing symptoms, as well.

When men have a heart attack, they experience the easily recognizable symptoms of crushing chest pain, shortness of breath, cold sweats, and pain radiating up the left jaw and down the left arm. Most women having a heart attack manifest far less dramatic symptoms; only 40% of women even have chest pain. Women may experience shortness of breath, weakness, unusual fatigue, flu-like symptoms of nausea, vomiting and cold sweats, dizziness or lightheadedness, irregular pain in the upper chest, back, in the arms, or neck or jaw pain. Many times, a woman's intuition, tells her "something is not right." If a woman is experiencing these symptoms for more than 10 minutes, and they are not going away when she lies down, then she should call 911 immediately. Time lost is heart muscle lost. While she's waiting for the ambulance to arrive, she should chew on an adult aspirin (325mg), or 4 baby aspirins (81mg x 4 = 324mg), if there are no adult aspirins around, to lower the risk of a blood clot.

Not only do women present with heart disease differently from men, but they also have different types of heart disease, as well. Men and women lay down cholesterol plaques differently, have differing issues with small vessel disease, and their hearts break and fail differently, as well.

CHOLESTEROL-PLAQUE DISTRIBUTION

Women lay down cholesterol plaques differently than men. Men's plaques deposit in clumps, whereas women's plaques are distributed more evenly (streaked) throughout the artery's walls. Women's angiographic studies (x-rays of blood vessels) may then be misinterpreted as "normal," so appropriate cardiac therapy may not be initiated.

ATRIAL FIBRILLATION (A FIB)

To stay alive, the heart needs to keep pumping to maintain blood circulating throughout the body. To keep blood flowing, capillaries drain into veins that drain into bigger veins, which drain into the body's two largest veins, the superior vena cava and the inferior vena cava. These cava veins return blood to the heart's right atrial chamber. The atria are the smaller upper chambers of the heart that pump blood into the larger ventricle chambers below. The heart's ventricles then contract to pump blood to the rest of the body. This requires synchronized electrical signals directing synchronized cardiac muscle contractions. If the ventricles cannot pump blood efficiently, heart failure occurs.

With atrial fibrillation (A fib), the heart's atrial chambers quiver rapidly and erratically, so they cannot squeeze blood reliably into the ventricles. Not only does this cardiac electrical malfunction cause an "irregularly irregular" heart rhythm, but blood also stagnates and clots in the atria. Pieces of this clot can break off and travel to other parts of the body. This traveling clot can lodge into an artery supplying the brain, causing a stroke, or it can lodge into an artery supplying a part of the bowel, causing bowel death. Patients with atrial fibrillation (A fib) may be placed on blood thinners to try to prevent blood clots from migrating. In many cases, people with atrial fibrillation (A fib) don't have any symptoms, while others experience heart palpitations (feeling that their heart is racing or fluttering), chest discomfort or shortness of breath. Because the heart is not pumping blood effectively, people with atrial fibrillation (A fib) may also experience fatigue or lack of energy, lightheadedness or exercise intolerance.

Atrial fibrillation (A Fib) is an irregular heart rate that becomes more common as people get older, disproportionately affecting more postmenopausal women than same-aged older men. Despite treatment for this irregular heart rhythm, postmenopausal women also have an increased risk of heart attacks, strokes and death secondary to atrial fibrillation (A fib), compared to same-aged older men.

CORONARY MICROVASCULAR DYSFUNCTION

Women are more likely than men to have coronary microvascular dysfunction, in which the blood vessel walls of the heart's tiny arteries are damaged or diseased. Standard tests, including traditional angiograms or cardiac catheterizations, can miss blockages in these smaller arteries. Specialized coronary reactive tests are required to properly evaluate these smaller blood vessels as they are exposed to different stimuli. If this cardiac condition is not diagnosed correctly, it cannot be treated properly, so the woman ends up with heart failure and dies.

BROKEN HEART SYNDROME

Broken heart syndrome, also known as stress-induced cardiomyopathy or takotsubo cardiomyopathy, can sometimes cause fatal heart damage to postmenopausal women. Extreme emotional stress, such as the death of a loved one, a family tragedy, or constant anxiety, can lead to a sudden onset of heart failure with electrocardiogram (ECG) changes and elevated cardiac enzymes mimicking an ischemic heart attack. Angiogram studies show clear coronary arteries supplying the heart, but demonstrate an abnormal bulging of the apex of the heart with abnormal ventricular wall motions.

An abnormal response to stress-related hormones such as adrenalin or norepinephrine may cause vasospasm of the tiny microvascular arteries in the heart, resulting in inadequate delivery of oxygen to the heart muscle. Fortunately, 95% of individuals with broken heart syndrome recover, and cardiac function improves over 2 months.

HEART FAILURE

Women's heart failure is different from men's heart failure. Gender-related differences in the anatomy and physiology of the heart muscle (myocardium) have been found. Heart failure with preserved ejection fraction or diastolic dysfunction occurs more commonly in women than in men.

Male heart failure occurs when a man with a history of blocked coronary arteries presents with shortness of breath, fluid in the lungs, low blood pressure and low left ventricular ejection fraction, indicating that the heart is failing to pump blood out to the rest of the body (systolic dysfunction).

On the other hand, a postmenopausal woman with heart failure presents with sudden onset shortness of breath, fluid backing up in her lungs and high, not low, blood pressure. Her echocardiogram (ultrasound of the heart) shows a normal left ventricular ejection fraction, and she has no evidence of blockages in the coronary arteries supplying her heart. A small stiff heart that is not pumping effectively is typical of "postmenopausal heart failure."

MORE HEART DIFFERENCES

Even before sustaining a heart attack, women are twice more likely then men to suffer from depression. After a heart attack, 60% of women will develop depression, compared with 20% of men, and depression doubles the risk for yet another heart attack. Nearly 10% of women have polycystic ovary syndrome (PCOS), and this ovarian hormone imbalance is a harbinger for diabetes and premature heart disease in young women. 20% of the population suffers from autoimmune diseases, such as lupus, rheumatoid arthritis, thyroiditis or multiple sclerosis, and 75% of those affected are women. Such autoimmune diseases damage the heart and blood vessels, increasing a woman's risk of heart attacks and strokes. 16% of women suffer from migraines, compared to 5% of men, and migraines with auras increase a person's risk of having a stroke.

1 in 12 women develops preeclampsia or other blood pressure problems during pregnancy. Preeclampsia is a gradual rise in blood pressure

combined with increasing amounts of protein in the urine, which can lead to seizures, liver damage and uncontrolled bleeding in a pregnant woman. It is a dangerous obstetrical condition that can be harmful to mother and baby, and it is treated by delivering the baby. A pregnancy complicated by preeclampsia doubles a woman's risk of having a stroke later on in life. A woman who develops gestational diabetes during her pregnancy has a 7-fold increased risk of going on to develop type 2 diabetes. Diabetes creates a higher cardiovascular risk for women than men, and diabetes doubles the risk of a second heart attack in women, but not in men.

Marital stress worsens the prognosis of heart disease more in women than it does in men. Not only do men and women communicate differently, their hearts malfunction differently, as well.

All in all, estrogen-deprived postmenopausal woman suffer more from debilitating and deadly cardiovascular problems than any other group. Appropriately timed and properly managed menopause hormone replacement therapy can maintain a woman's estrogen-edge over cardiovascular disease.

STROKES

Women face a higher lifetime risk of strokes than men. A stroke strikes 1 in 5 women, and 60% of female stroke victims will die from their stroke, while 60% of the survivors will have a permanent disability. 1 in 6 men develops a stroke with a mortality rate of 40%. Women are more likely than men to suffer a stroke as their first manifestation of cardiovascular disease, whereas men initially present with coronary heart disease.

80% of strokes are the ischemic variety, meaning a blood clot occludes an artery supplying a part of the brain, so delivery of oxygen and nutrients to that part of the brain is blocked, and brain tissue dies. This can occur spontaneously within an atherosclerotic diseased artery, or from atrial fibrillation (A fib) or congestive heart failure, where a piece of clot within the heart chamber can break off and travel to occlude a cerebral blood vessel that supplies the brain. 20% of strokes are hemorrhagic, meaning a damaged blood vessel bursts, so blood is no longer flowing to that part of the brain the vessel supplied, so brain tissue dies. 4 minutes without oxygen, and brain cells die.

In the case of a stroke, symptoms come on suddenly and require immediate attention:

- Numbness or weakness, usually in the face, arm or leg, and often on just one side
- Trouble walking, loss of balance or coordination
- Confusion, or trouble speaking or understanding
- Double or blurred vision
- A strong headache for no reason or feeling dizzy

While women experience the classic symptoms of stroke, they can also experience other symptoms that may be dismissed as something else, such as:

- Pain. Women are more likely to report pain as a symptom of their stroke, including chest pain, and sudden face or limb pain.
- Sudden nausea and vomiting, often accompanied by other more common symptoms of stroke.
- Hiccups. These involuntary contractions of the diaphragm are controlled by nerves in the brain that, when irritated, are associated with a stroke. It is unknown why this occurs in women but not in men.
- Extreme exhaustion. Women often experience a sudden fit of sleepiness, such as the urge to lie down and take a nap before having a stroke. Taking a nap is the worst thing to do when having a stroke since one's brain needs to stay active enough to get help.

If a woman is experiencing the sudden onset of any of these symptoms, she should call 911 immediately. Time lost is brain lost. Because 20% of strokes are the bleeding variety, it is recommended that people not take aspirin while they're waiting for the ambulance since aspirin can make a hemorrhagic stroke worse. The most effective stroke treatments are available only if the stroke is officially diagnosed within the first 3 hours of the first symptoms. Upon any suspicion of stroke, the woman should be brought to the Emergency Room immediately. A wait and see approach could be devastating. For a woman 65 years or older, regularly taking a low-dose baby aspirin (81mg) several days week helps decrease her risk of strokes and heart attacks by 20%. As a bonus, after being on aspirin for 5 or more years, a postmenopausal woman's risk of breast cancer, as well as her risk of colon cancer, diminish by 20%.

With or without estrogen therapy, postmenopausal women have more strokes than men, and strokes kill more women than men. The chance of suffering a stroke increases as a woman ages, particularly once she is over the age of 65, and strokes can be tragically incapacitating.

STROKES, OLDER WOMEN & ESTROGEN

The traditional standard-dose oral female hormone replacement therapy increases clot-associated stroke risk in older postmenopausal women over the age of 60. "Standard-dose" means the oral hormone pills usually prescribed to 50-something menopausal women, and traditional menopause hormones usually refer to conjugated equine estrogen (Premarin) or conjugated equine estrogen (Premarin) plus medroxyprogesterone (Provera) pills.

Once a woman reaches her mid-60s, she may no longer need the standard-dose of female hormones she was once prescribed in her 50s to alleviate bothersome menopausal symptoms. Just like the doses of her other medications are usually decreased as she moves into her elderly geriatric years, her estrogen replacement therapy dosing should be reduced, as well. An older postmenopausal woman can transition to either a lower oral estrogen dose or switch to a transdermal estrogen delivery system, such as estrogen skin patch, topical gel or skin spray. These dose reductions will reduce her risk of clot-related problems. She can retain the benefits of menopause hormone replacement while decreasing clot-related problems by switching from oral conjugated equine estrogen (Premarin) to FDA-approved, pharmaceutical-grade, bioidentical or "body"-identical low-dose oral micronized estradiol (Estrace) estrogen, which is associated with a lower risk of stroke. Also, transdermal hormone preparations, such as estrogen skin patches, topical gels or skin sprays, do not increase a woman's risk for blood clots or strokes, so they are safe estrogen options for older women, as well.

By coupling a touch of aspirin, and possibly a smidge of low dose statin, to a low dose bioidentical oral estradiol or a transdermal estrogen delivery system, the "geripause cocktail" provides an older postmenopausal woman with the many health benefits of estrogen with the clot-busting power of aspirin and cholesterol plaque-stabilizing influence of statins. This will protect an older woman's heart, her brain, her bones, her bladder and many other body parts.

Since 1994, all menopause hormone therapy users in Finland have been included in a national health insurance database, enabling detailed assessment of hormone therapy use and heart disease. A study assessed heart disease mortality from 1995 to 2009 in more than 290,000 women who had used menopause hormone therapy and compared them with same-aged women who had not taken estrogen replacement. Taking menopause hormone therapy for 1 to 8 years was associated with a 50% reduction in the rate of heart disease mortality. The hormone therapy-associated protection against heart disease mortality was more pronounced in women less than 60 years old.

In March 2015, researchers updated their Cochrane Database of Systematic Reviews on hormone therapy. They evaluated 19 randomized controlled trials involving 40,410 postmenopausal women. Women on oral menopause hormone therapy were compared to women taking a placebo (sugar pill). The average age of the women participating in most of the studies was over 60 years old, and the length of time they were on hormone therapy varied across the trials from 7 months to 10 years. In a subgroup analysis of the data, women who had initiated hormone replacement therapy within 10 years of menopause had 30% lower mortality from cardiac disease, and the incidence of coronary heart disease was reduced by 50%. By starting estrogen replacement therapy in a timely manner, there was no increased risk of stroke in women who embarked on menopause hormone therapy within 10 years of their final menstrual period.

KNOWING your NUMBERS

When it comes to preventing cardiovascular disease, a woman needs to know her numbers. A woman's risk for heart disease and strokes is determined by her age, menopausal status, family history, personal medical issues and life style. 80% of heart disease and strokes can be prevented with lifestyle changes. Risk factors for heart disease include:

FAMILY HISTORY

If a woman has a first-degree male relative (father or brother) diagnosed with coronary heart disease before age 55 or a first-degree female relative (mother or sister) with coronary heart disease before age 65, then she is at increased risk for heart disease, as well.

AGE

The risk for heart disease and strokes increases, as one gets older. The further a woman gets away from menopause the greater her risk. Before menopause, estrogen protects women from heart disease, so premenopausal women are much less likely than postmenopausal women to experience adverse cardiac events. An estrogen-deprived postmenopausal woman loses estrogen's edge over cardiovascular disease. At age 55, the lifetime risk of developing cardiovascular disease is equal for men and postmenopausal women, at which point heart attacks and strokes become more severe and more deadly in women.

SMOKING

More than 50% of all heart attacks in women under the age of 50 are tobacco-related.

When it comes to heart disease and strokes, smoking obliterates the estrogen advantage premenopausal women have over men. Women over the age of 35 who smoke should not take oral contraceptive pills (OCPs), because smoking increases their chance of having a stroke or heart attack.

SEDENTARY LIFESTYLE

When it comes to increased risk for heart disease, not exercising is just as bad as smoking, having high blood pressure or elevated cholesterol. Just 30 minutes a day of moderately intense physical activity will do the trick. A woman does not need to engage in strenuous workouts or pound her knee and hip joints jogging on hard asphalt for cardiac health. Brisk walking adequately strengthens the heart muscle, improves cholesterol levels, reduces stress, strengthens bones and controls weight. Moderate exercise is better than strenuous exercises at lowering blood pressure and building collateral vessels for improving blood flow to the heart. 10,000 steps a day keeps disease and disability away.

DIET

Poor dietary choices increase a woman's risk for adverse cardiovascular events. Eating foods found in the Mediterranean diet, and consuming about 1500 kcal of food a day, are heart healthy diet strategies for menopausal women. Food from plants does not contain cholesterol, and eating 7 fruits and vegetables a day is a heart-healthy, low-calorie way of procuring helpful anti-inflammatory anti-oxidants and user-friendly vitamins and minerals.

The Mediterranean diet involves eating primarily plant-based foods, such as fruits and vegetables, legumes, beans, whole grains, and seeds and nuts, particularly walnuts, almonds, and pistachios. A piece of whole grain bread is part of most meals. Fish, shellfish and poultry make up most of the protein intake. There are lots of chickens around, so eggs are eaten frequently. Red meat consumption is limited to once or twice a month. Dairy products are consumed in moderation, mostly as cheese and yogurt, and butter is used as a condiment. There is a little red wine consumed with meals, as well. Lard and saturated animal fats are replaced with the best oil on earth, extra-virgin olive oil. Herbs and spices, instead of salt, are used to flavor food. Since this food has such a high satiety index, there is very little processed sweets or dessert consumption. Remember, the more colorful the food is on the plate, the healthier the meal.

DIETARY FATS – the GOOD, the BAD, and the UGLY

Steering clear of chemically modified fats keeps arteries supplying the heart and brain clear of callous cholesterol plaques, as well. Naturally occurring fats are one of three general types:

- Saturated, (saturated with hydrogen), e.g., butter, lard or coconut oil
- Monounsaturated (one double bond in the fatty chain), e.g., olive oil or canola oil
- Polyunsaturated (two or more double bonds in the fatty chain) e.g.- omega-6 oils like sunflower or safflower oil, or omega-3 oils like fish and flaxseed oil.
- Partially hydrogenated fats or trans fats, on the other hand, are man-made fats that are derived by the forced chemical addition of hydrogen atoms into liquid polyunsaturated oils to make them solid at room temperatures. These chemically modified fats are harmful. Manufacturers use them in food processing because these fats stay solid at room temperature, so they are an economical way to keep flavors stable and extend the shelf life of packaged foods.

The chemical structure of these artificially hardened fats is different from either that of a naturally hard saturated fat (like butter) or unsaturated (mono- or poly-) natural oil. Saturated fats have a rigid straight molecular form. This straight configuration tends to "rigidify" the body structures into which they are incorporated, like blood vessels. This explains the association between saturated animal fats and atherosclerosis or hardening of the arteries.

Monounsaturated or polyunsaturated fats, on the other hand, have wavy or zigzag forms (called "cis" forms), so they are more flexible, and go with the flow, so they do not lead to atherosclerosis.

Partially hydrogenated fats also have bent molecular shapes, but they are bent in the mirror-opposite direction of naturally occurring unsaturated fats, so they are referred to as "trans" fats. Because partially hydrogenated or trans fats are bent the wrong way, they are difficult for the body to grab onto and metabolize properly. They are not incorporated into cell structures nor can they be excreted in the normal fashion. Since they can't go anywhere, they're left loitering around in the blood's circulation. Partially hydrogenated or trans fats are oxidized and incorporated into cholesterol plaques that narrow and harden arteries that supply the heart and brain. These bad fats accelerate atherosclerosis and significantly increase a woman's risk for cardiovascular disease. Partially hydrogenated or trans fats should be avoided.

Naturally occurring monounsaturated oils (olive oil and canola oil) and polyunsaturated oils (omega-3 and omega-6) increase "good" HDL-cholesterol ("H" for hurray), and decrease "bad" LDL-cholesterol ("L" for lousy), and are essential nutrients for health.

ALCOHOL

Alcohol consumption should be limited to no more than one drink a day. One drink is either 4 ounces of wine, 12 ounces of beer or 1.5 ounces of hard liquor. Any more than that increases a woman's risk of breast cancer, heart failure, and strokes.

OBESITY

1 out of 3 women is overweight (BMI 25 to 29.9) and 1 out of 3 women is obese (BMI 30 or greater). This means that only 1 out 3 women is sporting a healthy weight. This is a big problem for women's health.

A person's heart is only the size of their closed fist. The bigger and heavier a woman is, the harder it is for her heart to pump blood to the rest of the body. If the woman is carrying the weight around her abdomen (apple-shaped), she is at even higher risk of heart disease than a woman who's heavy in the hips and thighs (pear-shaped). Abdominal (visceral) fat is more metabolically damaging than subcutaneous fat. If a woman's waistline measures more than 35 inches, she is at increased risk for heart disease and strokes. Obesity puts a woman at risk for diabetes, cardiovascular disease, blood clots and breast cancer.

BLOOD PRESSURE

Blood pressure (BP) should be around 120/80. Once blood pressure reaches 140/90 or above, hypertension needs to be treated. Hypertension is defined as blood pressure (BP) readings repeatedly greater than or equal to 140/90. High blood pressure means the blood running through the arteries flows with too much force, and this puts more stress and strain on the heart. The increased shearing pressure on the walls of the blood vessels causes microscopic tears, and when the body repairs these tears, scar tissue traps loitering partially hydrogenated or trans fats, LDL cholesterol plaque, and white blood cells. This atherosclerotic process leads to hardened, narrowed arteries with blockages causing heart attacks and strokes.

1 out of 3 adults has hypertension, and half of them don't know it. Hypertension is a silent disease without symptoms; meanwhile, the person is sustaining permanent, irreversible organ damage, leading to a heart attack, stroke, blindness and kidney failure. In adults younger than 45 years old, hypertension is more common in men than in women. The prevalence becomes equal in both genders between ages 45 and 64 years. After age 65, women take the lead.

After 10 to 15 years of estrogen deficiency, postmenopausal arteries have narrowed and hardened from atherosclerotic damage. These distorted blood vessels increase an older woman's blood pressure, as well as increase her risk of heart attacks and strokes. By preventing atherosclerosis and relaxing blood vessels, estrogen helps a woman maintain her healthy blood pressure.

DIABETES

If a woman has diabetes, her chance of a heart attack or stroke triples. Diabetic women tend to be overweight or obese with cholesterol problems, and they are at greater risk for developing atherosclerosis and blood clots compared to their normal weight counterparts. Atherosclerosis is particularly aggressive and progresses significantly faster in women with diabetes than in women without diabetes. Elevated blood sugar is toxic to blood vessels and nerves, and diabetes increases triglycerides, a fatty substance circulating in the bloodstream. Elevated fatty triglycerides increase a woman's risk for cardiovascular disease far more than it does in men. After age 45, more women than men have diabetes, and diabetes is a more common cause of cardiovascular disease among women than among men.

Diabetes is diagnosed when:

-   Fasting blood (serum) sugar is ≥ 126 mg/dL
-   Random, or after eating, blood (serum) sugar is ≥ 200 mg/dL
-   Blood hemoglobulin A1C is ≥ 6.5%

Elevated blood sugars are particularly toxic to small blood vessels and nerves, which scar down and die. Capillaries damaged by diabetes limits blood circulation in tissues, and prevents wounds from healing properly.

CHOLESTEROL & LIPIDS

Prior to menopause, women tend to have lower cholesterol than men of the same age. The liver manufactures over 85% of the cholesterol in the blood and estrogen influences the liver's production of different types of cholesterol. Compared to men or postmenopausal women, a well-estrogenized woman is walking around with heart healthy cholesterol ratios.

Cholesterol is an essential component of every cell in the human body, so it needs to be delivered here, there, everywhere. Since cholesterol is a type of fat, it does not dissolve in the salty waters of the bloodstream. Carriers called lipoproteins transport cholesterol through the blood. The lipid or fatty part of lipoproteins surrounds the cholesterol, and the protein part provides a water-soluble shell for navigating through the salty bloodstream.

The two types of lipoproteins that carry cholesterol to and from cells are low-density lipoprotein (LDL) and high-density lipoprotein (HDL). Estrogen increases the liver's production of the "good" HDL-cholesterol ("H" for hurray) and reduces "bad" LDL-cholesterol ("L" for lousy) production. HDL-cholesterol is considered good because HDL is better for arteries than LDL-cholesterol. LDL transports cholesterol to the walls of the arteries, contributing to plaque formation and atherosclerosis. HDL acts as a scavenger, cleaning up LDL's messes and eliminating debris that can weasel its way into the lining of arterial walls, hardening and narrowing arterial passages.

Triglycerides are another type of fat, and they're used to store excess energy from the diet. Elevated triglycerides can be caused by a diet very high in carbohydrates, obesity, diabetes, inadequate physical activity, smoking or excess alcohol consumption. High levels of triglycerides in the blood are associated with aggressive atherosclerosis.

Fats circulating in the blood stream are collectively known as blood lipids. "Desirable" blood lipid levels for women are:

- Total cholesterol ... less than 200 mg/dl (over 240 mg/dl is high risk)
- LDL-cholesterol ... less than 130 mg/dl
- HDL-cholesterol ... over 50 mg/dl (over 60mg/dl protects against heart disease)
- Triglycerides ... less than 150 mg/dl

Although serum cholesterol is still considered an important risk factor for cardiovascular disease, cholesterol consumed in food is now thought to play a relatively insignificant role in determining blood levels of cholesterol. Recommendations to reduce dietary cholesterol have been a mainstay of U.S. food guidelines for years, starting with guidance from the American Heart Association in the 1960s. A better understanding of cholesterol metabolism has lead to a shift in the scientific view of dietary cholesterol in recent years. Reflecting this improved understanding, the Dietary Guidelines Advisory Committee, a group of experts appointed by the U.S. Department of Health and Human Services and U.S. Department of Agriculture, has recommended that limitations on dietary cholesterol be removed from the 2015 edition of Dietary Guidelines for Americans. The egg is glorious after all.

Although genetics and gender influence blood cholesterol levels, lifestyle choices have a tremendous impact on the quality and quantity of life we live. Statin medications can lower "bad" LDL-cholesterol levels and stabilize cholesterol plaques within the arteries, but statins have side effects such as muscle pain, nausea, and liver inflammation. There are no cardiac medications that significantly increase "good" HDL-cholesterol. Boosting HDL-cholesterol is accomplished through improved lifestyle activities, such as moderate exercise, better dietary choices, and not smoking. Estrogen replacement therapy increases a menopausal woman's HDL-cholesterol and lowers her LDL-cholesterol.

CIMT

The common carotid intima-media thickness (CIMT) is a measure of the inner wall thickness of the common carotid artery blood vessels supplying the brain. It is an FDA-approved ultrasound technique for evaluating atherosclerosis progression. The thicker the CIMT, the worse the atherosclerotic damage. Atherosclerosis of the coronary arteries supplying the heart leads to a heart attack, and atherosclerosis in the carotid arteries supplying the brain results in a stroke. The carotid artery in the neck is assessed using an ultrasound with computer-measured software.

CIMT is also a reflection of atherosclerosis occurring in the coronary arteries supplying the heart. Not only is the atherosclerotic burden in the carotid arteries supplying the brain the same as the atherosclerotic burden in the coronary arteries supplying the heart, the CIMT is an independent predictor of future cardiovascular events, including heart attacks, strokes, and cardiac death. CIMT evaluates how well a woman's arteries compares to other women her age. If her vascular age matches her chronological age or younger, then she has a lower risk for cardiovascular disease. If her vascular disease is older than her chronological age, then she needs to step up her game if she wants to decrease her risk of heart attacks and strokes. Fortunately, CIMT can identify atherosclerosis problems independent of other cardiac risk factors, and since CIMT can identify disease in its early stages before a woman has symptoms, the disease process can be slowed down with lifestyle changes and therapeutic interventions.

CACS

99% of the calcium in our bodies resides in our bones and teeth. The other 1% is essential to the functioning of the brain, the blood vessels, transmission of nerve impulses, for blood clotting and muscles contracting. As we age, we start depositing calcium in the wrong places. Kidney stones are more common in older people, calcium deposits occur in arteries of people older than 65 years old, and calcification of the breasts is seen in women over the age of 50.

Using a CT scan, calcification within cholesterol-plaques lining the coronary arteries supplying the heart can be quantified, producing a coronary artery calcium score (CACS). The higher the CACS, the more the coronaries are calcified. Although some calcification of the coronary arteries is a normal aspect of aging, more extensive coronary artery calcification reflects significant atherosclerotic damage with increased risk for heart attack. Menopause hormone therapy reduces a woman's calcified plaque burden in the arteries supplying her heart and brain.

CIMT and CACS are non-invasive, painless diagnostic modalities, and they are very useful tests for assessing any underlying atherosclerosis in women who may not have symptoms of cardiovascular disease. They are also used to monitor the effect of therapeutic interventions in slowing down arterial narrowing and calcification. More recent clinical trials involving menopause hormone therapy incorporate CIMT and CACS to measure the hormonal impact on atherosclerosis.

ESTROGEN'S EDGE

Prior to menopause, when estrogen, particularly estradiol, is flowing through a woman's heart and blood vessels, she is protected from cardiovascular disease. As she slides into menopause, however, physiological changes occur that increase her risk for heart disease and strokes. By the sixth decade of life, or after 10 to 15 years of estrogen deficiency, cardiovascular disease rates in women are not only equal to men of the same age, morbidity and mortality associated with heart attacks and strokes are much greater in women than in men.

When it comes to protecting the blood vessels that supply the heart and brain, estrogen is a many splendored thing. Estrogen lowers a woman's risk for hypertension, thus preventing damage to walls of arteries being pounded by high blood pressure. By increasing nitric oxide production, estrogen modulates vascular tone and lowers blood pressure. Through its actions on the brain's appetite and satiety centers, estrogen plays an important role in helping maintain healthy body weight. Estrogen is also responsible for directing fat accumulation away from a woman's abdominal (visceral) region to her hips and thighs. Abdominal (visceral) fat accumulation contributes to the production of inflammatory substances that damage blood vessels. Estrogen increases insulin sensitivity and lowers blood sugars, which helps protect blood vessels. Estrogen replacement therapy in a menopausal woman decreases her risk of developing diabetes by 25%, whereas full-strength statin drugs increase her risk of developing diabetes by 50%.

Estrogen's promotes favorable cholesterol and lipid levels by stimulating the liver's production of "good" HDL-cholesterol and decreasing levels of "bad" LDL-cholesterol. LDL-cholesterol gets incorporated into the cholesterol plaques lining and narrowing arteries. Through its antioxidant and anti-inflammatory effects on arterial walls, estrogen prevents atherosclerotic plaque build up.

Physiological levels of estrogen maintain favorable balances between blood clotting factors and prevent excess clot formation. Estrogen allows arteries to remain soft and flexible, so they can easily dilate and deliver needed blood flow to the heart, brain, and other organs. By hobbling destructive tissue mechanisms that bring on atherosclerotic changes in a woman's arteries, estrogen helps fend off cardiovascular disease, heart attacks and strokes in women. Prior to menopause, estrogen has been circulating in a woman's body for 40 years, protecting her blood vessels from the devastation of atherosclerosis. Once she loses estrogen, however, corrosion and destruction of her arteries begins. Menopausal hot flashes indicate that adverse vascular changes are already occurring among healthy appearing middle-aged women.

Simply because a woman is no longer reproducing does not mean that she should be deprived of estrogen's cardiovascular protection. In fact, a woman's body fares much better when she initiates estrogen replacement therapy during her early menopausal years, before atherosclerotic changes have marred and scarred her blood vessels. Women who start hormone therapy between ages 50 to 59, or within 10 years of menopause, decrease their risk of cardiovascular disease by 50%, compared to women who are not taking estrogen replacement. Initiating menopause hormone therapy in a timely manner does not increase a woman's risk for strokes, either.

Oral estrogen pills are absorbed through the intestinal tract and are delivered to the liver. The estrogen then stimulates the liver's increased production of proteins that cause blood clots. By avoiding the liver's first-pass effect, transdermal estrogen preparations, such as estrogen skin patches, topical gels or skin sprays, do not increase a woman's risk for blood clots or strokes. Replacing estrogen in a newly menopausal woman significantly decreases her "all-cause mortality," or her risk of dying from any and all causes, including breast cancer, by 30%.

Once a decade has gone by and menopause has become a distant memory, atherosclerosis may have progressed to the stage of hardened, narrowed arteries full of unstable, necrotic plaques. After the atherosclerotic damage has been done, it's too late to embark on estrogen replacement therapy for heart and brain protection. Using appropriately timed and properly managed hormone replacement therapy, a menopausal woman can keep estrogen's protective edge over aging arteries and significantly decrease her risk of cardiovascular disease. No other single medication takes care of a woman's heart, brain, and her thousands of miles of blood vessels, better than estrogen.

A WOMAN'S BRAIN- the FINAL FRONTIER

For many women, menopause means that their menses has stopped, and "mental pause" has occurred. Women may experience poor concentration with fuzzy thinking described as brain fog, or muddled mentation characterized as cobwebs in the brain. Loss of estrogen brings on "menopause moments," with episodes of forgetfulness involving word retrieval issues, such as not remembering a common word while conversing, losing one's train of thought while talking or not grasping someone's name. A menopausal woman may not be as proficient at multi-tasking as she use to be. She may feel overwhelmed and frazzled by events she previously took in stride.

Independent of hot flashes or night sweats, estrogen loss alters sleep architecture, so a menopausal woman has trouble falling asleep, staying asleep or waking up refreshed. She may experience more lightheadedness and dizziness, as well as intermittent loss of balance or clumsiness. Women who had never considered themselves emotional may experience mood swings, depression, anxiety, irritability, and crying spells. Some women find apathy and crushing fatigue unwanted menopausal companions.

Although less than 2% of women younger than 65 years old have dementia, as the years go by, a woman's risk of dementia or Alzheimer's disease escalates at triple the rate of a man's. Dementia is a general term for loss of memory and other intellectual abilities serious enough to hobble activities of daily living and result in dependency on others. Dementia is a disease; it is not a natural condition of aging. Alzheimer's disease is the most common form of dementia, accounting for 70% of dementia cases, with the remaining 30% a consequence of atherosclerosis, the narrowing and hardening of arteries that supply the brain. One in three 65-year-old women will go on to develop dementia. Although women comprise 75% of the population over 90 years old, half these women have dementia, compared to 1 in 4 men in this age group.

Even in healthy women, brain volume begins to decline as estrogen levels fall during the menopausal transition. This loss of brain tissue (atrophy) is particularly obvious in the hippocampus, parietal and frontal lobes of the brain, the areas that are primarily associated with memory and cognition. A similar loss in brain volume does not begin in men until a decade later, around age 60. Why do menopausal women lose brainpower?

When a woman goes through menopause, her estrogen levels dramatically plunge by 90%, so her brain and body sustain a traumatic hit from rapid estrogen loss. Men's testosterone levels, on the other hand, have been decreasing slowly and gradually with age. Starting at around 30 years old, a man's testosterone levels decrease by just 1% to 2% annually. Even if an older man's testosterone levels are 50% lower than what they were in his 20s, he still has a lot more testosterone in his system than a woman does. His body converts some of this testosterone to brain-sustaining estrogen. In adipose (fatty) tissue, the aromatase enzyme converts testosterone to estrone (E1) estrogen, which is then modified to brain-boosting estradiol (E2) estrogen. Men over the age of 60 have 3 times more estrogen circulating in their system than women of similar age. Because of their adipose (fatty) tissue's peripheral conversion of testosterone to estrogen, older men's brains have more estrogen than the brains of estrogen-deprived, older postmenopausal women. Although an older man's testosterone levels may be lower than what they use to be, he still has more testosterone to convert to estrogen than an older woman ever will, so his brain functions better longer. No wonder dementia is more common in older, estrogen- deprived women compared to older men.

There is no cure for Alzheimer's disease and no treatment prevents the disease from destroying brain function. A person may live anywhere from two to twenty years after being diagnosed with Alzheimer's disease. Those years are spent in an increasingly dependent state that exacts a staggering emotional, physical and economic toll on the individual and their loved ones. There is no real way to cope with one's downward dementia spiral, and there has never been a patient who recovered from Alzheimer's disease. It's one of the devastating tragedies of living beyond 65 years old. Fortunately, menopausal women can help decrease their risk of developing dementia with appropriately timed and properly managed estrogen replacement therapy.

BRAIN COMPOSITION

The brain remains the least understood of all the vital organs. Although the brain is only 2% of a person's body mass, it requires 25% of the body's oxygen and glucose supply. That's a tremendous amount of energy needed to fuel an organ. Unlike other organs that can rely on reserve fuel sources, such as fatty acids, or non-oxidative metabolic pathways, such as anaerobic metabolism, for sustenance during lean times, the brain cannot shift its metabolic pathways to utilizing alternate energy sources for survival. The brain needs a steady diet of glucose.

The brain is totally dependent on blood flow to survive. Without oxygen, a brain cell will die in 30 seconds, whereas it takes 3 hours of oxygen deprivation for a heart muscle to die. Because uninterrupted delivery of oxygen and glucose to the brain is vital to its existence, 1/3 of the brain is composed of blood vessels. To ensure that the brain never goes without its energy lifeline, glucose gets an unencumbered free pass into brain cells. Other tissues in the body require insulin to transport needed glucose into their cells.

25% of the body's cholesterol is in the brain, and the healthy brain contains more than 60% fat. Cholesterol insulates every brain cell's message deploying exit appendage (axon), so any process or medication that noticeably decreases cholesterol impedes the speed and efficiency in which messages travel down these axons.

With all this sugar and fat, the brain fits the profile of a glazed doughnut, yet this 3-pound convoluted mass of gray and white matter within our skull serves to control and coordinate all our mental and physical actions. Our brain determines everything we think, feel, dream, do and say. Our lives are only as good as our brain.

ATHEROSCLEROSIS DAMAGING the BRAIN

Among estrogen's many other glories, when it comes to brain function, estrogen is a many splendored thing. Through its cholesterol-lowering, anti-oxidative and anti-inflammatory capabilities, estrogen hampers atherosclerotic damage to the carotid arteries and cerebral blood vessels supplying the brain. Estrogen keeps these tributaries free of detrimental plaque buildup and prevents the arterial walls from narrowing and hardening. By binding to estrogen receptors on the cells lining the blood vessels' walls, estrogen stimulates the release of nitric oxide (NO), which causes vasodilation and increases blood flow to brain tissues.

Depending on the individual woman, it takes 10 to 15 years of estrogen deprivation for her arteries to be ravaged by atherosclerosis. Due to decreased blood flow to the brain, sustained reductions in oxygen and glucose delivery, as well as unreliable removal of metabolic waste products due to compromised capillary flow, brain function in an estrogen-deprived postmenopausal woman deteriorates. Estrogen keeps a woman's vascular channels flexible and dilated, and her brain's circulatory system free of detrimental debris.

Once a woman is 10 to 15 years beyond menopause, her blood vessels are burdened with atherosclerotic changes. Introducing estrogen hormone therapy to a postmenopausal woman aged 65 or older, or initiating estrogen replacement more than a decade beyond menopause can be problematic. At this late stage, oral estrogen pills may destabilize necrotic cholesterol plaques, causing a vulnerable plaque to crack open. A blood clot then forms across the crack. If the clot occludes the artery, blood flow is blocked, so tissue supplied by the blocked artery dies. If this clot happens in an atherosclerotic coronary artery supplying the heart, a heart attack occurs. If the clot forms in a cerebral artery supplying the brain, then a stroke or "brain attack" occurs.

At the dawn of menopause, however, blood vessels are still plaque free, elastic and flexible, so hormone therapy initiated within 10 years of menopause allows estrogen to continue its custodial magic of preventing atherosclerotic changes and maintaining healthy blood vessels.

BRAIN ARCHITECTURE

In addition to delivering on-going plumbing services to the brain's blood vessels, estrogen is involved in preserving the brain's cellular architecture and maintaining its inventory of neurotransmitters needed for brain cells to communicate with one another. This is how thoughts flourish, desires develop, memories are retrieved, and actions originate.

A thinking brain cell is known as a neuron. A neuron is an electrically excitable cell that processes and transmits information through electrical and chemical signals. Chemical signals from one neuron to another travel across synapses between these brain cells. A typical neuron is composed of a cell body with a nucleus, dendrites and an axon. Dendrites are multiple twig-like structures that arise from the cell body, branching multiple times, giving rise to a complex "dendritic tree." Dendrites receive messages from other neurons. Each neuron gives rise to just one axon, which transmits messages from the cell body to other neurons. The axon may branch hundreds of times to reach other neurons. All neurons are electrically excitable and maintain voltage gradients across their cell membranes by metabolically driven ion pumps. A cholesterol-rich myelin sheath provides insulation for the main axon emanating from a neuron. This allows for rapid transmission of electrical impulses down a brain cell's axon to reach its dendritic synapse. Upon reaching the synapse, the electrical message is converted to a chemical messenger that ferries the message across the synaptic junction between the axon's dendritic ends, to the receiving dendrite of the recipient brain cell. By transmitting messages from one neuron to another across synapses, these chemical messengers, referred to as neurotransmitters, allow brain cells to communicate with each other. Serotonin, dopamine, norepinephrine, and acetylcholine are neurotransmitters involved in thinking, feeling and moving.

Optimal brain functioning depends on all aspects of neurotransmissions performing up to speed. Although a person may appear idle, their brain is generating waves of activity all the time, even while sleeping.

Unlike other cells that multiply simply by dividing, only special types of stem cells give rise to neurons. In humans, the generation of neurons usually ends in adulthood, and the brain reaches full maturity by around age 25. So, we've got to hold on to the brain we've got.

HOT FLASHES

Lack of estrogen disrupts the body's thermostat located in the hypothalamus of a woman's brain. This causes thermal turmoil in 85% of menopausal women. These "body heat" episodes include hot flashes, night sweats, cold snaps, heat waves, or just feeling warmer than others. Such disturbances can occur once or twice a day or over a dozen times a day. They can occur for just a few years during the menopausal transition, or they can continue to exist for over a decade or more beyond a woman's final menstrual period.

Hot flashes, also referred to as hot flushes, and night sweats, are the most common culprits invading a menopausal woman's temperate tranquility. The sudden disruption generated by heat rising from a woman's core, radiating throughout her chest, and flushing up her neck and face, is not a desirable "hunka-hunka burning love" feeling. Rather, it is an overwhelming sensation of imminent spontaneous internal combustion, where clothes are ripped off, windows flung open, and a woman is tethered to a high-powered fan. Hot flashes can also be laced with apprehension, peppered with palpitations and drenched with sweat. Hot flashes are not energizing power surges; they are unwelcome and depleting stamina sappers. Night sweats disrupt sleep, and most women find it difficult to get back to sleep once awakened. Night after night of sleep deprivation leads to irritability, poor concentration, fatigue, apathy, and depressive symptoms.

Hot flashes and night sweats are detrimental to a menopausal woman's quality of life. Because the root cause of menopausal hot flashes is the lack of estrogen hormone, the most effective and reliable natural remedy for hot flashes is estrogen replacement therapy.

MINDFUL of EBB and FLOW, PEAKS and TROUGHS
PMS

Slumps in estrogen levels are connected to mood disorders in women. Although their blood serum hormone levels may be within the normal range, some women are more sensitive than others to the normal fluctuations of estrogen levels associated with monthly menstrual cycles. Diminished estrogen levels can lead to anxiety, irritability, feeling overwhelmed, melancholy, apathy, and sleep disturbances. These hormonal windows of psychological vulnerability occur when estrogen levels descend, such as before a woman's menstrual period, during the postpartum period and across the menopausal transition.

Most women cope with mild moodiness associated with waxing and waning estrogen levels. In 20% of women, however, such drops in estrogen levels can precipitate psychiatric problems requiring on-going therapy and psychotropic medications. For women already suffering from mental health issues, low-estrogen levels may exacerbate underlying psychiatric conditions.

85% of reproductive-aged women have at least 1 premenstrual symptom as part of their monthly cycles. These symptoms vary from woman to woman, and they can vary from month to month in the same woman. Acne, appetite changes, particularly chocolate and comfort carbs seeking behavior, fatigue, painful breasts, achiness, fluid retention and sleep disturbances, are all part of the premenstrual landscape. Fortunately, most women cope with mild versions of these symptoms and do not need treatment.

20% of women seek medical care to alleviate disruptive symptoms of premenstrual syndrome (PMS), and 5% of women suffer from premenstrual dysphoric disorder (PMDD).

PMDD is a severe extension of PMS, where extreme mood shifts can disrupt a woman's work or school activities, as well as damage her relationships. With PMDD, psychological symptoms dominate over physical issues, so selective serotonin reuptake inhibitor (SSRI) antidepressants, such as fluoxetine (Paxil, Sarafem), paroxetine (Paxil, Briselle) and sertraline (Zoloft), have emerged as first-line therapy.

Monophasic low-dose oral contraceptive pills (OCPs) contain the same dose of estrogen and progesterone in each hormone pill, so they provide a woman with a stable hormonal milieu throughout the month. These types of oral contraceptive pills (OCPs) are effective in alleviating garden-variety PMS symptoms.

PREGNANCY HIGHS

Pregnancy is associated with high levels of estrogen and progesterone hormones. During the pre-ovulatory or follicular phase of a woman's menstrual cycle, her ovarian follicles produce estrogen. Only after ovulation, when there is the potential for conception and pregnancy, does the ovarian corpus luteum manufacture the "pro-gestation or pro-pregnancy" progesterone hormone.

Blood serum levels of progesterone go from nothing prior to ovulation to a post-ovulation level of 20 ng/mL. With pregnancy, progesterone levels rise and remain at the post-conception level of 80 ng/mL for the first and second trimesters of pregnancy. During the 3rd trimester of pregnancy, progesterone levels surge to 300 ng/mL. Because progesterone's sole purpose is to help prepare and maintain the uterus and breasts for pregnancy, it does not stick around after the baby is born. 3 days after the baby is delivered, progesterone disappears, and this rapid drop in progesterone helps trigger lactation. Actual breast milk comes in a few days after colostrum does. Only after the next ovulation, when there is the potential for another pregnancy, will progesterone surface again.

A woman glows with pregnancy because her estrogen levels are soaring. A woman will produce more estrogen during just one pregnancy than she ever will throughout her entire non-pregnant life. Astonishingly, the amount of estrogen produced during the third trimester of pregnancy equals 100 years of menopausal hormone therapy. Blood serum estradiol levels during pregnancy are 30 times higher than non-pregnancy estrogen levels. Estradiol levels average around 150 pg/across most of a normal menstrual cycle. There is a very short preovulatory estradiol peak that can reach 400 pg/ml, but during a woman's menstrual period, estradiol levels drop down to menopausal troughs of 30 pg/ml.

Women enter the third trimester of their pregnancy with estradiol levels in the 6,000 to 7,000 pg/mL range. After the baby is born, mom's estrogen levels plunge rapidly, reduced to postpartum estradiol lows of 30 pg/mL. Within a week of delivering the baby, a new mom's estrogen levels have dropped to the same negligible estrogen levels found in a postmenopausal woman.

POSTPARTUM LOWS

During pregnancy, a woman is flying high on estrogen and progesterone, but once the placenta (afterbirth) is delivered, and the baby is sleeping soundly in the nursery, her hormones are descending rapidly, crashing and burning down to menopausal levels. No wonder 85% of women experience some shade of postpartum blues, which starts 3 to 5 days after the baby is born and lasts for 1 to 2 weeks.

20% of new moms develop postpartum depression requiring medical intervention, and 66% of women suffering from postpartum depression also have an underlying anxiety disorder. The risk of psychiatric problems soon after delivering a baby is greater in women who have suffered from mental health issues prior to their current pregnancy.

20% of women diagnosed with postpartum depression have bipolar disorder, and using antidepressants as the sole treatment for bipolar depression can worsen the course of the disease. Diagnosis depends on identifying the depressed phase, as well as the manic or hypomanic phase, so often there is a delay in correctly diagnosing this condition. The postpartum period, a time of very low estrogen, poses the greatest risk for new mania episodes in a woman's life.

Although the baseline risk for postpartum psychosis is 1 in 500, the risk rises to 1 in 7 for women who have suffered from a previous episode of postpartum psychosis. Postpartum psychosis is a psychiatric emergency, and inpatient treatment in a hospital is essential to ensure the safety of the mother and the baby. 5% of women suffering from postpartum psychosis are driven to kill their newborn or other children. Postpartum psychosis may be resistant to psychotropic medications, and if the patient is not responding to alternative interventions, electroconvulsive therapy (ECT) is considered.

When a new mother is trying to deal with psychological issues while simultaneously tending to a newborn, her fragile emotional state can interfere with bonding and may lead to attachment issues for mom and baby. Tragically, suicide accounts for about 20% of postpartum deaths and is the second most common cause of maternal mortality in postpartum women. Hemorrhage is the leading cause of death among new moms.

MOODY MENOPAUSE

What hormones giveth, lack of hormones can taketh away, and without estrogen, the brain loses crucial chemicals that nurture clear thinking, dreamy sleeping, and happy feelings. Independent of hot flashes, and despite living a perfect, stress-free life, estrogen loss constitutes a window of vulnerability to psychological issues for middle-aged, menopausal women.

Menopause is associated with higher rates of depression compared to other times in a woman's reproductive life. The Harvard Study of Moods and Cycles, the Seattle Midlife Women's Health Study, the Penn Ovarian Aging Study, the Massachusetts Women's Health Study and the Study of Women's Health Across the Nation (SWAN) show that the risk of depression doubles in women going through menopause. Despite 25% of women between the ages of 46 to 64 taking an antidepressant, this menopausal age bracket has the highest rate of completed suicides among women. Diagnosing depression in menopausal women can be challenging because the symptoms of depression and the normal symptoms of menopause overlap. Irritability, insomnia, fatigue, apathy, concentration difficulties, weight gain and libido changes are common symptoms of normal menopause, but they occur in clinically depressed individuals, as well.

A useful predictor of menopausal depression is a history of a mood disorder. Women who have suffered from postpartum depression, moderate to severe PMS, or have had intermittent or on-going psychiatric issues, may experience exacerbation of these problems during menopause. Panic attacks, obsessive-compulsive disorder, anxiety and bipolar mania may worsen or relapse during menopause. Estrogen loss due to menopause shifts brain chemicals, which can exacerbate mental health issues. 20% of women suffering from depression may also have an overlooked thyroid disease, so thyroid function should always be assessed when evaluating mood disorders in women.

The onset of schizophrenia in men occurs around ages 20 to 25, while in women initial onset occurs 5 to 10 years later. 40% of women with schizophrenia, however, do not manifest their disease until their late 40s. This second peak in the incidence of schizophrenia is not observed in men. Men suffering from schizophrenia fall ill more frequently and severely at a young age, and then less frequently and more mildly later in life. Women's menopausal schizophrenia illness is more difficult to treat and has a worse clinical course than what is observed in same-aged male patients. By regulating dopamine neurotransmitter systems in the brain, estrogen helps protect women from psychotic episodes.

NEUROTRANSMITTERS – the ULTIMATE COMMUNICATORS

In the absence of any real-life tragedies, melancholy or lack of joy in an otherwise healthy menopausal woman reflects low estrogen levels in the brain. Estrogen helps maintain the inventory of chemicals the brain depends on to transmit messages from one brain cell to another. Lack of estrogen depletes neurotransmitter supply and cripples communications between brain cells.

Serotonin, dopamine, norepinephrine, acetylcholine, and endorphins are neurotransmitters that influence emotions and expressions, moods and sentiment, sleep and dreams, learning and memory, pleasure and pain, posture and locomotion, movements and fine motor skills. Love, sex, and commitment are powered by neurotransmitters. Besides antibiotics used for infections, antidepressants and narcotics are the most commonly prescribed medications given to Americans, and two of these medications work on neurotransmitters.

Because of their impact on a range of activities connected to being human, neurotransmitters are powerbrokers in the brain. The serotonin neurotransmitter is involved with mood and attitudes; norepinephrine with attention and cognition; acetylcholine with learning and memory;

endorphins with pain and pleasure, and dopamine with motivation and rewards. Dopamine is also involved in lactation, locomotion, and coordinating movements.

Most substances that lead to addiction act by increasing dopamine levels. From a word origin standpoint, the similarity between the words "dopamine" and "dope" may be a phonic coincidence, but most addictive drugs impact dopamine and render the user dopey. Heroin, narcotics, cocaine, marijuana and alcohol all increase a person's sense of pleasure through their action on dopamine. Nicotine binds to nicotinic acetylcholine receptors that augment dopamine release. Cravings and addictions are propelled by brain sensations generated by neurotransmitters, and wicked withdrawal symptoms occur when brain cells are cut off from their supplier.

Antidepressants increase serotonin, norepinephrine or dopamine levels, either by preventing their reuptake, such as selective serotonin reuptake inhibitors (SSRIs), serotonin norepinephrine reuptake inhibitors (SNRIs), tricyclic antidepressants (TCAs) and tetracyclic antidepressants (TeCAs) which are SNRIs, or by preventing the enzymatic breakdown of these neurotransmitters, which is how monoamine oxidase inhibitors (MAOIs) work. Nausea, headaches, dry mouth, weight gain and sexual dysfunction are common side effects associated with antidepressants.

The SSRI antidepressants paroxetine (Paxil, Briselle), fluoxetine (Prozac, Sarafem) and sertraline (Zoloft) interfere with the breast protection effectiveness of tamoxifen (Nolvadex) used in breast cancer treatment and breast cancer prevention. Serotonin transporters are found in bone, and by affecting bone metabolism SSRIs increase the user's risk of osteoporosis-related fractures. First-generation (typical) antipsychotic medications block dopamine, while the newer second-generation (atypical) antipsychotic medications not only block dopamine receptors, they block a specific subtype of serotonin receptor, as well.

In the Women's Health Initiative Study of Cognitive Aging (WHISCA), elderly women with depression were followed for 5 years. Persistent depressive symptoms in older postmenopausal women were associated with cognitive impairment and dementia. The Women's Health Initiative Memory

Study (WHIMS) evaluated postmenopausal women, aged 65-79, for 7 ½ years, and found that antidepressant use was associated with a 70% increased risk of mild cognitive impairment (MCI), yet the most significant increase in antidepressant use is among women aged 65 years and older.

Mild cognitive impairment (MCI) is the transitional state between normal forgetfulness due to aging and the development of dementia. The progression rate from MCI to dementia is about 10% per year, with full conversion to dementia within 10 years. Among postmenopausal women participating in the Women's Health Initiative (WHI) Study, SSRI antidepressant use doubled a woman's risk of hemorrhagic and fatal strokes.

Parkinson's disease is a chronic and progressively degenerative brain disorder manifested by movement-related problems, such as rigidity, walking, more accurately, shuffling very slowly, trouble with balance, and tremor while resting. Eventually, thought processes become affected, depression develops and dementia occurs in the later stages of the disease. Symptoms of Parkinson's disease result from the death of dopamine-generating cells in the brain. Men are twice more likely than premenopausal women to develop Parkinson's disease. Women who have their ovaries removed prior to menopause, and subsequently do not receive estrogen replacement therapy, increase their risk of Parkinsonism by 70%.

MIGRAINES & MENOPAUSE

For many women suffering from headaches, decreased estrogen levels precipitate migraines. A mid-cycle migraine is due to the estrogen dip around the time of ovulation, and the premenstrual drop in estrogen can trigger a menstrual migraine. After delivering a baby, the vertical drop in estrogen levels can cause postpartum migraines. Declining estrogen levels generate more migraines in perimenopausal women, and menopausal women are more susceptible to migraine triggers.

Migraines in women are related to a complex interaction between the trigeminal or 5th cranial nerve, the brain's pain control centers and circulating levels of estrogen. When the trigeminal nerve is activated, neurotransmitters are released, causing vasodilation and extravasation (leakage of blood products) that result in an inflammatory response. This inflammatory reaction further stimulates the trigeminal nerve to transmit impulses back to the brain, where they are perceived as pain. Estrogen withdrawal lowers the trigeminal nerve's threshold for activation and interferes with the brain's processing of pain. Stabilizing a woman's estrogen environment decreases the frequency of migraines.

Brain cells communicate with each other through neurotransmitters, and in a woman's brain, neurotransmitters are influenced by estrogen. Whether stimulating enzymes that manufacture these chemicals, inhibiting enzymes that break them down, or implicated in the trafficking of brain chemicals here and there, estrogen is involved in neurotransmitter availability and brain cell-to-brain cell connectivity. Estrogen withdrawal during menopause can precipitate or compound mental health problems and exacerbate brain dysfunction.

Estrogen replacement therapy may be all most menopausal women need to cope with mild mood disorders. Some may require additional therapeutic interventions to navigate the psychological pitfalls of estrogen deficiency. Adding estrogen to a menopausal woman's psychotropic medication enhances treatment outcomes by accelerating response time to therapy and eliminating the need for increased dosing. This hormonal-pharmacological synergy achieves therapeutic results while minimizing side effects. Appropriate estrogen therapy helps menopausal women decrease their risk for mood disorders, psychiatric problems, cognitive impairment, and dementia.

DEMENTIA & ALZHEIMER'S DISEASE

Estrogen does more than just recalibrate the brain's hypothalamic thermostat or maintain neurotransmitter inventory. There are estrogen receptors in every nook and cranny of a woman's brain, so estrogen is involved with brain business at all levels. Estrogen receptors are particularly bountiful in brain structures that are important for cognitive functioning, such as the frontal lobe, parietal lobe, and hippocampus. Estrogen confers resilience against nerve damage and promotes brain cell survival through its antioxidative, anti-inflammatory and custodial actions.

Estrogen impacts brain cells by modulating synapses between neurons, protecting against apoptosis (preprogrammed cell death), maintaining the profile of dendritic branching and arborization, thwarting neurofibrillary tangles, and preventing the build-up of damaging debris in brain tissue. Without estrogen, brain circuits cross, messages are not transmitted, toxic amyloid deposits accumulate, tau proteins malfunction, and brain cells die. This leads to progressive and irreversible dementia. Earlier age at menopause is associated with a faster decline in a woman's cognitive capabilities, as well as increased deleterious brain changes associated with Alzheimer's disease. Brain imaging studies that compare aging women's brains to equally aged men's brains show that older women lose brain matter at a faster rate than their male counterparts. Obviously, estrogen is involved in maintaining brain health, brain architecture, and brain functioning.

Longitudinal research involves observing or following a group of subjects to study the long-term effects of a particular therapy. These studies compare the impact of taking or not taking a particular medicine for an extended period of time, often for more than a decade, so they provide helpful insight into lifespan issues. Longitudinal studies on menopausal women show that estrogen replacement therapy administered within 5 years of menopause, and used for at least 10 years, helps maintain brain function. The Baltimore Longitudinal Study of Aging (BLSA) which followed hundreds of menopausal women for 16 years, the Cache County Study, which followed thousands of menopausal women in Utah, and the Leisure World study, which followed thousands of women living in a retirement community in southern California, all indicate that women who use any menopause hormone therapy within 5 years of menopause, and stay on their estrogen replacement for 10 or more years, decrease their risk of Alzheimer's disease by 30-50%.

Over 95% of the time, dementia and Alzheimer's disease occur after the age of 65. If estrogen therapy is initiated when a woman is in her 60s, or a decade or more beyond menopause, it may be too late to help her brain. Once a postmenopausal woman's brain tissue has sustained permanent damage, estrogen cannot restore or revitalize dead or destroyed brain cells.

In the Women's Health Initiative Memory Study (WHIMS), post-menopausal women who were 65 or older when they started menopause hormone therapy experienced greater cognitive decline and dementia, compared to the placebo (sugar pill) group. In the WHIMS-MRI Study, magnetic resonance imaging (MRI) scans were used to assess the impact of menopause hormone therapy on brain anatomy. Brain scans revealed greater brain atrophy and tissue loss in older women who initiated menopause hormone therapy after age 65 than seen in women taking a placebo. On the other hand, brain MRI studies in younger menopausal women treated with hormone therapy reveal beneficial changes in brain morphology.

Initiating hormone therapy 10 to 15 years after menopause has long come and gone, does not resurrect a woman's brain architecture or rejuvenate cerebral function. It may even be detrimental to the remaining brain cells trying to survive. Estrogen cannot resuscitate dead brain cells or revive neurons pruned of their dendrites, poisoned by amyloid deposition or knotted up by neurofibrillary tangles. Quite frankly, nothing can, so preventive maintenance is the key to keeping the brain healthy.

Since dementia occurs at least 10 to 15 years after menopause, short-term estrogen use (4 to 7 years) during the early postmenopausal years is not long enough to show the benefits of estrogen's dementia protection. The Women's Health Initiative Memory Study of Younger Women (WHIMSY) studied whether giving oral conjugated equine estrogen (Premarin) 0.625mg hormone therapy to postmenopausal women aged 50 to 55 affected their cognitive function. Compared to women taking a placebo, these younger postmenopausal women on short-term hormone therapy showed no significant improvement in cognitive function, neither during the 7 years that they were actually taking the estrogen, nor during the 7 hormone-free years that they were subsequently followed. Both the Kronos Early Estrogen Prevention Study (KEEPS) and the Early versus Late Intervention Trial (ELITE) clinical trials also confirmed that using estrogen therapy for only a few years close to menopause neither improves, nor harms, cognitive function.

Short-term estrogen use does not vaccinate a menopausal woman against developing dementia later on. To have a mindful brain accompany a menopausal woman during the last 30 years of her life, estrogen replacement therapy and her brain need to be involved in a long-term relationship. Menopause hormone therapy needs to be started soon after a woman's ovaries stop producing estrogen, and estrogen replacement needs to be continued as long as she wants to retain her brain; otherwise, as the years of postmenopausal estrogen deficiency go by, a woman's brain goes bye-bye.

When any hormone deficiency exists, the hormone needs to be replaced in a timely manner, managed appropriately, and replacement continued until either the body starts manufacturing the hormone again, or until the patient passes away. Adjustments are made to the dosing and delivery of the hormones based on suitable clinical assessments. Insulin hormone therapy is not aborted at some arbitrary age, and thyroid hormone replacement is not simply abandoned because the person is too old for thyroid. On-going, properly managed estrogen replacement therapy is a woman's lifeline to keeping her brain intact and her personhood alive.

IT'S a NO-BRAINER

A menopausal woman's mind is a terrible thing to waste, and a woman's brain simply works better with estrogen on board. Initiating proper hormone replacement early in menopause and appropriately managing long-term estrogen therapy decreases a woman's risk of dementia by 30-50%. As brain cells' twist and buckle to the pathology of dementia, they lose their ability to respond favorably to estrogen. Initiating estrogen hormone therapy around age 60 or beyond, or a decade or more after menopause, is not helpful to brain function. Once dementia's distortion of brain cells has occurred, it's too late for estrogen. Sadly, by this time, a woman's cognitive skills are on a downward trajectory.

Estrogen's power is in the maintenance of neurons, and as part of the brain's custodial crew, estrogen does not engage in new construction. Estrogen does not give birth to new neurons, and at this point in human history, no therapeutic intervention lays down new brain matter. There are no medications that treat Alzheimer's disease or reverse dementia's relentless shuffle towards dependence, disability, and death.

Oxygen, glucose, and estrogen make up the holy trinity of brain survival. Healthy blood flow through patent carotid and cerebral arteries that are free of atherosclerotic damage is critical to the delivery of adequate oxygen and glucose to the cholesterol-rich brain. Maintaining the architectural and functional integrity of the brain's cellular mechanisms for data entry, message transmission, and subject integration is vital to its functions. Without infrastructure the brain deteriorates, and the grim corrosion of confusion and dementia set in. Fortunately, a menopausal woman can hold onto her brain with well-orchestrated hormone therapy.

Initiating estrogen replacement at the dawn of menopause, and appropriately managing hormone therapy for the long haul, not just for 5 to 10 years, will help keep a woman's brain intact and functioning. Limiting estrogen replacement to only short-term therapy will not vaccinate the woman against dementia in the future. Just like the brain needs adequate oxygen and glucose to stay alive, brain tissue needs on-going estrogen for proper maintenance. When it comes to leveraging the optimal protective effects of estrogen on a menopausal woman's brain, hormone therapy should be initiated early in menopause, when neurons and blood vessels are still healthy enough to respond to estrogen. As the years go by, the postmenopausal woman can stay on course with properly managed estrogen replacement therapy. Once a woman reaches 65 years old, adding a low-dose chewable baby aspirin (81mg) several times a week not only helps decrease an older woman's risk of strokes, heart attacks, breast cancer and colon cancer, it helps decrease dementia, as well. In an older postmenopausal woman, a touch of estrogen, a tweak of aspirin, and possibly a smidge of statin, is the perfect "geripause cocktail."

Miserably menopausal and then tragically demented is not a healthy way for a menopausal woman to spend the last 30 years of her life. With appropriately timed and well-orchestrated estrogen replacement therapy, not only does a woman travel comfortably to the sunny side of menopause, but her later years are pleasantly memorable, as well. Only estrogen provides this kind of brain protection power and improved quality of life to a menopausal woman. Nothing else compares to the wisdom of estrogen.

BLOOD CLOTS

For us to survive, our blood needs to clot. If we don't clot in time, we bleed to death. On the other hand, a blood clot in the wrong place could kill us. An unwelcome and unneeded blood clot that forms in a deep vein within the body is known as a deep vein thrombosis (DVT). Most of the time, the blood clot forms in a deep vein located in the leg, pelvis, and upper arm or shoulder region. Left untreated, a DVT can break off, travel down the bloodstream, and lodge in the lung's circulation. This is known as a pulmonary embolism (PE). A very large pulmonary embolism (PE) can block blood flow and compromise oxygen supply, which could result in heart failure. Early treatment of a DVT reduces the chance of developing a life-threatening pulmonary embolism (PE) to less than 1%.

A deep vein thrombosis (DVT) forms when the blood flow in the vein remains stagnant, or there is damage to the walls of the vein, or the blood is congealing and clotting too easily. Anyone can develop a DVT, but the main risk factors are:

- Immobilization, such as bed rest or sitting for long periods of time. Keep ankles rotating and toes wiggling while taking long car trips or plane rides. Walk around every 30 minutes.
- Spinal cord injury or paralysis.
- Limb trauma or orthopedic surgery
- Recent surgery that lasts more than an hour. Increased risk of blood clots lasts for 3 months after surgery.

- Cancer. Cancer may reduce the production of proteins that protect us from unwelcome blood clots.
- A coagulation or blood clotting abnormality (thrombophilia).
- A family or personal history of blood clots.
- Smoking.
- Obesity.
- Diabetes.
- Dehydration.
- Simply being over the age of 40.
- Oral contraceptive pills (OCPs) and menopause hormone therapy can also increase the risk of blood clots, but to a much lesser degree than pregnancy.
- For women, pregnancy, childbirth, and the post-partum period are particularly dangerous times for developing blood clots.

STATISTICS in PERSPECTIVE

- Merely by existing, a reproductive-aged woman's baseline risk of DVT is 1 in 1000.
- Simply by aging, the risk of DVT climbs. In women over age 80, the risk of DVT increases to 1 in 100.
- Oral contraceptive pills (OCPs), oral estrogen pills or selective estrogen receptor modulators (SERMs) such as tamoxifen (Nolvadex), raloxifene (Evista) or ospemifene (Osphena), or the combination of estrogen plus a SERM found in a tissue selective estrogen complex (TSEC), such as Duavee, increases a woman's risk of DVT from 1 in 1000 women to 3 in 1000. Triple the risk sounds like a lot, but the likelihood that a particular woman on oral hormone therapy will develop a DVT is very small, from 1 to 3 women among 1000.
- During pregnancy the risk of DVT increases by 6 times, from 1 in 1000 to 6 in 1000.
- Around the time of labor and delivery, and during the postpartum period, the risk of DVT is 10 times greater than when a woman

is not pregnant. The risk of a blood clot catapults from a non-pregnant woman's risk of 1 in 1000 to 10 in 1000 with a vaginal delivery. Having a Cesarean section further doubles that risk.

- The risk of maternal death associated with pregnancy is 1 in 10,000 women per year.

- While a woman is on birth control pills, her risk of dying from a blood clot to the lung is less than 1 in 100,000 women per year.

Because of soaring estrogen and progesterone levels encountered during pregnancy, the chance of developing a blood clot skyrockets. Not only does the blood itself clot much easier, ostensibly to help decrease blood loss during childbirth, but the pregnant uterus compresses pelvic veins, impeding blood flow, which further compounds a pregnant woman's risk of developing a DVT. In women, pregnancy overshadows everything and anything, in causing the greatest danger for blood clots.

HEREDITY & BLOOD CLOTS

Nearly 10% of the population has a genetic predisposition for forming these abnormal clots in their blood vessels. These conditions are known as thrombophilias, literally meaning, "clotting proclivity." This is in contrast to genetic conditions that cause a person to bleed too easily, such as hemophilia, literally meaning, "bleeding proclivity."

Factor V Leiden mutation, prothrombin G20210A mutation, antithrombin deficiency, protein C and protein S deficiencies, are types of thrombophilias that significantly increase a woman's risk of abnormal blood clots. For example, a woman with Factor V Leiden who takes oral contraceptive pills (OCPs) containing both estrogen-plus-progestin has a 35-fold increased risk of developing a DVT, compared to a 3-fold increased risk for a woman without thrombophilia. It is very risky for a woman with hereditary thrombophilia to either get pregnant or to embark on any hormone therapy. 1 out 3 women who experience a DVT has some hereditary thrombophilia.

For a woman without a familial predilection for deep vein thrombosis (DVT), or who is not suffering from any other condition predisposing her to blood clot formation, her personal chance of having a DVT while on oral estrogen hormone therapy is relatively low.

IT'S in the DELIVERY

In the Women's Health Initiative (WHI) hormone trials, where women took oral conjugated equine estrogen (Premarin) 0.625mg with or without the synthetic progestin, medroxyprogesterone (Provera) 2.5mg, most cases of blood clots occurred during the first couple of years of estrogen exposure, amongst the oldest (70 to 79 years old) participants, and in the heaviest women participating in the study.

Oral estrogen pills are absorbed through the intestines and are initially processed by the liver. During this "first-pass effect" estrogen stimulates the liver to produce more blood clotting factors, which increases the risk of developing DVTs. Estrogen replacement therapy administered through transdermal estrogen preparations, such as skin patches, topical gels or skin sprays, does not increase a woman's risk of blood clots. Transdermal estrogens are absorbed through the skin's capillaries, so they bypass the liver and enter the bloodstream directly. There is no augmented production of blood clotting proteins, so there is no increased risk of strokes or blood clots with estrogen skin patches. Also, the estrogen found in transdermal estrogen preparations is estradiol, which is identical to the estrogen produced by the woman's ovaries, so it is bioidentical or "body"-identical. Fewer blood clots develop while taking the bioidentical micronized oral estradiol (Estrace) compared to conjugated equine estrogen (Premarin) or other synthetic estrogens, whose chemical structure is not identical to the estrogen found naturally in a woman's body.

Obese women and women with diabetes are at increased risk of developing blood clots, just from being obese or having diabetes. Estrogen skin patches, or other transdermal estrogen preparations, provide these women with therapeutic options for menopause hormone therapy, without further increasing their risk for blood clots. Women who have been treated for a deep vein thrombosis (DVT) in the past, and do not have a hereditary thrombophilia, may also consider transdermal estrogens for menopause hormone therapy, as well.

Due to aging blood vessels, older women are at increased risk for adverse cardiovascular events (heart attacks and strokes), as well as developing abnormal blood clots. For women over the age of 65, taking low-dose chewable baby aspirin (81mg) regularly can help decrease their risk for clot-related strokes and heart attacks by 20%. Low-dose statins may help decrease the risk for blood clots, as well.

For older women who want to continue receiving the health benefits of estrogen replacement therapy, without increasing their baseline risk of stroke or blood clots, estrogen skin patches, topical gels or skin sprays, provide safe therapeutic options for estrogen delivery. By supplying a low dose of estrogen that bypasses the liver, these transdermal hormone delivery systems do not increase a woman's risk of stroke or blood clots. For older women who prefer to continue taking oral hormone pills, dropping the dose of oral estrogen from the standard dose of conjugated equine estrogen (Premarin) 0.625mg, or micronized estradiol 1mg, to half those levels, will help decrease the risk of stroke or blood clots associated with hormone therapy. Adding a touch of aspirin (clot buster), along with a smidge of statin (cholesterol plaque stabilizer), to an older woman's low dose estrogen replacement therapy, provides a clinically progressive combination for successful aging.

This "geripause cocktail" will keep an older woman's heart, brain, bones, bladder and vagina healthy, prevent her senses from withering, and decrease her risk of breast cancer and colon cancer, while simultaneously reducing her risk of dementia, osteoporosis, heart attacks, strokes and blood clots. Appropriately timed and properly managed estrogen replacement therapy will keep menopausal women of all ages healthy and relatively free of unwelcome blood clots.

MENOPAUSE HORMONE THERAPY – TYPE, TIME, and TIMING

Once it was finally established that a woman's bothersome menopausal symptoms were due to ovarian failure, initial attempts at replacement therapy involved desiccated and pulverized cow ovaries. Estrogen was not formally identified until 1925. Menopause hormone replacement therapy, and our understanding of the importance of estrogen for a woman's health have come a long way since then.

Menopause is a natural end to a woman's reproductive life cycle, but it should not be the end of her hormonal vitality. Just because she's outliving her ovaries, she should not be condemned to an existence marred by estrogen deficiency. Although a menopausal woman may no longer be able to get pregnant and reproduce, many well-designed clinical trials, as well as extensive research at the cellular, biochemical and genomic level, indicate that her mind, body and spirit benefit from appropriately timed and properly managed estrogen replacement therapy.

TIMING is EVERYTHING

Every woman needs estrogen to preserve anatomical integrity and maintain organ function prior to menopause, during menopause, and after menopause. Estrogen receptors are found throughout a woman's body, not just in her breasts and uterus, so estrogen is vital to a woman's vitality. For 40 years prior to menopause, all of her organs, from her brain to her Achilles' tendons, and everything in between, relied on her ovaries' production of estrogen. Without estrogen, a woman's metabolism slows down, tissue infrastructure breaks down and organ function spirals downward in a relentless decline towards disease and disability.

To maximize the health benefits derived from estrogen replacement therapy, hormone replacement therapy should be initiated within 10 years of menopause. Fortunately, for women who have not had a hysterectomy, Nature made the loss of ovarian hormones relatively simple to determine. Menopause signals the onset of ovarian hormone deficiency, and menopause occurs after 12 consecutive months of not having a menstrual period. If there are any questionable diagnostic issues, blood hormone levels can determine a woman's menopausal status.

When a hormone deficiency is diagnosed, the sooner the hormone is replaced, the less damage the body sustains. Hormone deficiency of any type leads to cellular injury, tissue damage and compromised organ functions, whether that deficient hormone is insulin, thyroid, estrogen or any other hormone. When hormone replacement therapy is delayed, tissue trauma and organ injury resulting from prior hormone neglect cannot be reversed. If one waits a decade or more before treating thyroid deficiency or insulin hormone deficiency, precious therapeutic time is lost, and the patient has already sustained permanent and irreversible organ damage. This holds true for menopausal estrogen deficiency, as well.

Once estrogen-deprived arteries become plagued by atherosclerosis, genitourinary systems fossilize, and brain cells tangle, initiating estrogen at this late juncture will not restore what was lost. Cavalierly embarking on hormone therapy at this late date could be detrimental. Judiciously re-introducing an older postmenopausal woman's system to her long-lost estrogen must be done meticulously with special precautionary measures. Although what's gone is gone, prudent estrogen replacement at this point may help slow down some of the deterioration otherwise exacerbated by ongoing estrogen deficiency.

No absolute contraindication to menopause hormone therapy has been established; however, there are certain clinical situations in which estrogen replacement should not be taken. Women with a history of breast cancer or uterine cancer are usually not prescribed estrogen. Abnormal uterine bleeding, or a questionable breast mass, needs to be evaluated prior to commencing any estrogen therapy. Like many other medications, estrogen is metabolized and broken down by the liver, so women with a severe active liver disease should not take hormones, and porphyria exacerbations may occur with oral estrogen therapy.

Barring any contraindications to taking hormones, estrogen replacement therapy is the most holistic, natural and physiologically correct method of addressing estrogen deficiency and treating bothersome menopausal symptoms. The closer to menopause a woman embarks on estrogen replacement, the sooner her bothersome symptoms resolve, and the better she protects her long-term health.

NURSES' HEALTH STUDY

One of the largest and longest observational studies on estrogen replacement therapy is the Nurses' Health Study. It involved 70,533 postmenopausal women who started hormone therapy soon after menopause and were followed for 20 years. The nurses were 30 to 55 years of age at enrollment in 1976, and those who were on hormone therapy took oral conjugated equine estrogen (Premarin). When all cardiovascular risk factors were considered, the risk of major adverse cardiac events, such as heart attacks or dying from coronary heart disease, was lower among current users of menopause hormone therapy, including short-term users, compared with women who never used estrogen replacement therapy. The mortality among nurses who used menopause hormone therapy was lower than among non-users, even after adjusting for dietary factors, alcohol intake, aspirin use, and exercise.

In addition, over the 20 years of follow-up, even after sustaining a major coronary heart disease event (heart attack or significant atherosclerosis), there was a trend for decreasing risk of recurrent coronary heart disease events with increasing duration of estrogen use, compared to women who were not on estrogen. On the other hand, postmenopausal women who were not using estrogen replacement therapy, and who then went on to suffer a heart attack, did not do so well when they embarked on menopause hormone therapy after their adverse cardiac event. Women in the Nurses' Health Study started estrogen replacement therapy close to menopause, and they benefited from years of long-term hormone therapy.

HERS & HERS II

Suspicion that estrogen-plus-progestin may not be all things to all postmenopausal women was confirmed by the Heart and Estrogen/Progestin Replacement Study (HERS) published in 1998, which was further reinforced with a follow-up study of the participants published in the summer of 2002 (HERS II).

HERS was the first, large, randomized placebo-controlled trial (RCT) to evaluate the efficacy of menopause hormone therapy in preventing heart attacks in women who already had clinical evidence of coronary heart disease. Coronary arteries supply blood to the heart muscle. All the women participating in the HERS trials had a history of a heart attack, coronary artery bypass surgery, percutaneous coronary revascularization or angiographic anatomical evidence of at least 50% occlusion of one or more of their major coronary arteries, prior to enrolling in the HERS clinical trial.

Nearly 2800 women across 20 clinical centers in the U.S. participated in the HERS hormone trials. With an average age of 67, these older women already had significant coronary heart disease and atherosclerosis before they were placed on estrogen-plus-progestin hormone therapy. They were randomized to receive either oral conjugated equine estrogen (Premarin) 0.625mg with the synthetic progestin, medroxyprogesterone (Provera) 2.5mg daily or a placebo (sugar pill) daily. The women were followed for 4.1 years. At the end of the study period, there was no overall reduction in risk of coronary artery disease with menopause hormone therapy, and there was no significant difference between the groups with respect to adverse cardiac events either: 172 women receiving menopause hormone therapy sustained either a non-fatal heart attack or died of heart disease, compared with 176 women who suffered the same, but who had been receiving placebo.

The risk of an adverse cardiac event was higher during the first year in the hormone therapy group compared to the placebo group, but then the risk decreased after the third and fourth years in the hormone group. To determine if this positive trend would continue, the women were followed-up for another 2.7 years in the HERS II trial.

In the HERS II follow-up study, lower rates of heart disease among women taking estrogen-plus-progestin hormone in year 5, 6 or 6.8 of hormone therapy did not persist. After 6.8 years of menopause hormone therapy, HERS II results indicated that estrogen did not reduce the risk of adverse cardiac events in postmenopausal women with established coronary artery disease. Initiating estrogen replacement therapy in an older woman, who had already sustained cardiovascular damage due to years of estrogen-deficiency, did not protect the older woman from another adverse cardiac event.

WHI Studies

The summer of 2002 was monumental in the world of menopause hormone replacement therapy. In the July 3, 2002, issue of The Journal of the American Medical Association (JAMA), results from the follow-up HERS II randomized controlled trial were published. Two weeks later, in the July 17, 2002, issue of JAMA, the principal results of the Women's Health Initiative (WHI) trial assessing the risks and benefits of estrogen-plus-progestin in healthy postmenopausal women were published.

WHI studies confirmed that, even in "healthy" women without evidence of heart disease, embarking on hormone therapy long after menopause has come and gone, is not beneficial for a woman's cardiovascular system. On the other hand, hormones protected women from osteoporosis-related fractures no matter how old they were when they initiated menopause hormone therapy.

The HERS II & WHI principal trial results, released back-to-back within two weeks of each other in July 2002, challenged the world of traditional menopause hormone therapy. Then, in the spring of 2004, the results of the estrogen-alone arm of the WHI menopause hormone trial were publicized. It appeared that postmenopausal women, who had had a hysterectomy and then years later started conjugated equine estrogen (Premarin) without a progestin, did not experience less heart disease than women taking a placebo (sugar pill). Both the summer 2002 and spring 2004 WHI hormone trials had been stopped prematurely, due to increased risk of breast cancer, blood clots, and strokes.

By the late 1900s, 50% of all postmenopausal women were harnessing the health benefits of estrogen replacement therapy. After the HERS II and WHI hormone trial results were published at the beginning of the 21st century, only 5% of were taking hormones. Traditional menopause hormone therapy was no longer considered a beacon for healthy aging. For women over the age of 50, the HERS and WHI hormone trials nearly extinguished the lights on treating ovarian hormone deficiency with appropriate menopause hormone replacement therapy.

To everything there is a season, and this holds true for menopause hormone therapy, as well. Further analysis of the data and follow-up evaluations confirmed that the health benefits of estrogen replacement therapy are maximized, while any risks are minimized, by timing therapy appropriately. The "timing hypothesis" suggests that there is a window of opportunity, shortly after menopause, in which hormone therapy has a beneficial effect on coronary heart disease and brain function. On the other hand, delaying hormone replacement therapy for a decade or more beyond menopause, is not that helpful, and in some women may be detrimental.

We know that a "one size fits all" dress is flattering to no one, and further research confirms that just one type and dose of estrogen replacement therapy is not adequate for menopausal women of various ages with different physiological dispositions. Clinical methods employed for managing other types of hormone deficiency need to be applied to replacing ovarian hormones in a menopausal woman. Similar to medical approaches utilized to address thyroid hormone replacement in hypothyroidism, insulin hormone replacement in diabetes or aldosterone hormone replacement in adrenal insufficiency, menopause hormone therapy should be properly managed according to a woman's clinical needs and therapeutic goals.

The WHI hormone therapy trial involved over 27,000 women, aged 50 to 79 years, with an average age of 63 years old, who were recruited into the study across 40 U.S. clinical centers. Women who had a hysterectomy were randomized to receive either oral conjugated equine estrogen (Premarin) 0.625mg daily or a placebo pill daily and were followed for 6.8 years. Women who had a uterus were randomized to receive either oral conjugated equine estrogen 0.625mg with the synthetic progestin, medroxyprogesterone 2.5mg (Prempro) daily or a placebo pill daily and were followed for 5.6 years.

In the WHI studies, women who initiated hormone therapy close to menopause reduced their risk for coronary heart disease, as well as reduced their risk for diabetes, compared to women not taking hormones. By delaying estrogen therapy, older postmenopausal women increased their risk for heart disease. Analysis of the WHI hormone therapy trials showed that in postmenopausal women aged 50 to 59 years, hormone replacement therapy significantly reduced heart disease and total mortality.

When averaged, both HERS and WHI studies involved similar aged women (HERS was 67, WHI was 63); however, the women in the HERS study already had clinically evident cardiovascular disease, prior to initiating any menopause hormone therapy. Only 3.5% of the women participating in the WHI hormone trials were between the ages of 50 to 54, and over 70% were over the age of 60. The women of WHI did not have obvious or documented cardiovascular disease, so they were considered "average" healthy postmenopausal women, although 70% were overweight or obese, 40% were past tobacco smokers with 10% still smoking at the time they enrolled in WHI, and 40% were currently being treated for hypertension. These women may have been average, but they certainly were not that healthy when they started menopause hormone therapy.

The risk of coronary heart disease is lower in women who start estrogen replacement therapy within 10 years of menopause compared to women who do not take estrogen. It takes about 10 to 15 years of estrogen deficiency for atherosclerosis to take root and damage a woman's blood vessels' architecture and functional reserves. As years of estrogen deprivation go by, the blood vessels supplying a woman's heart become laden with calcified cholesterol plaques, as inflammation and oxidation mar and scar her blood vessels. Her damaged arteries harden and narrow in this unrelenting process known as atherosclerosis.

It takes years of subclinical atherosclerotic changes to occur before a woman develops outward symptoms of coronary heart disease, such as a heart attack, irregular heart rhythm, or in some cases, sudden death. Embarking on oral estrogen therapy after atherosclerosis has already taken hold could destabilize vulnerable cholesterol plaques, and precipitate blood clots across these cracked and jagged cholesterol plaques. If this clot blocks a coronary artery supplying the heart muscle, a heart attack occurs.

In contrast, during a woman's freshly menopausal years, at least within 10 years of her final menstrual period, her arteries are still soft and flexible and relatively free of cholesterol plaques. Starting estrogen replacement therapy during this window of biological opportunity hampers atherosclerotic changes and protects a woman's blood vessels from the ravages of estrogen deprivation.

Computerized axial tomography (CAT or CT) visualization of calcified plaque in the coronary arteries is a marker of atherosclerosis and is predictive of future risk of adverse cardiovascular events, such as heart attacks or sudden death. In a substudy of the WHI trial using the oral conjugated equine estrogen (Premarin) 0.625mg therapy for 7.4 years, it was found that, among women aged 50 to 59 years old, the coronary artery calcium score (CACS) was lower among women receiving estrogen replacement compared to women taking placebo (sugar pill).

Once arteries have been damaged by atherosclerosis, estrogen cannot repair or reverse these vascular damages on its own. At this late juncture, estrogen replacement therapy can no longer redeem arteries scarred and marred by atherosclerosis. It will take the joint effort of multiple medications, blood thinners and possibly cardiac catheterization with stent placement to maintain blood flow through severely narrowed atherosclerotic passages.

The appropriateness and safety of initiating a menopausal woman's estrogen replacement therapy soon after she develops ovarian hormone deficiency, that is, during her early menopausal years, has been further confirmed by other randomized controlled trials, as well. The DOPS, KEEPS, and ELITE trials are among these recent studies.

DOPS

In the Danish Osteoporosis Prevention Study (DOPS), over 1000 recently menopausal women, aged 45 to 58 years, who were perimenopausal or had ceased menstrual bleeding within the past 2 years, were randomized to receive either oral menopause hormone therapy or a placebo for 10 years. The "body"-identical or bioidentical oral micronized 17beta-estradiol was the estrogen used in the study, and for those women with a uterus, oral progestin, norethisterone acetate, was added to the estradiol therapy. The study was mainly designed to evaluate the effects of hormone therapy on osteoporosis fracture prevention, but analysis of coronary heart disease outcome measures were also conducted. The planned duration of the study was 20 years, from 1990 to 2010; however, the hormones were stopped after about 10 years, owing to adverse reports from other trials in the early 2000s. The women who had participated in the trial were followed for cardiovascular disease, death and cancer occurrence for up to 16 years.

When compared to women taking a placebo pill, those women who started menopause hormone therapy within 2 years of menopause, and then took the hormones for 10 years, reduced their risk of heart attack, heart failure and total mortality from all causes by 50%. Early initiation and prolonged hormone replacement using this type of menopause hormone therapy did not increase a woman's risk of breast cancer, nor did it increase her risk for having a stroke.

KEEPS

In the Kronos Early Estrogen Prevention Study (KEEPS), the women enrolled were on average 53 years old (ranging from 42 to 58), and hormone therapy was initiated within 3 years of menopause in all participants. They were randomized to receive either conjugated equine estrogen (Premarin) 0.45mg/day or transdermal estradiol skin patch 0.05mg/day or a placebo.

Women who had not had a hysterectomy added micronized oral progesterone 200 mg for 12 days each month to their estrogen replacement. The women were followed for 4 years.

On hormone therapy, the women's bothersome menopausal symptoms such as hot flashes, night sweats and sleep disturbances were alleviated, and they experienced benefits to mood and sexual function, as well. Overall, those women on menopause hormone therapy experienced improved quality of life compared to the women on placebo. There was no significant difference in the common carotid artery intima-media thickness (CIMT) measured by high-resolution B-mode ultrasound or coronary artery calcium score (CACS) measured by CT scan, between the estrogen users and non-users. CIMT and CACS are markers of heart disease risk: the thicker the wall of the carotid artery supplying the brain or the more calcified the coronary arteries supplying the heart, the worse the atherosclerosis (hardening and narrowing) of the woman's arteries, and the greater her risk for strokes and heart attacks.

After 4 years of menopause hormone therapy, rates for heart attacks, stroke and blood clots were not significantly different between those women who received menopause hormone therapy compared to those who received placebo. For women this close to menopause, there may not be a significant difference in arterial architecture between women taking estrogen replacement therapy compared to women taking placebo. It takes 10 to 15 years of estrogen deficiency to develop damaging atherosclerotic changes in the blood vessels of a postmenopausal woman. The KEEPS trial further confirmed that there are no adverse outcomes to starting estrogen hormone therapy close to menopause. Since estrogen replacement therapy alleviated bothersome menopausal symptoms, the women taking hormones experienced an improved quality of life.

ELITE

The Early versus Late Intervention Trial with Estradiol (ELITE) was designed soon after the WHI results were initially released to test the timing hypothesis. The women enrolled in the ELITE trial were stratified into two subgroups: women within 6 years of menopause (average age 55, and they were on average less than 4 years beyond menopause), and women 10 or more years beyond menopause (average age 64, and they were about 14 years beyond menopause).

The women within each age subgroup were randomized to receive either daily treatment with oral estrogen (1 mg micronized 17beta-estradiol) or placebo. For women who had not had a hysterectomy, those who received the daily estrogen pill applied micronized progesterone gel intravaginally for 12 days each month, while those who were taking the daily placebo pill applied a placebo gel intravaginally for 12 days each month. The primary endpoint was the rate of change of the common carotid intima-media thickness (CIMT) measured every 6 months for 6 years. The thicker the CIMT, the worse the atherosclerosis changes.

During the 6 years of follow-up, there was really no difference between the rates of increase in the CIMT among older women who did not take hormones compared to older women who had delayed initiating hormone therapy until they were well beyond menopause. In contrast, the women who began hormone therapy within 6 years of menopause showed 40% less increase in their CIMT compared to menopausal women who did not take hormone replacement therapy. Women who took estrogen therapy early in their menopausal years experienced significantly less atherosclerosis and less damage to the arteries supplying their brain, compared to older women who delayed initiating hormone therapy until a decade past menopause.

DEMENTIA and HORMONE TIMING

If a menopausal woman waits too long to start her estrogen replacement therapy, not only does she increase her risk of cardiovascular disease, she increases her risk of dementia and Alzheimer's disease, as well. The atherosclerotic process that damages blood vessels and causes heart disease is also associated with cognitive decline in elderly postmenopausal women.

The Women's Health Initiative Memory Study (WHIMS) is an ancillary study of the Women's Health Initiative (WHI) hormone therapy trials. WHIMS evaluated women aged 65 to 79 years, who had been randomized to receive either menopause hormone therapy or placebo. In the WHI studies, an increased risk of dementia was observed in women aged 65 or older, who had delayed taking hormone therapy until a decade more after menopause. In the estrogen-plus-progestin arm of the WHI hormone trial, elderly women who were 75 and older when they initiated menopause hormone therapy experienced vascular dementia, the type of dementia due to decreased blood flow to the brain, but not increased risk of developing Alzheimer's dementia. The estrogen-alone arm of the WHI hormone trial contained older, obese women, with established atherosclerotic damage to the blood vessels supplying the brain. Their trend for increased risk of dementia reflects the challenges of initiating estrogen replacement therapy decades after menopause.

Recent observational trials suggest that starting estrogen replacement during the early menopausal years reduces the risk of dementia by 30%. A prospective study of 2000 postmenopausal women in Utah concluded that a reduction in the risk of Alzheimer's disease required long-term estrogen replacement therapy, initiated at least 10 years before the symptoms of dementia appear. Furthermore, a meta-analysis evaluating 10 clinical trials found no increase in the risk of dementia or Alzheimer's disease in women who had a history of ever using menopause hormone therapy compared to non-hormone users.

Once an estrogen-deprived menopausal woman sustains damaging changes to her brain, such as pruning of the branches of her brain cells, amyloid deposition and tau disruptions, oxidation damages, or depleted acetylcholine neurotransmitters, estrogen replacement cannot reconstitute what the brain has already lost. Estrogen is part of the maintenance and repair crew of a woman's brain, so estrogen is not involved in the new construction of brain architecture.

The favorable effects of hormone therapy on cognition and reducing the risk of Alzheimer's disease are limited to women who initiate estrogen replacement therapy close to menopause and stay on estrogen long-term. The brain needs estrogen. To leverage estrogen's brain protection power, estrogen replacement therapy should be initiated within 10 years of menopause, before irreversible brain damage linked to estrogen deficiency occurs. 1 out of 5 women will develop disabling dementia, and 66% of seniors living with Alzheimer's disease are women. Appropriate estrogen replacement therapy decreases a woman's risk of developing dementia by 30%. No other agent offers this kind of brain-protecting power.

Within a decade of menopause, women lose 20% of their bone density, and as the years of estrogen deprivation unravel, they continue to lose 1 to 2% of bone mass annually, year after year. Once 30% of bone density is lost, osteoporosis-related fractures are a common occurrence in postmenopausal women 65 years and older. Without estrogen, 50% of postmenopausal women will sustain an osteoporosis-related fracture. On the other hand, estrogen replacement therapy reduces the incidence of these crippling and deadly fractures by 50%. Over 70% of women over the age of 70 suffer from urinary incontinence. A woman's bladder needs estrogen to function properly. The longer her bladder is deprived of estrogen, the more damaged its function.

Without skipping a beat, estrogen replacement therapy started close to menopause reduces a woman's risk of heart disease, heart failure and cardiac death by 50% and decreases her risk of dementia by 30%. 45% of women will die of cardiovascular disease, either a heart attack or a stroke, compared to 3% of women who will succumb to breast cancer. 10 times more women die from cardiovascular disease than breast cancer. Cardiovascular disease really is the "big C" for women. Estrogen replacement therapy does not cause breast cancer. In postmenopausal women, estrogen replacement therapy decreases mortality from all-causes, such as death due to cardiovascular disease, breast cancer, diabetes, dementia, osteoporosis, wound infections, etc., including decreasing the fatality rate among women who had used menopause hormone therapy prior to being diagnosed with breast cancer. Appropriately timed and properly managed menopause hormone therapy channels estrogen's heart healthy and brain preserving power.

WHAT'S YOUR TYPE? – Synthetic vs. Bioidentical ("Body"-identical)

Hormones whose chemical structures are identical to the hormones produced naturally by a woman's body are considered bioidentical or "body"-identical.

All hormones are synthesized in a lab, and irrespective of the raw material from which they are made, as long as the final hormone's chemical structure matches the hormone found naturally in a woman's body, it is considered bioidentical. The target estrogen to replace in menopause hormone therapy is estradiol, also known as 17beta-estradiol. Estradiol is the most potent of all the estrogens, and it is the main estrogen that a woman's ovary produces during her reproductive years. Natural progesterone is a solo act known simply as progesterone. Synthetic progestogens whose chemical structures are not identical to natural progesterone are referred to as progestins.

For bioidentical oral estradiol and progesterone to be absorbed through the intestinal tract, they need to be "micronized," that is, the hormone crystals need to be broken down to really small, microscopic pieces. Oral micronized estradiol (Estrace), the estradiol used in transdermal estrogen preparations, and oral micronized progesterone (Prometrium) are FDA-approved, pharmaceutical grade bioidentical hormones. Oral micronized estradiol (Estrace) was FDA-approved in 1984, and oral micronized progesterone (Prometrium) received approval in 1998.

FDA-approved, pharmaceutical-grade, bioidentical oral hormone therapy pills were not widely available to menopausal women until the very end of the 20th century. When postmenopausal women were being enrolled in the WHI studies in the early 1990s, conjugated equine estrogen (Premarin) and synthetic medroxyprogesterone (Provera) were the predominant hormones galloping across menopause therapy's pharmaceutical landscape. Although pregnant mares' urine is a natural source of hormones, conjugated equine estrogen (Premarin) contains 10 different estrogens, most of them alien to a woman's body. A human female does not need all those different estrogens in her system. When it comes to hormone therapy for women, the more similar the replacement hormone's chemical structure is to the target hormone being replaced, the more biologically compatible and wholesome the menopause hormone therapy.

Findings from the WHI Observational Study, which tracked 94,000 women's use of estrogen replacement therapy for 10 years, indicate that there is a difference in stroke risk between various types of oral estrogen.

The study found that women taking bioidentical micronized oral estradiol (Estrace) had a lower risk of stroke than women using conjugated equine estrogen (Premarin).

In the Danish Osteoporosis Prevention Study (DOPS), menopausal women were randomized to take either bioidentical oral micronized estradiol or a placebo for 10 years. Women taking the oral micronized estradiol hormone did not experience an increased risk of stroke. In the WHI estrogen-alone trial, women randomized to take conjugated equine estrogen (Premarin) for 6.8 years sustained a 30% increased risk of stroke when compared to women taking a placebo. Conjugated equine estrogen (Premarin) interferes with vascular cells production of nitric oxide (NO), which then limits the blood vessels' capacity to relax and dilate. Micronized estradiol does not interfere with the circulation's ability to expand and increase blood flow. Conjugated equine estrogen (Premarin) is also associated with a greater risk of developing deep vein thrombosis or blood clots (DVTs) when compared to bioidentical oral micronized estradiol (Estrace).

When it comes to menopause hormone therapy, "body"-identical or bioidentical micronized progesterone is better tolerated than replacement regimens containing synthetic progesterones, identified as progestins. The type of progesterone a menopausal woman uses can influence her risk for breast cancer. Synthetic progestins are less breast-friendly than micronized progesterone. Observational studies report that estrogens coupled to synthetic progestins have more impact on increasing breast cancer risk than estrogen coupled with micronized progesterone.

The E3N-EPIC French cohort clinical study, which involved over 80,000 menopausal women followed for 8 years, found an increased risk of breast cancer associated with exposure to synthetic progestins, but not with exposure to bioidentical oral micronized progesterone. The addition of bioidentical oral micronized progesterone (Prometrium) to estrogen therapy maintains the favorable impact of estrogen on cholesterol lipid profiles, whereas synthetic progestin somewhat blunts this benefit. Oral micronized progesterone can have a calming, sedating effect, so taking it at night allows menopausal women to sleep even better.

The more compatible the hormone replacement is to a woman's physiology, the healthier the therapeutic outcomes. We now have plant-derived, FDA-approved, pharmaceutical-grade female hormone replacement hormones whose chemical structures are identical to the hormones found naturally in a woman's body.

Conjugated equine estrogen (Premarin) was the workhorse of estrogen replacement for over half a century, and it helped us arrive at a better understanding of the nuances involved with appropriate menopause hormone therapy. Containing a variety of different estrogens, conjugated equine estrogen (Premarin) is natural to a horse, but it is alien to a woman's body. "Body"-identical or bioidentical estradiol preparations are naturally more compatible with a menopausal woman's hormone physiology. The horse and buggy gave way to modern modes of transportation. With the advent of FDA-approved, bioidentical pharmaceutical preparations available for menopause hormone replacement therapy, it's time to retire the pregnant mares.

PILL or PATCH

Menopause hormone therapy can be administered in a variety of ways. As long as bioequivalent doses are given, estrogen delivered by various routes can relieve menopausal symptoms and prevent long-term health problems exacerbated by estrogen deficiency. There are estrogen oral pills, transdermal estrogens such as estrogen skin patches, topical gels, estrogen skin spray, estrogen pellets that are implanted under the skin, estrogen vaginal suppositories or vaginal creams, as well as vaginal estrogen rings. Different routes of administration have different metabolic effects, which provides flexibility in dosing and preparations, to accommodate each menopausal woman's hormonal needs.

Like all oral medications, estrogen pills go through the liver's first-pass effect. Non-oral hormone preparations, such as the estrogen in skin patches, are absorbed directly into the bloodstream, bypassing the liver. Both oral estrogen and estrogen skin patches have beneficial effects on a menopausal woman's cardiovascular system, and there is no increased breast cancer risk whether estrogen replacement is taken orally or delivered through transdermal estrogen preparations, such as estrogen skin patches.

Non-oral estrogens do differ from estrogen pills in certain respects, however. Unlike oral estrogen pills, transdermal estrogen preparations (estrogen patch, topical gel or spray) neither elevate fatty triglycerides nor do they increase bile's cholesterol saturation, so transdermal preparations do not cause gallbladder problems. By avoiding the liver's first-pass effect, estrogen skin patches do not stimulate the liver's production of clotting factors, so estrogen patches do not increase a woman's risk for blood clots. Low-dose estrogen patches (delivering 50mcg of estradiol or less per day) do not increase a woman's risk for strokes, either. Oral estrogen encourages the liver's production of sex hormone binding globulin (SHBG) which lower's testosterone availability, whereas estrogen patches allow testosterone to roam free, which can help boost libido.

In the past, menopausal women with various medical conditions were excluded from enjoying the benefits of estrogen replacement therapy. With transdermal estrogen preparations, obese menopausal women, diabetics and women with a history of non-familial deep vein thrombosis (DVT) can safely benefit from estrogen replacement therapy. Non-oral estrogens, such as estrogen skin patches, do not increase the risk of stroke, blood clots or gallbladder disease. The availability of different types of hormone preparations further expands therapeutic options for menopausal women.

ESTROGEN-Alone vs. ESTROGEN-plus-PROGESTIN Therapy

Differences between the results of the two arms of the WHI hormone trial point to differences in the risk-to-benefit profile of estrogen-alone therapy versus estrogen-plus-progestin therapy. Since this is such an important aspect of menopause hormone therapy, let's quickly review the principal results of the WHI study.

There were two arms to the WHI Hormone Therapy Trial: one arm involved postmenopausal women who had had a hysterectomy in the past, randomized to taking a conjugated equine estrogen (Premarin) 0.625mg pill daily or a placebo pill for 6.8 years, and the other arm involved postmenopausal women who still had their uterus, randomized to taking a Prempro pill daily or a placebo pill for 5.6 years. Prempro is a combination pill containing conjugated equine estrogen (Premarin) 0.625mg plus the synthetic progestin, medroxyprogesterone (Provera) 2.5mg.

Upon enrollment, the average age of the women participating in the WHI trials was 63 years old, the ages ranged from 50 to 79. Both the estrogen-alone and the estrogen-plus-progestin hormone therapy regimens reduced a postmenopausal woman's risk of diabetes and decreased her risk of suffering an osteoporosis-related fracture. Both hormone regimens involved estrogen pills, and since oral estrogens go through the first-pass effect of stimulating the liver's production of clotting factors, both the oral estrogen-alone therapy and the oral estrogen-plus-progestin therapy were associated with increased risk of blood clots, strokes and gallbladder disease.

However, when breast cancer risk or the risk of heart disease were assessed, there were definite advantages to being in the estrogen-alone group compared to the estrogen-plus-progestin group. WHI data from the intervention phase of the estrogen-plus-progestin trial showed an increased relative risk of heart disease that was highest during the first year of therapy, and an increased relative risk of breast cancer compared to women taking placebo. In contrast, the estrogen-alone group experienced no increase in risk of heart disease or breast cancer. In fact, women who took estrogen-alone had less chance of developing breast cancer than the women who took a placebo (sugar pill). After stopping menopause hormone therapy, the women participating in the WHI trials were followed for over a decade. Not only was there a decrease in the chance of being diagnosed with breast cancer in the estrogen-alone group, but there was also a reduction in breast-cancer mortality, long after stopping the estrogen therapy. In contrast, combined estrogen-plus-progestin was associated with a slightly increased risk of invasive breast cancer in the 11 years' long-term follow-up of the WHI randomized and observational studies.

Estrogen does not initiate or cause breast cancer. Estrogen replacement may stimulate the growth of preexisting breast tumor cells allowing a woman's breast cancer to be diagnosed sooner. Only after taking the oral conjugated equine estrogen (Premarin) 0.625mg for over 15 years, is there a slightly increased risk of being diagnosed with breast cancer. Made from the urine of pregnant mares, conjugated equine estrogen (Premarin) contains 10 different estrogens, most of them alien to a woman's system. Despite taking these horse-derived estrogens, breast cancer risk is not increased until nearly two decades of therapy.

From the onset of puberty, and through the next 40 years of her life, a woman's ovaries are constantly producing estrogen, specifically estradiol. Although estradiol production fluctuates during the menstrual cycle, her body is continually bathed in estrogen. On the other hand, the only time the ovary manufactures progesterone is after ovulation, and as its "pro-ges-tation" name implies, progesterone's sole purpose is to prepare a woman's uterus and breasts for pregnancy. If conception does not occur, the progesterone level drops back down to zero, menstrual bleeding occurs, and another follicle/oocyte (egg) lines up for ovulation.

Once a woman's ovaries are depleted of estrogen-producing follicles/oocytes (eggs), she becomes menopausal. Since a menopausal woman no longer ovulates, she cannot get pregnant naturally. Unlike progesterone, estrogen has been an on-going integral part of a woman's biology and will continue to preserve her health and vitality through menopause and beyond. With menopause, there is no chance of pregnancy, so there is no need for a menopausal woman to be exposed to a hormone whose sole purpose is to prepare her body for pregnancy.

Progesterone is added to estrogen replacement therapy simply to protect a menopausal woman's uterus. Estrogen stimulates the endometrial lining of the uterus to proliferate and grow and grow. Unchecked, this tissue over-growth (endometrial hyperplasia) can lead to abnormal uterine bleeding, endometrial polyps and uterine cancer. Progesterone stops this overgrowth and protects the uterus from endometrial uterine cancer. Women who have had a hysterectomy do not need progesterone's uterine protection when they go on estrogen replacement therapy.

Clinical studies show that menopause hormone therapy that couples estrogen therapy with daily low dose progesterone, known as "continuous" hormone regimens, provide adequate uterine protection. When the endometrial lining of the uterus is continuously exposed to progesterone, estrogen cannot stimulate the lining to grow. On the other hand, hormone regimens involving daily estrogen with intermittent progesterone, such as taking higher doses of progesterone two weeks every month, may still allow some endometrial tissue to grow. As long as there is estrogen in a postmenopausal woman's system, her uterus does better with daily progesterone protection.

Although estrogen stimulates breast cell proliferation, it is the progesterone component of hormone therapy that is associated with slightly increasing a menopausal woman's absolute risk of breast cancer by less than 1% (0.8% to be exact). As the "pro-gestation" hormone preparing the breasts for pregnancy, progesterone increases the breasts' milk-producing glandular tissue, which increases breast density and tissue heterogeneity. This is problematic for older, non-pregnant breasts, which should be fatty and minimally dense. Breast tissue density can be determined only by mammograms, and it is not related to breast size or how firm breasts may feel. Not only does increased breast tissue density render mammograms trickier to interpret, but increased heterogeneity and breast density on mammograms are also linked to increased risk of developing breast cancer.

Oral micronized progesterone (Prometrium) effectively protects the uterus and has less adverse effects on menopausal breast tissue than synthetic progestins. Although oral micronized progesterone (Prometrium), which is "body"-identical or bioidentical to a woman's natural progesterone, is better than exposing a woman's body to synthetic progestin, a progestational agent of any kind in a postmenopausal woman is prickly to her physiology.

An alternative to the estrogen-plus-progesterone hormone therapy for menopausal women with a uterus is a tissue selective estrogen complex (TSEC). A TSEC couples estrogen hormone with a selective estrogen receptor modulator (SERM) agent. The SERM acts like progesterone to protect the endometrial lining of the uterus. Duavee is a TSEC that is a combination pill containing conjugated estrogen (Premarin) 0.45mg coupled to the SERM, bazedoxifene 20mg, which has been FDA-approved to treat hot flashes and prevent osteoporosis in menopausal women who have not had a hysterectomy.

Many women are not comfortable adding a SERM chemical to their estrogen therapy to accomplish uterine protection, but they would still like to have their breasts emancipated from unnecessary progesterone exposure. This can be accomplished using a progestin-containing intrauterine device (IUD). The Mirena/Liletta IUD contains 52mg of the progestin, levonorgestrel, and can be utilized as a vehicle for safely delivering progesterone to only where it's needed, the endometrial lining of the uterine cavity. Imperceptibly housed within the uterus, the progestin IUD releases a very low dose of levonorgestrel progestin into the uterine cavity, and this prevents the endometrial tissue from overgrowing in response to estrogen therapy. The Mirena/Liletta IUD is replaced every 5 to 7 years in a gynecologist's office, where the actual procedure takes 10 minutes. The procedure is comfortable when the prostaglandin, misoprostol (Cytotec), is used to help soften and dilate the cervix. With a progestin IUD providing worry-free uterine protection, a menopausal woman can enjoy all the benefits of estrogen replacement therapy without exposing her breasts, or the rest of her body, to extraneous progesterone. For a menopausal woman who has not had a hysterectomy, this truly is easy, breezy estrogen replacement therapy.

PREMATURE MENOPAUSE & BEYOND

We now have a much better understanding of the what, when, where and how of menopause hormone therapy. Without a doubt, the 1% of women who experience premature ovarian failure or go through "premature menopause" before the age of 40 should be placed on estrogen replacement therapy. The 10% of women who go through "early menopause," that is, they stop having menstrual periods between the ages of 40 to 45, should also proceed with hormone replacement therapy. Like any other hormonal condition, ovarian hormone deficiency should be treated with appropriately dosed hormone replacement therapy.

Women who experience menopause before the age of 45 usually need higher doses of estrogen replacement to alleviate bothersome menopausal symptoms and achieve therapeutic hormone levels. Due to drops in testosterone production, young menopausal women may need a touch of testosterone added to their hormone replacement regimen, as well. Without adequate hormone replacement therapy, younger menopausal women will suffer heart attacks, strokes, dementia and osteoporosis earlier than their well-estrogenized, non-menopausal counterparts.

Once a woman who experienced early or premature menopause turns 50-ish, she's now in step with the majority of women who are going through menopause between the ages of 46 to 56. When she reaches her early 50s, she should not simply abandon her hormones. An aging hypothyroid patient does not abandon her thyroid hormone replacement once she gets older, nor does a diabetic abort her insulin injections just because she's approaching her senior years. The now middle-aged woman just needs to have the hormone doses and preparations used for treating her ovarian insufficiency adjusted to be physiologically in line with a 50-something menopausal woman.

When a woman reaches her mid-60s and beyond, estrogen dosing and hormone preparations can be reduced further to accommodate for aging. Just a little bit of on-going estrogen therapy, along with a touch of aspirin, and possibly a smidge of statin, goes a very long way to keeping an older, geripausal woman active and independent.

ESTROGEN – GOING for the GOLD

Unlike any other prescription medicine or any other remedy, hormones are part of a woman's intrinsic biological make-up and are fundamental to her continued health and happiness. Estrogen is part of a woman's original design since the beginning of time. A menopausal woman can no longer reproduce naturally, but loss of ovarian hormone production is not a signal that her heart, brain and the rest of her body no longer need estrogen to function properly for the last few decades of her life.

A menopausal woman lives better and healthier when her estrogen hormone is replaced appropriately. We now have the right hormone preparations available, in the right doses, given at the right time, to help maintain a menopausal woman's vitality for decades. We can also integrate blood hormone levels with clinical outcomes to further fine-tune hormone replacement therapy.

From head-to-toe and everywhere in between, estrogen has been taking care of a woman's body for 40 years prior to menopause, so why not keep up the good work for her last 30 years? Thanks to predictable nutrition, modern sanitation, and contemporary obstetrical care, populations of women now live into their 80s, yet menopause still occurs around age 51. Back in the late 1800s, the impact of ovarian failure on a woman's long-term health was a non-issue, since the average lifespan was 49 years. Prior to the early 1900s, populations of women did not consistently live long enough to make it through menopause. Nature had neither planned for a woman to live past her reproductive years nor for a woman to outlive her ovaries.

For many older postmenopausal women living without the health benefits of estrogen, life is an existence cluttered with multiple pharmaceutical medicines and their drug-drug interactions and uncomfortable side effects, frequent trips to doctors, dentists and other therapists, multiple medical and surgical procedures, and finally shuffling down a melancholy path to despondent infirmity.

In going for the gold to health and happiness with menopause hormone therapy, we now know to:

1) Initiate estrogen replacement therapy within 10 years of menopause.
2) Use "body"-identical or bioidentical hormones that are FDA-approved, pharmaceutical-grade preparations. The estrogen should be estradiol, also known as 17beta-estradiol, and the progesterone should be bioidentical progesterone, not a synthetic progestin. For better absorption through the intestinal tract, the bioidentical hormones are reduced to tiny pieces, that is, they are micronized. The hormone replacement pills are known as oral micronized estradiol and oral micronized progesterone. Generics are fine, but the compounding of hormones should be reserved for situations where a

woman is either allergic to components of prefabricated hormones, or the specific hormone is not available.

3) Consider transdermal hormone preparations, such as estrogen skin patches, topical gels or skin sprays, for diabetic menopausal women or women at increased risk for blood clots, strokes, elevated triglycerides or gallbladder issues. Because the liver's first-pass effect is by-passed by non-oral estrogen preparations, these methods deploy lower doses of hormones than oral pills to achieve therapeutic goals. Transdermal estrogen hormone preparations provide all the benefits of oral estrogen replacement therapy without increasing a woman's risk for blood clots or strokes, and they do not cause triglyceride elevations or gallbladder problems. This is particularly applicable in older or heavier women who, even without hormones of any kind, are at increased risk for blood clots, strokes, and metabolic issues, compared to their younger or leaner counterparts.

4) Try to limit a menopausal woman's progesterone exposure just to her uterus. If progesterone is needed, bioidentical progesterone is preferred over synthetic progestin to minimize progesterone's adverse impact on a woman's breast tissue, cholesterol levels and moods. When possible, a progestin IUD is a viable therapeutic vehicle for limiting delivery of progesterone only to where it is needed, inside the uterus.

Once a woman reaches her half-century mark, she looks across the vista spanning the next 30 years of her life. It is no longer a matter of quantity, but the quality of the future years of her life that come into focus. Will she be vital and relevant or debilitated and burdensome? Will she be healthy and independent enough to enjoy living through her golden years or will she be warehoused in a nursing home somewhere?

Nothing alleviates menopausal symptoms like menopause hormone therapy. Nothing prevents tissue damage exacerbated by estrogen deficiency like estrogen replacement therapy. No other single substance, no other single pharmaceutical agent, or no other single anything, natural or otherwise, protects a woman's heart, brain, bones, bladder and vagina like estrogen, specifically estradiol, can. Controversial issues regarding menopause hormone therapy have been resolved, and compelling perspectives on estrogen's beneficial impact on a woman's quality of life, both during her symptomatic menopausal years, as well as throughout her elderly future, have been elucidated. Mastering menopause through appropriately timed and well-orchestrated hormone replacement therapy is the key to healthy aging and dignified longevity.

GERIPAUSE COCKTAIL

How we age matters. After all, it's not just quantity, but quality of life counts, as well. Life expectancy has increased more in the past 50 years than it had in the previous 200,000 years of human existence. Women who reach age 65 can expect to live another 20 years, and those who reach age 75 can expect to live an additional 13 years. Although women may live longer than men, they don't seem to be living as well.

Among people age 75 or older, women are 60% more likely than men to need help with one or more activities of daily living (ADLs), such as eating, bathing, dressing or just getting around the house. 70% of women age 75 years or older are widowed, divorced or never married, compared to only 30% of men in the same age group. 75% of residents living in a nursing home are women. Frailty and infirmity do not need to be a woman's inevitable consequence of longevity. The most effective strategy for successful aging involves healthy lifestyle choices and maintenance of a harmonious hormonal environment.

Urinary incontinence, dementia, and hip fractures land women in nursing homes, and these crippling conditions could have been avoided with appropriately timed and properly managed estrogen replacement therapy. Comparatively speaking, no other medication, intervention or therapy packs the punch of vitality and dignity that the simple estrogen molecule provides a postmenopausal woman.

There is a lot more to estrogen's influence on a woman's anatomy and physiology besides its impact on her breasts and uterus, so estrogen deficiency compounds hardships associated with aging. A woman's mind, body and spirit need estrogen, and nothing takes care of estrogen deficiency like estrogen replacement. Well-orchestrated menopause hormone therapy reduces an older woman's risk of heart disease, breast cancer, diabetes, dementia, osteoporosis, incontinence, blindness, tooth loss, shape-shifting, skin wrinkling and sexual dysfunction. To minimize organ damage exacerbated by estrogen deficiency, a menopausal woman should start hormone therapy soon after her ovaries stop producing estrogen, and hormone replacement should continue as long as she wants to maintain her quality life and age with dignity.

When taking care of geriatric patients, that is, patients who are over the age of 65, careful attention is given to proper dosing of their medications. Dosing needs to be adjusted to accommodate for the aging body's reduced capacity to metabolize medicine. Similar to the reduced dosing of her other medications, an older woman's hormone dosages will also need to be adjusted. This may involve lowering hormone doses or adjusting hormone preparations. In addition, adding a touch of low-dose baby aspirin (81 mg), and if needed, a smidge of low dose statin, helps prevent blood clots in aging blood vessels. This "geripause cocktail" allows a woman to garnish the benefits of long-term estrogen replacement therapy safely, well into her geriatric years.

MENOPAUSE + LONGEVITY = GERIPAUSE

For most women, degenerative conditions occur at least a decade after menopause. Compared to her same-aged, but well-estrogenized contemporaries, an estrogen-deprived postmenopausal woman is far more vulnerable to chronic and debilitating diseases. Despite riding the geriatric merry-go-round of taking more and more pharmaceuticals, coping with medication side-effects and drug-drug interactions, as well as being subjected to numerous medical and surgical procedures, most estrogen-deprived postmenopausal women lapse into infirmity.

Although all this clinical activity keeps the health care industry busy and profitable, it is a painful and debilitating existence for the little old lady shuffling from one medical office to another, from one rehab facility to another, and from one hospitalization to another, only to end up languishing in a nursing home somewhere.

Looking at reality-based numbers on women's health issues, we see that 45% of women will die from cardiovascular disease, 1 out of 5 women will develop dementia or Alzheimer's disease, 1 out of 2 women will sustain an osteoporosis-related fracture, and 70% of postmenopausal women over the age of 70 are incontinent. A woman's lifetime risk of breast cancer is 1 out of 8, but only 3% of women will die from breast cancer. Statistics show that more women will die from heart attacks, strokes, dementia or hip fractures than will ever succumb to breast cancer, yet women are far more afraid of breast cancer than they are of any other diagnosis. Fortunately, we now know that estrogen replacement therapy does not cause breast cancer.

A DECADE HAS GONE BY

If hormone therapy is not started within 10 years of menopause, a woman loses estrogen receptors and tissue responsiveness, so she will not experience all the benefits of timely hormone replacement therapy. At this point, she faces the stark reality of disease and disability exacerbated by on-going estrogen deficiency.

What happens to a woman who overlooked estrogen replacement therapy during her early menopausal years? Once she is a decade or more beyond menopause, a woman approaches late menopause or the "geripause" years, from Greek *geron* meaning "old one." Because menopause occurred a long time ago, and due to vascular damage sustained from years of estrogen deficiency, it may be too late or too risky for many geripausal women to initiate hormone therapy.

An estrogen-deprived, older postmenopausal woman's blood vessels may already be riddled with calcified cholesterol plaques, so simply giving her the standard dose of oral estrogen pills can increase her risk of developing blood clots across her hardened and narrowed atherosclerotic arteries. This could precipitate a heart attack or stroke. Starting estrogen therapy this late after menopause will not improve brain cells already tarnished by corrosive processes leading to dementia and Alzheimer's disease. Without estrogen, her body's collagen infrastructure has crumbled, so her bladder sags and her vagina has collapsed. Initiating estrogen replacement at this point cannot reverse these changes, it can only slow down further deterioration, somewhat.

This is similar to what happens when a diabetic patient is not taking insulin hormone therapy properly, or a hypothyroid patient has not been taking thyroid hormone replacement regularly. Any permanent damage that has already occurred due to hormone deficiency will not be reversed when, finally, adequate insulin is administered or suitable thyroid hormone levels are achieved. Replacing hormones at this point only helps slow down the rate of decline associated with hormone deficiency.

Reacquainting an estrogen-deprived, older postmenopausal woman's body to her female hormones will not reconstitute what she has already lost. Introducing low-dose estrogen hormone therapy at this late date may help salvage some bone density, muscle strength, vaginal tissue and bladder function. Even if estrogen replacement was not part of a woman's early menopausal years, it does not necessarily mean that hormone therapy has to disappear forever. If an older woman has already experienced a heart attack, sustained a stroke, or suffers from dementia or Alzheimer's disease, then it is considered too late for her to ever embark on estrogen replacement therapy.

BACK to ESTROGEN

Although it is trickier, and slightly riskier, to initiate female hormone therapy a decade or more after a woman's body has been deprived of her ovarian hormones, her relationship with estrogen can be reestablished very judiciously and very carefully. As always, thoughtful and collaborative consideration for the risks versus benefits of hormone therapy for each woman has to be assessed given her own medical needs and personal outlook. Since drug-related problems occur more frequently in the older patient population, special precautions need to be taken when prescribing and dosing any and all medications in this age group.

Any adverse cardiac or cerebral circulation problems associated with initiating hormone therapy 10 or more years after menopause results from estrogen's up-regulation of destabilizing mechanisms that disrupt necrotic cholesterol plaques within an older woman's atherosclerotic arteries. This means that introducing estrogen to an older woman's damaged blood vessels may cause a vulnerable cholesterol plaque in a diseased artery to crack open, and then a blood clot forms across this opening. If the blood clot blocks arterial flow to the heart muscle, a heart attack occurs. If the blood clot blocks arterial flow to a part of the brain, a "brain attack" or stroke occurs.

Just through sheer aging alone, an estrogen-deprived older woman is already at increased risk of developing a heart attack, stroke or a blood clot, so there is no need to tip the scales further with a synthetic oral estrogen given at too high a dose for her. Simply administering the standard dose and type of hormones used in a younger, freshly menopausal woman to an older woman far beyond menopause increases the geripausal woman's risk of developing blood clots. Furthermore, older women who have been estrogen-deprived for many years often experience side effects when standard doses of estrogen are initiated. Breast tenderness can be particularly disturbing. "Standard dose" is the dose of hormones used in a 50-something, newly menopausal woman. In geripausal women lower estrogen doses achieve therapeutic goals and any further adjustments can be made as clinically warranted.

If a woman has been hormone-deprived for a decade or more after menopause and wants to pursue estrogen therapy, a sensibly-sequenced geripause cocktail gently reacquaints her system to estrogen replacement, while simultaneously decreasing her risk for having a clot-related cardiovascular event. This involves prudent pretreatment with a cholesterol plaque stabilizer (low-dose statin), along with a clot buster (chewable baby aspirin, 81mg), prior to initiating any low-dose "body"-identical or bioidentical female hormone replacement therapy. A low-dose transdermal estrogen preparation (patch, gel or spray) is the preferred estrogen, and if a woman has not had a hysterectomy, she will also need micronized progesterone added for uterine protection.

Since statins take about 3 to 6 months to stabilize cholesterol plaques and prevent them from cracking open, an older woman, or a woman estrogen-deficient for more than a decade, will need to be on a low dose statin medication, along with a chewable low-dose baby aspirin (81mg), for 3 to 6 months, prior to starting any female hormone therapy. Then, a low-dose estrogen skin patch, and if she has a uterus, low dose oral micronized progesterone, are added to the statin and baby aspirin therapy. The clot-busting power of a chewable low-dose baby aspirin (81mg) reduces the risk of heart attacks and strokes in women over the age of 65. Furthermore, regularly taking aspirin for 5 or more years decreases a woman's risk of breast cancer, as well as decreases her risk of colon cancer. Menopause hormone therapy is not detrimental to a statin-treated woman, and any regression of atherosclerotic cholesterol plaques takes a couple of years of statin therapy.

Aging with dignity is not just a function of estrogen. It is a combination of lifestyle choices, existing health issues, and genetics. After being estrogen-deficient for over a decade, the gentle, geripause cocktail approach to initiating female hormone therapy in a carefully selected, appropriately informed and highly motivated postmenopausal woman allows her the option of salvaging some of the residual health benefits of estrogen therapy relevant to her personal needs. No medication of any kind or clinical intervention of any type is totally risk-free, so each woman needs to be evaluated and managed on a case-by-case basis. At this late stage of estrogen deprivation, embarking on low dose estrogen therapy will not restore what an older postmenopausal woman has already lost. A modicum of estrogen, judiciously sprinkled across her geripausal years, may help ease some of her hardships exacerbated by further hormone deficiency.

TANTALIZING TELOMERES

Intriguingly, the fountain of youth may flow from the ends of our DNA strands. Located at the end of each chromosome, telomeres are small sections of DNA that help preserve genetic information. Like the plastic tips on shoelaces, they prevent chromosomal fraying and tangling when a cell replicates. Sheltered from genetic degradation, telomeres maintain cellular integrity as cells divide and replace themselves. Each time a cell divides telomeres get shorter and shorter, and after about 60 cell replications, the shortened stump of a telomere prevents further cell division. As a normal biological process of aging, the cell then stops dividing and ultimately dies. Telomeres are considered the biological clock of the cell.

Excessive shortening of telomeres is found in genetic disorders or syndromes of accelerated aging, such as dyskeratosis congenita and progeria. Pruned telomeres are also associated with heart disease, cancers, Alzheimer's disease, and mortality of elderly people older than 65 years. Telomere length is an indicator of how rapidly cells age. Since lengthy telomeres are linked to living longer, interventions directed at curbing the shortening of telomeres may slow aging and age-related diseases. Telomerase is the cellular enzyme that prevents the shortening of telomeres. Activating telomerase maintains telomere length and slows down the aging process. Although scientists are years away from being able to lengthen telomeres in humans, practical strategies that activate telomerase will help a woman hang onto her telomeres. Avoiding sugar-sweetened sodas and greater adherence to the Mediterranean diet are associated with longer telomeres. Physical activity and minimizing stress are beneficial to telomere length, as well.

Females live longer than males in many animal species, including humans. At birth, telomere length is the same in baby girls and baby boys, but by adulthood telomeres are longer in women than in men. The effects of estrogen probably cause this discrepancy between the genders and estrogen's positive impact on maintaining telomeres can be explained on the basis of the mitochondrial theory of aging. Mitochondria are DNA-containing, specialized compartments found in every cell of the body, except red blood cells. Considered the powerhouse of the cell, mitochondria are responsible for creating 90% of the energy needed by the body to sustain life. As energy factories, mitochondria generate oxygen, as well as free radicals that are damaging to telomeres and other cellular structures. The oxidative damage of mitochondrial DNA is 4 times greater in males than in females.

Estrogen binds to estrogen receptors within cells and stimulates cellular pathways that produce antioxidant enzymes to protect telomeres. Telomere lengths are longer in postmenopausal women on long-term female hormone replacement therapy than in postmenopausal women deprived of estrogen. By increasing the expression of longevity-associated genes, including those encoding for telomerase and other antioxidant enzymes, estrogen helps women live better longer.

In SUMMARY - QUALITY of LIFE

Although civilization as we know it has been around for 6,000 years, it has only been within the past century that the majority of women are reaching menopause and outliving their ovaries. Of course, as outliers on the bell curve of aging, there were a few women who lasted into their 70s and 80s in the past, but the widespread occurrence of populations of women spending a third of their lives in the postmenopausal, estrogen-deprived state is a recent phenomenon in human history. These days, a woman who makes it into her 50s can expect to live into her 80s and beyond. Although life expectancy has increased significantly, the average age for menopause remains at 51 years old. Since Nature had not planned for women to survive beyond their reproductive years, extended longevity brings diseases and ailments exacerbated by estrogen deficiency. Mankind has prolonged the quantity of years lived. Now, womankind has to determine the quality of those extended years.

AGING and MENOPAUSE

Aging is the natural progression of deteriorating structure and diminishing function that occurs with the passage of time. Defined by the final menstrual period in a woman's life, menopause is a normal, natural event of aging. Because menopause simply represents the end of the reproductive phase of a woman's life, it need not be the beginning of inevitable decline and disability exacerbated by estrogen deficiency. For most women menopause usually occurs naturally between the ages of 46 to 56. For others, menopause simply comes earlier or is brought on by an infection, illness, surgery, chemotherapy or radiation.

Regardless of how or when a woman becomes menopausal, her ovaries were aging long before she was even born. A female fetus will have her lifetime's greatest number of ovarian follicles/oocytes (eggs) at 4 to 5 months of pregnancy, about 6 million eggs. When she is born, there's already been a 66% reduction in the number of eggs, down to 2 million. By puberty, a teenage girl has lost another 85% of her eggs, so she is down to 300,000. From this diminished reservoir, only 450 eggs will ovulate during a woman's reproductive years. This continual decline in a woman's ovarian egg reserves is in stark contrast to male sperm production. From puberty onward, and as long as he lives, a man continuously produces millions of fresh sperm, about 100 million sperm per day. Even postmortem, sperm retrieval within 36 hours after a man is dead can provide motile, fertile sperm.

A woman, on the other hand, is born with all the eggs she will ever have, and her biological clock just keeps winding down. Loss of follicles/oocytes (eggs) and declining fertility occurs naturally and is not interrupted by pregnancies or oral contraceptive pills (OCPs). When a woman reaches her mid-to-late 30s, her chance of getting pregnant diminishes. Destined for ovarian obsolescence, this persistent decline of follicles/oocytes (eggs) continues until menopause. Once ovarian follicles/oocytes (eggs) are depleted, her menstrual cycles stop. She cannot get pregnant naturally, and her ovaries no longer produce adequate amounts of female hormones. A menopausal woman is a woman with ovarian hormone deficiency.

From head-to-toe, and all the organs in between, estrogen is an influential component of a woman's cellular design. For 40 years prior to menopause, the estrogen generated by her ovaries, specifically estradiol (E2), kept a woman healthy and happy. Since estrogen is involved in over 400 functions in a woman's body, losing estrogen will have adverse consequences on a woman's health and quality of life. 85% of menopausal women will feel the uncomfortable symptoms of estrogen loss immediately while a few sail through menopause without a glitch. Each woman's perspective and response to this universal gynecological event is influenced by whether she experiences troublesome symptoms, the culture she lives in, her lifestyle, and her personal attitude towards possible treatment options.

The fact that all women are affected by menopause sooner or later should not deter us from treating it, any more than the commonality of tooth decay, arthritis or cataracts, would deter us from treating these age-related, life-diminishing eventualities. Menopause is a hormone deficiency state, and just as other hormone deficiency conditions are treated with appropriate hormone replacement therapy, menopause should also be addressed accordingly. People with thyroid deficiency receive thyroid hormone replacement. Diabetics who lack insulin hormone are treated with insulin shots or have an insulin pump. Men with low testosterone receive testosterone replacement. Biological reality dictates that if a gland fails to produce a hormone involved in maintaining physiological well-being, then that hormone needs to be replaced; otherwise, tissues degenerate, organs deteriorate and disabilities cripple one's spirit.

Fading estrogen levels are a treatable part of aging. Normal aging is associated with poor vision, decreased hearing, receding gums, bad hearts, creaky joints, clogged blood vessels, leaky bladders, confused brains, and increased cancers. We treat all these conditions to improve a person's quality of life, to prevent disability and to increase longevity. We don't withhold hearing aids, joint replacements or cancer treatments in older people just because these problems normally occur in elderly individuals.

Estrogen loss causes more than a menopausal collage of bothersome hot flashes, sleep disturbances, vaginal dryness, fatigue and mood swings. Among other debilitating conditions exacerbated by estrogen deficiency, a woman's estrogen loss leads to weight gain and shape-shifting, skin thinning and increased wrinkling, tooth loss and decreased hearing, stiff joints and weak muscles, libido loss, cardiovascular disease, diabetes, depression, dementia, osteoporosis and urinary incontinence. Coping with just one of these ailments is difficult enough; but when a woman becomes menopausal, all these problems intensify and collectively chip away at her body and spirit.

Since menopause is a naturally occurring event, a woman may resign herself to the notion that Nature should just take its course and avoid hormone replacement therapy. The sobering reality is that Nature was not planning on women consistently living beyond menopause. Humans, however, have developed sustaining behaviors for strength and longevity, and we now realize that women need estrogen as part of their strategy for optimal aging. Alternatively, a woman may rationalize that since her mother cruised through menopause without hormones, and since her grandmother also seemed okay without estrogen replacement, then she does not need menopause hormone therapy either. The genetic reality is that a woman possesses half of her mother's DNA and only a quarter of her grandmother's genetic constitution. Given the previous generation's reticence on matters pertaining to their bodies, it is difficult to know what they really suffered when they transitioned through "the change."

With or without bothersome menopausal symptoms, all postmenopausal women are subject to the destructive impact of 10 or more years of estrogen deprivation. Exacerbated by estrogen deficiency, women's "old age" chronic diseases and debilitating conditions manifest themselves a decade or more after menopause. What was once considered unavoidable aging in women is mitigated with appropriate estrogen replacement therapy.

The ROOT CAUSE

The root cause of bothersome menopausal issues is estrogen deficiency, so the most effective and physiologically natural approach to treating menopausal symptoms is hormone replacement therapy. Many women, however, try a medley of complementary and alternative strategies to stymie troublesome symptoms and fend off menopausal meltdown. Women may muscle, meditate or march their way through hot flashes and sleep deprivation. They may marinate in herbs, munch on soy, or meander through their menopausal journey. These endeavors may help a menopausal woman feel better, but they do not prevent organ damage caused by menopausal estrogen deficiency.

Women who exercise adequately, eat well, minimize alcohol consumption, maintain a healthy weight, and avoid tobacco and other toxic substances, decrease their risk of cancer and chronic diseases. Improved lifestyle measures are critical to disease avoidance, but without estrogen's tissue-maintenance power, hormone loss leads to bodily harm.

Preserving a decent quality of life is not just a matter of navigating the symptomatic menopausal years. It's looking 10 to 15 years down the road, to around age 65 and the years beyond. That's when the corrosive consequences of estrogen loss clearly manifest themselves. Heart disease, dementia, Alzheimer's disease, osteoporosis, strokes, dropped bladders, obliterated vaginas and cancers do not immediately occur the day after menopause. There is a delay of about a decade or so, from the onset of menopause to the manifestation of chronic diseases and troublesome conditions of aging. It takes years of estrogen deprivation for tissue architecture to be destroyed, organ function to deteriorate, and disease to settle in. By then, however, it may be too late for estrogen. Estrogen's role is maintenance and prevention, not resurrection of dead or dying cells.

Menopause is the failure of ovaries to produce hormones. As such, it induces an unhealthy, estrogen-deficient state. But, like any other hormone affliction, simply replacing the deficient hormone is neither a miracle cure nor an elixir of youth. Utilizing appropriate hormone preparations and replacing a menopausal woman's estrogen in a timely manner will not stop her from aging, nor will it prevent diseases and cancers she is genetically-driven to develop. Hormones cannot neutralize decades of poor lifestyle choices either. Without estrogen, however, a menopausal woman's body will break down, regardless of everything else that is done to keep things patched up. Modern medicine is marvelous at doling out new pharmaceuticals, surgical devices and high-tech gadgets to the aging patient population. These interventions are important in our therapeutic armamentarium, but for a menopausal woman's true sustainability, hormone harmony needs to be achieved.

SUMMER of 2002

In 1991, the National Institutes of Health (NIH) launched the Women's Health Initiative (WHI) study to determine the effects of estrogen and progestin on the main health threats to older women: heart disease, dementia, cancer and osteoporosis. The WHI hormone trial included over 27,000 healthy postmenopausal women between ages 50 to 79, with an average age of 63. When the women enrolled in the study, 70% were over age 60, 70% were overweight or obese, 50% were current or past tobacco smokers, and nearly half were being treated for hypertension. Only 3.5% of the women in WHI were between the ages of 50 to 54. Women with bothersome menopausal symptoms were excluded from participating in the WHI trials, since there was concern that they would drop out of the study to seek therapeutic relief of their symptoms.

The principal results of the WHI randomized controlled trial (RCT) on the risks and benefits of menopause hormone therapy using oral conjugated equine estrogen (Premarin), with or without the synthetic progestin, medroxyprogesterone (Provera), were released in the summer of 2002 and the spring of 2004. Menopause hormone therapy was shown to decrease the risk of osteoporosis-related fractures, decrease the risk of developing diabetes and decrease the risk of colon cancer. Taking estrogen-only decreased a woman's risk of breast cancer, but the estrogen-plus-progestin combination slightly increased a woman's risk of breast cancer. Overall, traditional hormone replacement therapy, using certain types of hormones, appeared to increase the risk of heart attacks, strokes, dementia, gallbladder problems and blood clots. There was no significant difference in the risk of dying from any causes between women taking menopause hormones compared to women taking a placebo (sugar pill).

In the WHI trials, the majority of women who embarked on hormone therapy were 12 or more years beyond menopause, so more than likely they had subclinical (asymptomatic) atherosclerotic hardening and narrowing of the arteries supplying their heart and brain. Also, the WHI participants were considered "healthy," despite carrying extra weight, smoking and having hypertension. In and of themselves, each of these problems contributes to atherosclerosis, with or without estrogen. At this late juncture in a postmenopausal woman's life, estrogen cannot neutralize years of lifestyle assaults, reverse established medical problems or resurrect estrogen-deprived, permanently damaged tissue.

The WHI participants' ages spanned across a canyon of three decades. A 50-year-old freshly menopausal woman is obviously physically and physiologically different from a 79-year-old postmenopausal woman who has sustained years of estrogen deficiency. Nonetheless, when the principal findings of the WHI hormone trials were initially publicized, all these women were bunched together and sweeping conclusions regarding menopause hormone therapy were drawn. Because the majority of the WHI participants were well beyond menopause, because only a single type of hormone preparation was utilized (an oral estrogen pill that was derived from the urine of pregnant mares [Premarin], along with a synthetic progestin), and because women with bothersome menopause symptoms were excluded from participating in the hormone trials, principal results from the WHI study painted a very broad, very negative, and very gloomy picture of menopause hormone therapy.

The lumped and clumped conclusions initially released from the WHI hormone trials were in contrast to previous research and clinical studies on menopause hormone therapy. These earlier hormone studies had observed positive, healthy effects of estrogen replacement therapy in menopausal women. Tremendous anxiety and confusion followed these initial WHI reports, and many women stopped taking hormones. Although stratification of WHI's results by women's ages reconciled some of the controversial issues related to menopause hormone therapy, additional clarification was needed to balance all the benefits of estrogen replacement therapy with any possible risks. The hormone intervention arms of the WHI trials wrapped up more than a decade ago. More detailed analysis of the raw data and follow-up studies have further expanded and refined our understanding of the valuable health benefits of appropriately timed and properly managed menopause hormone therapy.

TYPE, TIME, & TIMING

A woman can expect to spend a third of her life beyond menopause. Beginning in her 60s, the unpleasant impact of chronic diseases emerges, adversely affecting both the quality and quantity of her life, as well as the quality of the lives of loved ones around her. The ravages of obesity, diabetes, cardiovascular disease, osteoporosis, osteoarthritis, Alzheimer's disease, incontinence, and cancer, are mainly felt a decade or so after menopause has come and gone.

Fortunately for women, menopause opens a window of opportunity for prevention strategies that promote successful aging and enhance longevity. Coupled with opportune lifestyle choices, nothing takes care of a menopausal woman better than well-orchestrated estrogen replacement therapy. Initiating menopause hormone therapy at the right time is critical to maximizing therapeutic goals and preventing chronic diseases. Estrogen-based hormone therapy established within 10 years of menopause results in far greater rewards for a woman's mind, body and soul, than delaying its inauguration.

Introducing hormone therapy in an older postmenopausal woman, or a woman who is a decade or more past menopause, cannot undo damage already inflicted by aging and exacerbated by estrogen deficiency. Furthermore, cavalierly initiating menopause hormone therapy in an older woman who has been estrogen-deprived for a decade or more can worsen dementia, and destabilize necrotic cholesterol plaques in atherosclerotic blood vessels, leading to strokes and heart attacks.

When a woman who has been taking menopause hormone therapy reaches her mid-60s, either decreasing the dose of her estrogen replacement therapy and/or switching her hormone medicine from an oral estrogen to a transdermal estrogen preparation (estrogen skin patch, topical gel or skin spray), should be considered. Also, adding a touch of aspirin, and possibly a smidge of statin, creates a sensible geripause cocktail that minimizes any clot-related risks associated with oral estrogen replacement therapy in an older woman. Judicious management of hormones allows an older, postmenopausal woman to continue benefiting from the long-term use of low-dose estrogen replacement therapy. Starting hormone therapy during the early menopausal years, and continuing properly managed estrogen replacement into a woman's older years, offers a menopausal woman the best chance of avoiding the pitfalls of disease and disability compounded by estrogen deficiency.

Instead of using synthetic hormones that deviate from what is naturally found in a woman's body, it is best to replace ovarian hormones with FDA-approved, pharmaceutical-grade "body"-identical or bioidentical hormone preparations. These are chemically identical to the hormones produced naturally by a woman's body, so they do not have the drawbacks associated with synthetic hormones. Transdermal estrogen preparations contain bioidentical estradiol, and the estrogen is absorbed through the skin's capillaries directly into the bloodstream. Since transdermal hormones avoid the liver's first-pass effect, estrogen skin patches or topical estrogen gels, or sprays, do not increase a woman's risk for strokes, blood clots or gallbladder issues, nor do they increase a woman's fatty triglycerides.

Over 70% of women over the age of 70 have urinary incontinence. A woman who lives into her 80s has a 1 in 3 risk of developing Alzheimer's disease, and a 1 in 8 chance of being diagnosed with breast cancer. A woman's risk of dying from breast cancer is 1 in 36, so she is more likely to succumb to another debilitating disease, long before breast cancer takes her. Only 3% of women die from breast cancer, whereas over 45% of women die from cardiovascular disease (heart disease and strokes), and 50% of women sustain an osteoporosis-related fracture. 20% of women with a hip fracture die within a year of their injury, and 50% of the survivors end up spending the rest of their lives in a nursing home. The top 3 reasons older women end up in nursing homes are urinary incontinence, dementia and hip fractures, afflictions that could have been prevented with appropriate estrogen replacement therapy.

Among its many other benefits, menopause hormone therapy significantly decreases a woman's risk of cardiovascular disease, dementia and osteoporosis, while simultaneously maintaining her bladder control and vaginal tissue integrity. Estrogen replacement therapy does all this without increasing a woman's risk of breast cancer.

Adding a synthetic progestin to a menopausal woman's estrogen therapy, however, slightly increases her absolute risk of breast cancer by less than 1% (0.8%, to be exact). This risk is less than the increased breast cancer risk associated with obesity or alcohol consumption. Although it is only a marginally increased risk, when possible, it is prudent to minimize progesterone's impact on menopausal breast tissue.

When it comes to menopause hormone therapy, progesterone's sole purpose is protection of the uterus from estrogen stimulating the overgrowth of the endometrial uterine lining. Menopausal women who have had a hysterectomy do not need progesterone with their estrogen replacement therapy. If a woman with a uterus takes estrogen-only therapy, she increases her risk of endometrial tissue overgrowth, which can lead to uterine cancer, so she needs to have progesterone, or a substance that acts like progesterone, delivered to her uterus. This can be in the form of progesterone pills, vaginal progesterone gel, a tissue selective estrogen complex (TSEC) containing estrogen coupled to a selective estrogen receptor modulator (SERM) that protects the uterus, or a progestin-containing intrauterine device (IUD).

CRUMBLING ELDERLY YEARS

Fortunately, a menopausal woman will not die immediately from lack of estrogen. Regrettably, as the years go by, she will suffer from chronic diseases and infirmities exacerbated by estrogen deficiency.

By the time a woman is diagnosed with life-diminishing conditions, such as heart disease, stroke, dementia, hip fracture, macular degeneration of the retina, urinary incontinence with diaper dependence, etc., it will be too late for estrogen replacement therapy to slow down her downward spiral. At this point, powerful pharmaceutical drugs with their litany of side effects and drug-drug interactions will be prescribed and a procession of surgical and medical procedures performed, as the postmenopausal woman rides the health care merry-go-round of endless doctor appointments, dental chairs, therapy sessions, laboratory tests and radiological scans.

Feeble, frail and fearful, an estrogen-deprived elderly woman ends up languishing in a nursing home, with intermittent trips to the hospital. There is nothing cozy or radiant about golden years gone wretched and rusty. We will all die of something eventually, but why not try to optimize the quality of the last 30 years of a woman's life?

COMFORTABLE GOLDEN YEARS

Estrogen replacement therapy has been used to alleviate hot flashes, treat vaginal dryness and prevent osteoporosis for over 70 years. It has an impressive track record for safely taking care of millions of menopausal women around the world. Estrogen replacement therapy does not cause breast cancer. Appropriate hormone replacement therapy, and the operative word is "appropriate," does not significantly increase a woman's risk of strokes or blood clots, either. Nothing takes care of a woman like estrogen.

Not only is estrogen replacement therapy the most natural and physiologically correct treatment for bothersome menopausal symptoms, extended follow-up and long-term studies show a 30% reduction from all causes of death (heart disease, strokes, blood clots, breast cancer, dementia, and osteoporosis) among women who initiate hormone therapy while they are less than 60 years old or within 10 years of menopause, and then stay on hormone therapy long-term.

Contemporary hormone delivery systems and innovative therapeutic regimens allow menopausal women of all ages to benefit from custom-tailored hormone replacement therapy. From brain cells to skin cells, and every cell in between, estrogen naturally and holistically supports all the organs in a woman's body and preserves her physical, mental, sexual and spiritual well-being. Nothing, absolutely nothing, takes care of a menopausal woman the way appropriately timed and properly managed estrogen replacement therapy can. Mastering menopause through hormone harmony and wholesome lifestyle choices allows a woman to journey to the sunny side of menopause and provides her with a pleasant path to dignified aging with meaningful longevity.

REFERENCES

Chapter 1: The ERA of WHI

- Rossouw JE, Anderson GL, Prentice RL, et al. Writing Group for the Women's Health Initiative Investigators. Risks and benefits of estrogen plus progestin in healthy postmenopausal women: principal results from the Women's Health Initiative randomized controlled trial. *JAMA* 2002 July 17; 288(3):321-33.
- Women's Health Initiative Screening Committee. Effects of conjugated equine estrogen in postmenopausal women with hysterectomy: the Women's Health Initiative randomized controlled trial. *JAMA* 2004 Apr 14;291(14):1701-12.
- Vickers MR, Martin J, Meade TW; WISDOM study team. The women's international study of long-duration oestrogen after menopause (WISDOM): a randomized controlled trial. *BMC Womens Health.* 2007 Feb 26;7:2.
- Hays J, Ockene JK, Brunner RL, et al. Women's Health Initiative Investigators. Effects of estrogen plus progestin on health-related quality of life. *N Engl J Med.* 2003;348(19):1839-54.
- Jarvstrat Lotta, Septz Holm ACE, Lindh-Astrand L, Hoffmann MK, Fredrikson MG, Hammar ML. Use of hormone therapy in Swedish women aged 80 years and older. *Menopause* 2015 March;22(3):275-278.

- Hoffmann M, Hammar M, Kjellgren KI, Lindh-Astrand L. Changes in women's attitudes towards and use of hormone therapy after HERS and WHI. *Maturitas.* 2005 Sep 16; 52(1): 11-7.
- Lindh-Astrand L, Bixo M, Hirschberg AL, Sundstrom-Poromaa I, Hammar M. A randomized controlled study of taper-down or abrupt discontinuation of hormone therapy in women treated for vasomotor symptoms. *Menopause* 2010 Jan-Feb; 17(1):72-9.
- Fournier A, Fritel X, Panjo H, Zins M, Ringa V. Health characteristics of women beginning postmenopausal hormone therapy: have they changed since the publication of the Women's Health Initiative? *Menopause* 2014 Jul; 21(7):687-93.

Chapter 3: MENOPAUSE – TYPES and TIMING

- Lahdepera M., Lummaa V., Helle S., Tremblay M., Russell A.F. (2004). "Fitness benefits of prolonged post-reproductive lifespan in women." *Nature* (6979): 178-81. doi:10.1038/nature02367
- Hawkes, K. (2003). "Grandmothers and the evolution of human longevity." *Am J Hum Biol* 15 (3): 380-400
- Voland, E. and Beise, J. (2002). "Opposite effects of Maternal and Paternal Grandmothers of Infant Survival in Historical Krummhorn." MPIDR WP 2001-026
- He C, Kraft P, Chen C. "Genome-wide association studies identify loci associated with age at menarche and age at natural menopause." *Nature Genetics* 41 (6) (2009): 724-28
- Mikkola TS, Clarkson TB, Estrogen replacement therapy: atherosclerosis and vascular function, *Cardiovasc Res* 53:605, 2002.
- Herrington DM, Espeland MA, Crouse JR, III, Robertson J, Riley WA, McBurnie MA, Burke GL, Estrogen replacement and brachial artery flow-mediated vasodilatation in older women, *Arteriorscl Tromob Vasc Biol* 21:1955, 2001.
- Zandi PP, Carlson MC, Plassman BL, Welsh-Bohmer KA, Mayer LS, Steffens DC, Breitner JCS, for the Cache County Memory

Study Investigators, Hormone replacement therapy and incidence of Alzheimer disease in older women. The Cache County Study, *JAMA* 288:2123, 2002.

- Hodis HN, Mack WJ. Postmenopausal hormone therapy in clinical perspective. *Menopause* 2007; 14:944-957.
- Rossouw JE, Anderson GL, Prentice RL, et al. Risks and benefits of estrogen plus progestin in healthy postmenopausal women: principal results from the Women's Health Initiative randomized control trial. *JAMA* 2002;288:321-333.
- Canonico M, Oger E, Plu-Bureau G; Estrogen and Thromboembolism Risk (ESTHER) Study Group. Hormone therapy and venous thromboembolism among postmenopausal women: impact of the route of estrogen administration and progestogens: the ESTHER study. *Circulation* 2007;115:840-845.

Chapter 5: LIFESTYLE – LIVE LONG and AGE WELL

- Mosca L, Mochari-Greenberger H, Dolor RJ, et al. Twelve-year follow-up of American women's awareness of cardiovascular disease risk and barriers to heart health. *Circ Cardiovascular Qual Outcomes* 2010;3:120-127.
- Pai JK, Manson JE. Acceleration of cardiovascular risk during the late menopausal transition. *Menopause* 2013;20:1-2.
- Collins P, Rosano G, Casey C, et al. Management of cardiovascular risk in the perimenopausal woman: a consensus statement of European cardiologists and gynecologists. *Climacteric* 2007;10:508-526.
- Perk J, De Backer G, Gohlke H, et al. European guidelines on cardiovascular disease prevention in clinical practice (version 2012): the Fifth Joint Task Force of the European Society of Cardiology and Other Societies on Cardiovascular Disease Prevention in Clinical Practice (constituted be representatives of nine societies and by invited experts). *Atherosclerosis* 2012;223:1-68.

- Mosca L, Benjamin EJ, Berra K, et al. Effectiveness-based guidelines for the prevention of cardiovascular disease in women – 2011 update: a guideline from the American Heart Association. *J Am Coll Cardiol* 2011;57:1404-1423.

Chapter 6: COMPLEMENTARY and ALTERNATIVE THERAPIES

- Newton KM, Reed SD, LaCroix AZ, Grothaus LC, Ehrlich K, Guiltinan J. Treatment of vasomotor symptoms with black cohosh, multibotanicals, soy, hormone therapy, or placebo: a randomized trial. *Ann Intern Med.* 2006 Dec 19;145(12):869-79.
- Rada G et al. Non-hormonal interventions for hot flushes in women with a history of breast cancer. Cochrane Database Syst Rev. 2010 Sep8;(9)CD004923.
- Nelson HD et al. Non-hormonal therapies for menopausal hot flashes: systematic review and meta-analysis. *JAMA.* 2006 May 3;295(17) 2057-71.
- Bair YA, Gold EB, Zhang G, et al. Use of complementary and alternative medicine during the menopause transition: longitudinal results from the Study of Women's Health Across the Nation (SWAN). *Menopause.* 2008;15:32-43.
- Peng W, Adams J, Sibbritt D, Frawley J. Critical review of complementary and alternative medicine use in menopause: focus on prevalence, motivation, decision-making, and communication. *Menopause.* 2014; Vol.21, No.5, pp. 536-548
- MacLennan AH, Henry D, Hills S, Moore V, Oral estrogen replacement therapy versus placebo for hot flushes. *Climacteric.* 2001 Mar; 4(1):58-74.
- Newton KM, Buist DS, Keenan NL, Anderson LA, LaCroix AZ. Use of alternative therapies for menopause symptoms; results of a population-based survey. *Obstet Gynecology* 2002;100:18-25.

- Lethaby A, Marjoribanks J, Kronenberg F, Roberts H, Eden J, Brown J. Phytoestrogens for menopausal vasomotor symptoms. *Cochrane Database Syst Rev* 2013 Dec 10;12:CD001395.
- Lagari VS, Levis S. Phytoestrogens for menopausal bone loss and climacteric symptoms. *J Steroid Biochem Mol Biol.* 2014 Jan;139:294-301.
- Pearce J, Hawton K, Blake F, Barolow D, Rees M, Fagg J, Keenan J, Psychological effects of continuation versus discontinuation of hormone replacement therapy by estrogen implants: a placebo-controlled study, *J Psychosom Res* 42:177, 1997.
- Cornwell T, Cohick W, Raskin I. Dietary phytoestrogens and health. *Phytochemistry* 2004;65(8):995-1016.
- Messina M, McCaskill-Stevens W, Lampe JW. Addressing the soy and breast cancer relationship: Review, commentary, and workshop proceedings. *J Natl Cancer Inst* 2006;98(18):1275-1284.
- Nedrow A, Miller J, Walker M, Nygren P, Huffman LH, Nelson HD. Complementary and alternative therapies for the management of menopause-related symptoms. A systematic review. *Arch Intern Med* 2006;166:1453-1465.
- Sacks FM, Lichtenstein A, Van Horn L, Harris W, Kris-Etherton P, Winston M. Soy protein, isoflavones, and cardiovascular health. An American Heart Association Science Advisory for Professionals from the Nutrition Committee. *Circulation* 2006;113:1034-1044.
- Messina M. Soy foods, isoflavones, and the health of postmenopausal women. *Am J Clin Nutr* 2014 June 4;100(Supplement 1)423S-430S.
- Li L, Lv Y, Xu L, Zheng Q. Quantitative efficacy of soy isoflavones on menopausal hot flashes. *Br J Clin Pharmacol* 2014 Oct 15. doi: 10.1111/bcp.12533.
- Quaas AM, Kono D, Mack WJ, Hodis HN, Felix JC, Paulson RJ, Shoupe D. Effect of isoflavone soy protein supplementation on endometrial thickness, hyperplasia and endometrial cancer risk in

postmenopausal women: a randomized control trial. *Menopause* 2013 Aug;20(8):840-4.

- Moriyama CK, Oneda B, Bernardo FR, et al. A randomized, placebo-controlled trial of the effects of physical exercises and estrogen therapy on health-related quality of life in postmenopausal women. *Menopause* 2008;15:613-618.

- Joshi S, Khandwe R, Bapat D, Deshmukh. Effect of yoga on menopausal symptoms. *Menopause Int* 2011;17:78-81.

- Goldstein S, Espie M, Druckmann R. Does Relizen, a non-hormonal treatment for vasomotor symptoms inhibit the CYP2D6 enzyme system? Poster presentation at 25th Annual Meeting of the North American Society, Oct 2014, Washington, DC with abstract in *Menopause* 2014 Dec;21(2):1322.

- Winther K, Rein E, Hedman C. Femal, an herbal remedy made from pollen extracts, reduces hot flushes and improves quality of life in menopausal women: a randomized, placebo-controlled, parallel study. *Climacteric* 2005 Jun;8(2):162-70.

- Rossouw JE, Anderson GL, Prentice RL, LaCroix AZ, Kooperberg C, Stefanick ML, Jackson RD, Beresford SA, Howard BV, Johnson KC, Kotchen JM, Ockene J; Writing Group for the Women's Health Initiative Investigators. Risks and benefits of estrogen plus progestin in healthy postmenopausal women: principal results from the Women's Health Initiative randomized controlled trial. *JAMA* 2002 July17;288(3):321-33.

Chapter 8: ESTROGEN RECEPTORS – HERE, THERE and EVERYWHERE

- Helguero LA, Faulds MH, Gustafsson JA, et al. Estrogen receptors alpha (ER-alpha) and beta (ER-beta) differentially regulate proliferation and apoptosis of the normal murine mammary epithelial cell line HC11. *Oncogene* 2005;24:6605-6616.

- Barkhem T, Carlsson B, Nilsson Y, Enmark E, Gustafsson J, Nilsson S. Differential response of estrogen receptor alpha and estrogen receptor beta to partial estrogen agonists/antagonists. *Mol Pharmacol.* 1998;54:105-112.

- Li L, Neaves WB. Normal stem cells and cancer stem cells; the niche matters. *Cancer Res.* 2006 May;66(9):6458.

- Cristofanilli M et al. Circulating tumor cells, disease progression, and survival in metastatic breast cancer. *N Engl J Med.* 2004;351:781-791.

- Warnock JK, Swanson SG, Borel RW, Zipfel LM, Brennan JJ. Combined esterified estrogens and methyltestosterone versus esterified estrogens alone in the treatment of loss of sexual interest in surgically menopausal women. *Menopause* 2005;12(4): 359-60.

- Davis SR, van der Mooren MJ, van Lunsen RH, et al. Efficacy and safety of a testosterone patch for the treatment of hypoactive sexual desire disorder in surgically menopausal women: a randomized, placebo-controlled trial. *Menopause* 2006;13(3)5:387-396.

- Shifren J, Davis SR, Moreau M, et al. Testosterone patch in the treatment of hypoactive sexual desire disorder in naturally menopausal women: results from the INTIMATE NMI study. *Menopause* 2006;13(5):770-779.

- Parker, WH, Feskanich D, Broder MS, Chang E, Shoupe D, Farquhar CM, et al. Long-term mortality associated with oophorectomy compared with ovarian conservation in the Nurse's Health Study. *Obstet Gynecol* 2013;121(4):709-16.

- Parker WH, Broder MS, Chang E, et al. Ovarian conservation at the time of hysterectomy and long-term health outcomes in the Nurses' Health Study. *Obstet Gynecol* 2009;113:1027-1037.

- Rivera CM, Grossardt BR, Rhodes DJ, et al. Increased cardiovascular mortality after early bilateral oophorectomy. *Menopause* 2009;16:15-23.

- Appiah D, Winters SJ, Hornung CA. Bilateral oophorectomy and the risk of incident diabetes in postmenopausal women. *Diabetes Care* 2014 Mar;37(3):725-33.
- Rocca W, Bower JH, Maraganore D, et al. Increased risk Parkinsonism in women who underwent oophorectomy before menopause. *Neurology* 2008;70:200-209.
- Rocca W, Bower J, Maraganore D, et al. Increased risk of cognitive impairment and dementia in women who underwent oophorectomy before menopause. *Neurology* 2007;69:1074-1083.
Rocca W, Grossardt B, Geda Y, et al. Long-term risk of depressive and anxiety symptoms after early bilateral oophorectomy. *Menopause* 2008;15:1050-1059.
- Mucowski SJ, Mack WJ, Shoupe D, Kono N, Paulson R, Hodis HN. Effect of prior oophorectomy on changes in bone mineral density and carotid artery intima-media thickness in postmenopausal women. *Fertil Steril* 2014 Arp;101(4)1117-22.
- Jacoby VL, Grad D, Wactawski-Wende J, et al. Oophorectomy vs ovarian conservation with hysterectomy; cardiovascular disease, hip fracture, and cancer in the Women's Health Initiative Observational Study. *Arch Intern Med* 2011;171:760-768.
- Ridker PM, Cook NR, I-Min L, Gordon, D, Gaziano M, Manson JE, Hennekens CH and Buring JE. A randomized trial of low-dose aspirin in the primary prevention of cardiovascular disease in women. (Women's Health Study). *N Engl J Med* 2005 Mar 31;352:1293-1304.

Chapter 9: GLANDS, GLANDS, GLANDS

- Stuenkel CA. Subclinical thyroid disorders. *Menopause: The Journal of the North American Menopause Society* 2015 Feb;22(2):231-233.
- Aggarwal N, Razvi S. Thyroid and aging or the aging thyroid? An evidence-based analysis of the literature. *J Thyroid Res* 2013;2013:481287.

- Sowers M, Luborsky J, Purdue C, et al. Thyroid stimulating hormone (TSH) concentrations and menopausal status in women at the mid-life: Study of Women Across the Nation (SWAN). *Clin Endocrinol (Oxf)* 2003;58:340-347.
- Hyland KA, Arnold AM, Lee JS, Cappola AR. Persistent subclinical hypothyroidism and cardiovascular risk in the elderly: the cardiovascular health study. *J Clin Endocrinol Metab* 2013;98:533-540.
- Taylor PN, Razvi S, Pearce SH, Dayan CM. Clinical review: A review of the clinical consequences of variation in thyroid function within the reference range. *J Clin Endocrinol Metab* 2013;98:3562-3571.
- Giri A, Edwards TL, LeGrys VA, Lorenz CE, Funk MJ, Schectman R, Heiss G, Robinson JG, Hartmann KE. Subclinical hypothyroidism and risk for incident ischemic stroke among *postmenopausal* women. *Thyroid* 2014 Aug;24(8):1210-7.
- LeGrys VA, Funk MJ, Lorenz CE, Giri A, Jackson RD, Manson JE, Schectman R, Edwards TL, Heiss G, Hartmann KE. Subclinical hypothyroidism and risk for incidental myocardial infarction among postmenopausal women. *J Clin Endocrinol Metab.* 2013 Jun;98(6):2308-17.
- Garber JR, Cobin RH, Gharib H, et al. American Association of Clinical Endocrinologists and American Thyroid Association Taskforce on Hypothyroidism in Adults. Clinical practice guidelines for hypothyroidism in adults: cosponsored by the American Association of Clinical Endocrinologists and the American Thyroid Association. *Endocr Pract* 2012;18:988-1028.

Chapter 11: DANCING with HORMONES

- Hankinson, SE, Colditz GA, Hunter DJ, et al. A quantitative assessment of oral contraceptive use and risk of ovarian cancer. *Obstetrics and Gynecology* 1992; 80(4):708-714.
- Franco, Eduardo L., Duarte-Franco, Eliane. Ovarian cancer and oral contraceptives. *The Lancet* Jan 26, 2008, Vol. 371:277-278.

- Armstrong, Carrie. Practice Guidelines: ACOG Guidelines on Noncontraceptive Uses of Hormonal Contraceptives. *Am Fam Physician* 2010 Aug 1;82(3):288-295
- Halbreich U, Borenstein J, Pearlstein T, Dahn LS. The prevalence, impairment, impact and burden of premenstrual dysphoric disorder (PMS/PMDD). *Psychoneuroendocrinology* 2003;28 (Suppl 3):1-23
- Perkonigg A, Yonkers KA, Pfister H, et al. Risk factors for premenstrual dysphoric disorder in a community sample of young women: the role of traumatic events and posttraumatic stress disorder. *J Clin Psychiatry* 2004;65:1314-1322.
- Treloar SA, Heath AC, Martin NG. Genetic and environmental influences on premenstrual symptoms in an Australian twin sample. *Psychol Med* 2002;32:25-38.
- Masho SW, Adera T, South-Paul J. Obesity as a risk factor for premenstrual syndrome. *J Psychosom Obstet Gynaecol* 2005;26:37-47.
- Bailey JW, Cohen LS. Prevalance of mood and anxiety disorders in women who seek treatment for premenstrual syndrome. *J Womens Health Gend Based Med.* 1999;8:1181-1184.
- Ford O, Lethaby A, Mol B, Roberts H. Progesterone for premenstrual syndrome. *Cochrane Database Syst Rev.* 2006;(4):CD003415.
- Hammarback S, Backstrom T. Induced anovulation as treatment of premenstrual tension syndrome: a double-blind cross-over study with GnRH-agonist versus placebo. *Acta Obstet Gynecol Scand.* 1988;67:159-166.
- Inoue Y, Terao T, Iwata N, et al. Fluctuating serotonergic function in premenstrual dysphoric disorder and premenstrual syndrome; findings from neuroendocrine challenge tests. *Psychopharmacology* 2007;190:213-219.
- Wyatt KM, Dimmock PM, O'Brien PM. Selective serotonin reuptake inhibitors for premenstrual syndrome. *Cochrane Database Syst Rev.* 2002;(4):DC001396.
- Beaber, Elisabeth F, Buist, Diana SM, Barlow, William E., Malone, Kathleen E., Reed, Susan D., and Li, Christopher I. Recent

oral contraceptive use by formulation and breast cancer risk among women 20 to 49 years of age. *Cancer Research.* 2014 Aug 1;74(15):4078-89.

- Grodin, JM, et al. Source of estrogen production in postmenopausal women." *Journal of Clinical Endocrinology and Metabolism* 1973;19(1):207-214.

- Peragallo Urrutia R, Coeytaux RR, McBroom AJ, Gierisch JM, Havrilesky LJ, Moorman PG, Lowery WJ, Dinan M, Hasselblad V, Sanders GD, Myers ER. Risk of acute thromboembolic events with oral contraceptive use: a systematic review and meta-analysis. *Obstet Gynecol* 2013 Aug;122(2 Pt 1):308-9.

- Galson, Steven K. Prevention of deep vein thrombosis and pulmonary embolism. *Public Health Rep.* 2008 July-Aug;123(4):420-21.

- Deitelzweig SB, Johnson BH, Lin J, Schulman KL. Prevalence of clinical venous thromboembolism in the USA: current trends and future projections. *Am J Hematol.* 2011 Feb;86(2):217-20

- Freeman AL, Pendleton RC, Rondina MT. Prevention of venous thromboembolism in obesity. *Expert Rev Cardiovas Ther.* 2010 Dec;8(12):1711-21.

Chapter 12: HORMONES: LET'S GET BIOCHEMICAL

- Holinka CF, Brincat M, Coelingh Bennink HJT. Preventive effect of oral estetrol in a menopausal hot flush model. *Climacteric* 2008; 11(Suppl 1):15-21.

- Coelingh Bennink HJT, Singer C, Simoncini T, Genazzani A, Kubista E. Estetrol, a pregnancy-specific human steroid, prevents and suppresses mammary tumor growth in a rat model. *Climacteric* 2008; 11:29.

- Coelingh Bennink HJT, Heegaard AM, Visser M, Holinka CF, Christiansen C. Oral bioavailability and bone-sparing effects of estetrol in an osteoporosis model. *Climacteric* 2008; 11(Suppl 1):2-14.

- Heegaard AM, Holinka CF, Kenemans P, Coelingh Bennink HJT. Estrogenic uterovaginal effects of oral estetrol in the modified Allen-Doisy test. *Climacteric* 2008; 11(Suppl 1):22-28.
- Coelingh Bennink HJT, Skouby S, Bouchard P, Holinka CF. Ovulation inhibition by estetrol in an in vivo model. *Contraception* 2008; 77: 186-190.
- Sowers MR< Crawford S, McConnell DS, et al. Selected diet and lifestyle factors are associated with estrogen metabolites in a multiracial/ethnic population of women. *J Nutri.* 2006;136(6):1588-1595.
- Campbell KL, Westerlind KC, Harber VJ, Bell GJ, Mackey JR, Courneya KS. Effects of aerobic exercise training on estrogen metabolism in premenopausal women: a randomized controlled trial. *Cancer Epidemiol Biomarkers Prev.* 2007;16(4):731-739.
- Mackey RH, Fanelli TJ, Modugno F, Cauley JA, McTigue KM, Brooks MM, Chlebowski RT, Manson JE, Klug TL, Kip KE, Curb JD, Kuller LH. Hormone therapy, estrogen metabolism, and risk of breast cancer in the Women's Health Initiative Hormone Therapy Trial (WHI-HT). *Cancer Epidemiol Biomarkers Prev.* 2012 Nov; 21(11): 2022-32.
- Dallal CM, Tice JA, Buist DS, Bauer DC, Lacey JV Jr, Cauley JA, Hue TF, Lacroix A, Falk RT, Pfeiffer RM, Fuhrman BJ, Veenstra TD, Xu X, Brinton LA; B-FIT Research Group. Estrogen metabolism and breast cancer risk among postmenopausal women: a case-cohort study with B-FIT. *Carcinogenesis* 2014 Feb;35(2):346-55.
- Fuhrman BJ, Schairer C, Gail MH, Boyd-Morin J, Xu X, Sue LY, Buys SS, Isaacs C, Keefer LK, Veenstra TD, Berg CD, Hoover RN, Ziegler RG. Estrogen metabolism and risk of breast cancer in postmenopausal women. *J Natl Cancer Inst.* 2012 Feb22; 104(4):326-39.
- LaCroix AZ Lotchen J, Anderson G, Brzyski R, Cauley JA, Cummings SR, Gass M, Johnson KC, Ko M, Larson J, Manson JE, Stefanick ML, Wactawski-Wende J. Calcium plus vitamin D

supplementation and mortality in postmenopausal women: the Women's Health Initiative calcium-vitamin D randomized controlled trial. *J Gerontol A Biol Sci Med Sci.* 2009 May;64(5):559-87.

- Prentice RL, Pettinger MB, Jackson RD, Wactawski-Wende J, LaCroix AZ, Anderson GL, Chlebowski RT, Manson JE, Van Horn L, Vitolins MZ, Datta M, LeBlanc ES, Cauley JA, Rossouw JE. Health risks and benefits from calcium and vitamin D supplementation: Women's Health Initiative clinical trial and cohort study. *Osteoporosis* 2013 Feb;24(2):567-80.

- Scheffers CS, Armstrong S, Cantineau AE, Farquhar C, Jordan V. Dehydroepiandrosterone (DHEA) for women in the peri- or postmenopausal phase. *Cochrane Database Syst Rev.* 2015 Jan 22;1:CD011066. [Epub ahead of print]

- Chowdhury R, Kunutsor S, Vitezova A, Oliver-Williams C, Chowdhury S, Kiefte-de-Jong JC,

- Khan H, Baena CP, Prabhakaran D, Hoshen MB, Feldman BS, Pan A, Johnson L, Crowe F, Hu FB, Franco OH. Vitamin D and risk of cause specific death: systematic review and meta-analysis of observational cohort and randomized intervention studies. *BMJ* 2014 Apr 1;348:g1903.

- Alfawaz H, Tamim H, Alharbi S, Aljaser S, Tamimi W. Vitamin D status among patients visiting a tertiary care center in Riyadh, Saudi Arabia: a retrospective review of 3475 cases. *BMC Public Health* 2014 Feb 13;14:159.

- Al-Mogbel ES. Vitamin D status among Adult Saudi Females visiting Primary Health Care Clinics. *Int J Health Sci (Qassim)* 2012 Jun;6(2):116-26.

Chapter 13: BIOIDENTICALS vs. SYNTHETICS

- Boothby LA, Doering PL. Bioidentical hormone therapy: a panacea that lacks supportive evidence. *Curr Opin Obstet Gynecol* 2008;20:400-407.

- Holtorf K. The bioidentical hormone debate: are bioidentical hormones (estradiol, estriol, and progesterone) safer or more efficacious than commonly used synthetic versions in hormone replacement therapy? *Postgrad Med* 2009;121:73-85.

- Lewis JG, McGill H, Patton VM, Elder PA. Caution on the use of saliva measurements to monitor absorption of progesterone from transdermal creams in postmenopausal women. *Maturitas* 2002;41:1-6.

- Garafalakis M, Hickey M. Role of androgens, progestins and tibolone in the treatment of menopausal symptoms: a review of the clinical evidence. *Clin Interv Aging* 2008 Mar; 3(1) 1-8.

- Erel CT, Senturk LM, Kaleli S. Tibolone and breast cancer. *Postgrad Med J.* 2006 Oct; 82(972):658-662.

- Cummings SR, Ettinger B, Delmas PD, Kanemans P, Stathopoulos V, Verweij P, Mol-Arts M, Kloosterboer L, Mosca L, Christiansen C, Bilezikian J, Kerzberg EM, Johnson S, Zanchetta J, Grobbee DE, Seifert W, and Eastell R for the Long-Term Intervention on Fractures with Tibolone (LIFT) Trial Investigators. The effects of tibolone in older postmenopausal women. *N Engl J Med.* 2008 Aug 14;359(7):697-708.

- Bundred NJ, Kenemans P, Yip CH, Beckmann MW, Foidart JM, Sismondi P, Schoultz BV, Vassilopoulou-Sellin R, Galta RE, Lieshout EV, Mol-Arts M, Planellas J, Kubista E. Tibolone increases bone mineral density but also relapse in breast cancer survivors: The Livial Intervention following Breast Cancer: Efficacy, Recurrence and Tolerability Endpoints (LIBERATE) trial bone substudy. *Breast Cancer Res.* 2012 Jan17;14(1):R13.

- Mirkin S, Amadio JM, Bernick BA, Pickar JH, Archer DF. 17beta-estradiol and natural progesterone for menopausal hormone therapy: REPLENISH phase 3 study design of a combination capsule and evidence review. *Maturitas* In press uncorrected proof accessed March 21, 2015. DOI: http://dx.doi.org/10.1016/j.maturitas.2015.02.266.

Chapter 14: HORMONES: PHYTO's, MYCO's, XENO's and DESIGNER NON-STEROIDALS

- Ozen S, Darcan S. Effects of environmental endocrine disruptors on pubertal development. *Journal of Clinical Research in Pediatric Endocrinology* 2011;3(1):1-6.

- Roy JR, Chakraborty S, Chakraborty TR. Estrogen-like endocrine disrupting chemicals affecting puberty in humans- a review. *Medical Science Monitor* 2009;15(6):RA137-145.

- Lovekamp-Swan T, Davis BJ. Mechanisms of phthalate ester toxicity in the female reproductive system. *Environmental Health Perspectives* 2003;111(2):139-45.

- Bolli A, Bulzomi P, et al. Bisphenol A impairs estradiol-induced protective effects against DLD-1 colon cancer cell growth. *International Union of Biochemistry and Molecular Biology Life* 2010;62(9):684-87.

- Sengupta P, Banerjee R. Environmental toxins: Alarming impacts of pesticides in male infertility. *Human & Experimental Toxicology* 2014 Oct;33(10):1017-1039.

- Rozati R, Reddy PP, Reddanna P, Mujtaba R. Role of environmental estrogens in the deterioration of male factor fertility. *Fertil Steril* 2002 Dec;78(6):1187-94.

- Dhaliwal LK, Suri V, Gupta KR, Sahdev S. Tamoxifen: An alternative to clomiphene in women with polycystic ovary syndrome. *J Hum Reprod Sci.* 2011 May;4(2):76-9.

- Pinkerton JV, Thomas S. Use of SERMs for treatment in postmenopausal women. *J Steroid Biochem Mol Biol* 2014 Jul;142C:142-154.

- Goetz M, Schaid DJ, Wickerham DL, Safgren S, Mushiroda T, Kubo M, Batzler A, Costantino J, Vogel V, Paik S, Carlson E, Flockhart D, Wolmark N, Nakamura Y, Weinshilbourm RM, Ingle JN, Ames M. Evaluation of CYP2D6 and efficacy of tamoxifen and raloxifene in women treated for breast cancer chemoprevention:

results from the NSABP P1 and P2 clinical trials. *Clini Cancer Res* 2011 Nov31;17(21):6944-51.

- Pinkerton JV, Stanczyk FZ. Clinical effects of selective estrogen receptor modulators on vulvar and vaginal atrophy. *Menopause* 2014 Mar;21(3):309-19.

- Vogel VG. The NSABP Study of Tamoxifen and Raloxifene (STAR) trial. *Expert Rev Anticancer Ther.* 2009 Jan;9(1):51-60.

- Barrett-Connor E, Mosca L, Collins P, Geiger MJ, Grady D, Kornitzer M, McNabb MA, Wenger NK for the Raloxifene Use for The Heart (RUTH) Trial Investigators. Effects of raloxifene on cardiovascular events and breast cancer in postmenopausal women. *N Engl J Med* 2006; 355:125-137.

- Kangas L, Unkila M. Tissue selectivity of ospemifene: pharmacologic profile and clinical implications. *Steroids* 2013 Dec 11;78(12-13):1273-80.

- Berga SL. Profile of ospemifene in the breast. *Reprod Sci.* 2013 Oct; 20(10): 1130-6.

- Howlader N, Noone AM, Krapcho M, Garshell J, Miller D, Altekruse SF, Kosary CL, Yu M, Ruhl J, Tatalovich Z, Mariotto A, Lewis DR, Chen HS, Feuer EJ, Cronin KA (eds). SEER Cancer Statistics Review. 1975-2011. (http://seer.cancer.gov/csr/1975_2011/). National Cancer Institute. Bethesda MD, http://seer.cancer.gov/csr/1975_2011_/browse_csr.php?sectionSEL=23&pageSEL=sect_23_table.10.html. (http://seer.cancer.gov/csr/1975_2011/browse_csr.php?sectionSEL=23&pageSEL=SECT_23_table.10.html based on November 2013 SEER data submission, posted to the SEER Web site, April 2014.

- Lobo RA. Where are we 10 years after the Women's Health Initiative (WHI)? *J Clin Endocrinol Metab* 2013 May;98(5):1771-80.

- Mirkin S, Komm BS. Tissue-selective estrogen complexes for postmenopausal women.

- *Maturitas.* 2013 Nov;76(3):213-20.

- Moore AA, Pinkerton JV. Conjugated estrogen plus bazedoxifene – a new approach to estrogen therapy. *OBG Management* 2014 Oct;26(10):52-54.

Chapter 15: PROGESTERONE: PILLS, VAGINAL GELS or IUD

- Manson JE, Chlebowski RT, Stefnick ML, et al. Menopausal hormone therapy and health outcomes during the intervention and extended poststopping phases of the Women's Health Initiative (WHI) randomized trials. *JAMA* 2013;310(13):1353-1368.
- The Writing Group for the PEPI Trial. Effects of hormone replacement therapy on endometrial histology in postmenopausal women: The Postmenopausal Estrogen/Progestin Interventions (PEPI) Trial. *JAMA* 1996;275(5):370-375.
- Anderson GL, Limacher M, Assaf AR, et al. Effects of conjugated equine estrogen in postmenopausal womem with hysterectomy: the Women's Health Initiative randomized controlled trial. *JAMA* 2004 Apri 14;291(14):1701-12.
- Stefanick ML, Anderson GI, Margolis KL, et al: WHI Investigators. Effects of conjugated equine estrogens on breast cancer and mammography screening in postmenopausal women with hysterectomy. *JAMA* 2006;295(4):1647-1657.
- Fournier A, Berrino F, Clavel-Chapelon F. Unequal risks for breast cancer associated with different hormone replacement therapies: results from the E3N cohort study. (published correction appears in *Breast Cancer Res Treat* 2008;107(2):307-308). *Breast Cancer Res Treat* 2008;107(1):103-111.
- Fournier A, Berrino F, Riboli E, Avenel V, Clavel-Chapelon F. Breast cancer risk in relation to different types of hormone replacement therapy in the E3N-EPIC cohort. *Int J Cancer* 2005 Apr 10;114(3):448-54.
- Lobo RA. Where are we 10 years after the Women's Health Initiative (WHI)? *J Clin Endocrinol Metab* 2013 May;98(5):1771-80.
- Archer DF, Dorin M, Lewis V, Schneider DL, Pickar JH. Effects of lower doses of conjugated equine estrogens and medroxyprogesterone acetate on endometrial bleeding. (Design: The Women's Health, Osteoporosis, Progestin, Estrogen (Women's HOPE) Study) *Fertil Steril* 2001 Jun;75(6):1080-7.

- Cicinelli E, de Ziegler D, Bulletti C, Mateo MG, Schonauer LM, Galantino P. Direct transport of progesterone from vagina to uterus. *Obstet Gynecol* 2000;95:403-406.
- Levine H, Watson N. Comparison of the pharmacokinetics of Crinone 8% administered vaginally versus Prometrium administered orally in postmenopausal women. *Fertil Steril* 2000 Mar;73(3):516-21.
- Warren MP, Biller BM, Shangold MM. A new clinical option for hormone replacement therapy in women with secondary amenorrhea: effects of cyclic administration of progesterone from the sustained-release vaginal gel Crinone (4% and 8%) on endometrial morphologic features and withdrawal bleeding. *Am J Obstet Gynecol* 1999;180(1 Pt 1): 42-8.
- Cicinelli E, de Ziegler D, Galantino P, Pinto V, Barba B, Morgese S, Schonauer S. Twice-weekly transdermal estradiol and vaginal progesterone as continuous combined hormone replacement therapy in postmenopausal women. *Am J Obstet Gynecol* 2002 Sep;187(3): 556-560.
- Pinkerton JV, Abraham L, Bushmakin AG, et al. Evaluation of the efficacy and safety of bazedoxifene/conjugated estrogen for secondary outcomes including vasomotor symptoms in postmenopausal woman by years since menopause in Selective estrogens, Menopause and Response to Therapy (SMART) trials. *J Womens Health (Larchmt)* 2014;23(1):18-28.
- Archer DF. Delivery of therapeutic agents to the target tissue. *Menopause* 2011;18(10): 1040-1041.
- Kim ML, Seong SJ. Clinical applications of levonorgestrel-releasing intrauterine system to gynecologic diseases. *Obstet Gynecol Sci* 2013 Mar;56(2):67-75.
- Varma R, Soneja H, Bhatia K, Ganesan R, Rollason T, Clark TJ, Gupta JK. The effectiveness of a levonorgestrel-releasing intrauterine system in the treatment of endometrial hyperplasia – a long-term follow-up study. *Eur j Obstet Gynecolo Reprod Biol.* 2008 Aug;139(2):169-75.

- Chin J, Konje JC, Hickey M. Levonorgestrel intrauterine system for endometrial protection in women with breast cancer on adjuvant tamoxifen. *Cochrane Database Syst Rev.* 2009 Oct;(4):CD007245.

- Kaunitz AM, Meredith S, Inki P, Kubba A, Sanchez-Ramos L. Levonorgestrel-releasing intrauterine system and endometrial ablation in heavy menstrual bleeding: a systematic review and meta-analysis. *Obstet Gynecol* 2009 May;113(5):1104-16.

- Ergun B, Kuru O, Sen S, Kilic Y. Comparison between roller-ball endometrial ablation and levonorgestrel intrauterine system in the treatment of abnormal uterine bleeding. *J Turk Soc Obstet Gynecol* 2011;8(4):259-63.

- Soonboonporn W, Panna S, Temtanakitpaisan T, Daewrudee S, Soontrapa S. Effects of the levonorgestrel-releasing intrauterine system plus estrogen therapy in perimenopausal and postmenopausal women: systematic review and meta-analysis. *Menopause* 2011;18(10): 1060-1066.

- Wu JP, Pickle S. Extended use of the intrauterine device: a literature review and recommendations for clinical practice. *Contraception* 2014 Jun;89(6):495-503.

- Kaislasuo J, Suhonen S, Gissler M, Lahteenmake P, Heikinheimo O. Intrauterine contraception: incidence and factors associated with uterine perforation – a population-based study. *Hum Reprod* 2012;27(9):2658-2663.

- Sivin I, Stern J, Coutinho E, Mattos CER, El Mahgoub S, Diaz S, Pavez M, Alvarez F, Brache V, Thevinin F, Diaz J, Faundes A, Diaz MM, McCarthy T, Mishell Jr DR, Shoupe D. Prolonged intrauterine contraception: a seven-year randomized study of the levonorgestrel 20 mcg/day and the copper T380 Ag IUDs. *Contraception* 1991 Nov;44(5):473-80.

- Lundstrom E, Soderqvist G, Svane G, Azavedo E, Olovosson M, Skoog L, von Schoultz E, Von Schoultz B. Digitized assessment of mammographic breast density in patients who received low-dose intrauterine levonorgestrel in continuous combination with oral estradiol valerate: a pilot study. *Fertil Steril* 2006 Apr;85(4):989-95.

Chapter 16: HOT! HOT! HOT!

- Freedman RR, Physiology of hot flashes. *Am J Hum Biol* 2001; 13:453-464
- Greene RA. Cerebral blood flow. *Fertil Steril* 2000;73:143
- Kronenberg F, Hot flashes: epidemiology and physiology. *Ann NY Acad Sci.* 1990; 592:52-86.
- Avis NE, Crawford SL, Greendale G, Bromberger JT, Everson-Rose SA, Gold EB, Hess R, Joffe H, Kravitz HM, Tepper PG, Thurston RC; for the Study of Women's Health Across the Nation (SWAN). Duration of menopausal vasomotor symptoms over the menopause transition. *JAMA Intern Med.* Published online February 16, 2015. doi: 10.1001/jamainternmed.2014.8063.
- Rodstrom D, Bengtsson C, Lissner L, Milsom I, Sundh V, Bjorkelund C. A longitudinal study of the treatment of hot flushes: the population study of women in Gothenburg during a quarter of a century. *Menopause* 2002;9:156-61.
- Vikstrom J, Spetz Holm A, Sdsjo G, Marcusson J, Wressle E, Hammar M. Hot flashes still occur in a population of 85-year old Swedish women. *Climacteric* 2013;16:453-459.
- Politi MC, Schleinitz MD, Col NF, Revisiting the duration of vasomotor symptoms of menopause: a meta-analysis, *J Gen Intern Med* 2008; 23: 1507-1503
- Col NF, Guthrie JR, Politi M, Dennerstein L, Duration of vasomotor symptoms in middle-aged women: a longitudinal study, *Menopause* 2009; 16:453.
- Utian WH, Shoupe D, Bachmann G, Pinkerton JV, Pickar JH. Relief of vasomotor symptoms and vaginal atrophy with lower doses of conjugated equine estrogens and medroxyprogesterone acetate. *Fertil Steril.* 2001 Jun;75(6):1065-79.

- Sarrel, MD, Portman D, Lefebvre P, Lafeuille MH, Grittner AM, Fortier J, Gravel J, Duh, MS, Aupperle PM. Incremental direct and indirect cost of untreated vasomotor symptoms. *Menopause* 2015 March;22(3):260-266.

- Whiteley, J, Wagner JS, Bushmakin A, Kopenhafer, L, Dibonaventura M, Racketa J. Impact of the severity of vasomotor symptoms on health status, resource use, and productivity. *Menopause* 2013;20:518.524.

- Thurston RC, El Khoudary SR, Sutton-Tyrrell K, et al. Are vasomotor symptoms associated with alterations in hemostatic and inflammatory markers? Findings from Study of Women's Health Across the Nation (SWAN). *Menopause* 2011;18:1044-1051.

- Joffe H, Massler A, Sharkey KM. Evaluation and management of sleep disturbance during the menopause transition. *Semin Reprod Med.* 2010;28:404-421

- Reed SD, Ludman EJ, Newton KM, Grothaus LC, LaCroix AZ, Nekhlyudov L, et al. Depressive symptoms and menopausal burden in the midlife. *Maturitas* 2009;62:306-310.

- Woods NF, Smith-DiJulio K, Percival DB, Tao EY, Mariella A, Mitchell S. Depressed mood during the menopausal transition and early postmenopause:observations from the Seattle Midlife Women's Health Study. *Menopause.* 2008;15:223-232.

- Thurston, RC, Sutton-Tyrrell K, Everson-Rose SA, Hess R, Matthews KAl Hot flashes and subclinical cardiovascular disease: findings from the Study of Women's Health Across the Nation (SWAN) Heart Study. *Circulation* 2008;118:1234-1240

- Herber-Gast G, Mishra, G. Early severe vasomotor menopausal symptoms are associated with diabetes. *Menopause* 2014;21(8)855-860.

- Rossouw JE, Prentice RL, Manson JE, Wu L, Barad D, Barnabei VM, et al. Postmenopausal hormone therapy and risk of cardiovascular disease by age and years since menopause. *JAMA* 2007;297:1465-1477.

- Crandall CJ, Tseng CH, Crawford SL, Thurston RC, Gold EB, Johnston JM, et al. Association of menopausal vasomotor symptoms with increased bone turnover during the menopausal transition. *J Bone Miner Res.* 2010.
- Huang Y, Malone K, Cushing-Haugen KL, Daling J and Li, C. Relationship between menopausal symptoms and the risk of postmenopausal breast cancer. *Cancer Epidemiology Biomarkers & Prevention* 2011;20(2)1-10.
- Avis NE, Ory M, Matthews KA, Schocken M, Bromberger J, Colvin A. Health-related quality of life in a multiethnic sample of middle-aged women: Study of Women's Health Across the Nation (SWAN). *Med Care* 2003;41:1262-1276.
- Nappi RE, Lachowskly M. Menopause and sexuality: prevalence of symptoms and impact on quality of life. *Maturitas* 2009;63:138-141
- Newton KM, Buist DS, Keenan NL, Anderson LA, LaCroix AZ. Use of alternative therapies for menopause symptoms; results of a population-based survey. *Obstet Gynecology* 2002;100:18-25.
- Rada G et al. Non-hormonal interventions for hot flushes in women with a history of breast cancer. Cochrane Database Syst Rev. 2010 Sep8;(9)CD004923.
- Nelson HD et al. Non-hormonal therapies for menopausal hot flashes: systemic review and meta-analysis. *JAMA.* 2006 May 3;295(17) 2057-71.
- Bair YA, Gold EB, Zhang G, et al. Use of complementary and alternative medicine during the menopause transition: longitudinal results from the Study of Women's Health Across the Nation (SWAN). Menopause. 2008;15:32-43.
- Peng W, Adams J, Sibbritt D, Frawley J. Critical review of complementary and alternative medicine use in menopause: focus on prevalence, motivation, decision-making, and communication. *Menopause.* 2014; Vol.21, No.5, pp. 536-548

- MacLennan AH, Henry D, Hills S, Moore V, Oral estrogen replacement therapy versus placebo for hot flushes. *Climacteric.* 2001 Mar; 4(1):58-74.
- Pearce J, Hawton K, Blake F, Barolow D, Rees M, Fagg J, Keenan J, Psychologocial effects of continuation versus discontinuation of hormone replacement therapy by estrogen implants: a placebo-controlled study, *J Psychosom Res* 42:177, 1997.
- Winther K, Rein E, Hedman C. Femal, a herbal remedy made from pollen extracts, reduces hot flushes and improves quality of life in menopausal women: a randomized, placebo-controlled, parallel study. *Climacteric.* 2005 Jun;8(2):162-70.
- Goldstein, S et al. Poster presentation, "Relizen's effect on the isoenzyme CYP2D6." at annual meeting of North American Menopause Society, Oct 2014, Washington, DC.
- Ak E, Bulut SD, Bulut S, et al. Evaluation of the effect of selective serotonin reuptake inhibitors on bone mineral density: an observational cross-sectional study. *Osteoporosis Int.* 2014 Sep 4 (Epub ahead of print). doi:10.1007/s00198-014-2859-2).
- Moura C, Bernatsky S, Ambrahamowicz M, et al. Antidepressant use and 10-year incident fracture risk: the population-based Canadian Multicentre Osteoporosis Study (CaMoS). *Osteoporosis Int.* 2014;25(5):1473-1481.
- Bruyere O, Reginster J-V. Osteoporosis in patients taking selective serotonin reuptake inhibitors: a focus on fracture outcome. *Endocrine* 2014 Aug 5 (Epub ahead of print). doi: 10.1007/s12020-014-0357-0.

Chapter 17: SLEEP, GLORIOUS SLEEP

- Xu, Q, Lang, C. Examining the relationship between subjective sleep disturbance and menopause: a systematic review and meta-analysis.

Menopause: The Journal of the North American Menopause Society 2014 Dec;21(12):1301-1318.

- Netzer NC, Eliasson AH, Strohl KP. Women with sleep apnea have lower levels of sex hormones. *Sleep Breath.* 7(1):25-29, March 2003
- Toffol E, et al. Melatonin in perimenopausal and postmenopausal women: Associations with mood, sleep, climacteric symptoms, and quality of life. *Menopause.* Vol 22, Issue 5,
- May 2014
- Schernhammer ES, Laden F, Speizer FE, Willett WC, Hunter DJ, Kawachi I, Colditz GA. Rotating Night Shifts and Risk of Breast Cancer in Women Participating in the Nurses' Health Study. *Journal of the National Cancer Institute* 2001. 93(20): 1563-1568.
- Feychting M, Osterlund B, Ahlbom A. Reduced cancer incidence among the blind. *Epidemiology.* 1998 Sep; 9(5):490-4.
- Hansen J. Increased breast cancer risk among women who work predominantly at night. *Epidemiology.* 2001 Jan; 12(1):74-7.

Chapter 18: MIRROR, MIRROR: SKIN, HAIR, and SHAPE-SHIFTING

- Emmerson E, Hardman MJ. The role of estrogen deficiency in skin aging and wound healing. *Biogerontology* 2012 Feb;13(1):3-20.
- Verdier-Sevrain S, et al. Biology of estrogens in skin: implications for skin aging. *Experimental Dermatology* 2006;15:83-94.
- Sator PG, Sator MO, Schmidt JB, Nahavandi H, Radakovic S, Huber JC, Honinsmann H. A prospective, randomized, double-blind, placebo-controlled study on the influence of hormone replacement therapy on skin aging in postmenopausal women. *Climacteric* 2007 Aug;10(4):320-4.
- Dunn LB, Damesyn M, Moore AA, Reuben DB, Greendale GA. Does estrogen prevent skin aging? Results from the First National Health and Nutrition Examination Survey (NHANES- I). *Arch Dermatology* 1997 Mar'133(3)339-42.

- Handel AC, Lima PB, Tonolli VM, Mio LDB, Miot HA. Risk factors for facial melasma in women: a case-control study. *The British Journal of Dermatology* 2014;171(3):588-594.
- Ronkainen PH, Kovanen V, Alen M, Pollanen E, Palonen EM, Ankarberg-Lindgren C, Hamalainen E, Turpeinen U, Kujala UM, Puolakka J, Kaprio J, Sipila S. Postmenopausal hormone replacement therapy modifies skeletal muscle composition and function: a study of monozygotic twin pairs. *J Appl Physiol* 2009 Jul;107(1):25-33.
- Sipila S. Body composition and muscle performance during menopause and hormone replacement therapy. *J Endocrinol Invest.* 2003 Sep;26(9):893-901.
- Michael YL, Gold R, Manson JE, Keast EM, Cochrane BB, Woods NF, Brzyski RG, McNeeley SG, Wallace RB. Hormone therapy and physical function change among older women in the Women's Health Initiative (WHI): a randomized controlled trial. *Menopause* 2010 Mar;17(2):295-302.

Chapter 19: WHAT about WEIGHT?

- Balkau B, Deanfield JE, Despres JP, Bassand JP, Fox KA, Smith SC Jr, et al. International Day for the Evaluation of Abdominal Obesity (IDEA): a study of waist circumference, cardiovascular disease, and diabetes mellitus in 168,000 primary care patients in 63 countries. *Circulation* 2007;116:1942-51.
- Toth, MJ, Tchernof A, Sites CK, Poehlman ET. Effect of menopausal status on body composition and abdominal fat distribution. *Int J Oes Relat Metab Disord* Feb 2000. 24(2):226-31.
- Samieri C, Sun Q, Townsend MK, Chiuve SE, Okereke OI, Willet WC, Stampfer M, Grodstein F. The association between dietary patterns at midlife and health in aging: an observational study. *Ann Intern Med* Nov 2013. 159 (9):584-91.

- Huang G, Wang D, Zeb I, Budoff MJ, Harman SM, Miller V, Brinton EA, El Khoudary SR, Manson JE, Sowers MR, Hodis HN, Merriam GR, Cedars MI, Taylor HS, Naftolin F, Lobo RA, Santoro N, Wildman RP. *Atherosclerosis* 2012 Mar;221(1):198-205.
- Bertaso AG, Bertol D, Duncan BB, Foppa M. Epicardial fat: definition, measurements and systematic review of main outcomes. *Arq Bras Cardiol.* 2013 Jul;101(1):e18-28.
- Fourkala, Evangelia-Ourania et al. Association of skirt size and postmenopausal breast cancer risk in older women: a cohort study within the UK Collaborative Trial of Ovarian Cancer Screening (UKCTOCS). *BMJ Open* 2014 Sep 24, (doi:10.1136/bmjopen-2014-005400).

Chapter 21: SEXUAL FEELING

- Brody S. The relative health benefits of different sexual activities. *J Sex Med* 2010;7:1336-1361.
- Davison SL, Bell RJ, LaChina M, Holden SL, Davis SR. The relationship between self-reported sexual satisfaction and general well-being in women. *J Sex Med* 2009;6:2690-2697.
- Chao JK, Lin YC, Ma MC, et al. Relationship among sexual desire, sexual satisfaction, and quality of life in middle-aged and older adults. *J Sex Marital Ther* 2011;37:386-403.
- Hawton K, Gath D, Day A. Sexual function in a community sample of middle-aged women with partners: effects of age, marital, socioeconomic, psychiatric, gynecological, and menopausal factors. *Arch Sex Behav* 1994;23:375-395.
- Morley JE, Tolson DT. Sexuality and aging. In: Alan J, Sinclair AJ, Morley JE, Vellas B, eds. *Pathy's Principles and Practice of Geriatric Medicine,* 5th ed. New York, NY; Wiley Blackwell, 2012:99-102.
- Simon J, Klaiber E, Wiita B, Bowen A, Yang HM. Differential effects of estrogen-androgen and estrogen-only therapy on vasomotor symptoms, gonadotropin secretion, and endogenous androgen

bioavailability in postmenopausal women. *Menopause* 6:138-146, 1999.

- Basson R, Schultz WW. Sexual sequelae of general medical disorders. *Lancet* 2007;369:409-424.

- Dasgupta R, Wiseman OJ, Kanabar G, Fowler CJ, Mikol DD. Efficacy of sildenafil in the treatment of female sexual dysfunction due to multiple sclerosis. *J Urol* 2004;171:1189-1193; discussion 1193.

- Brody S, Kruger TH. The post-orgasmic prolactin increase following intercourse is greater than following masturbation and suggests greater satiety. *Biol Psychol.* 2006 Mar;71(3):312-5.

- Turna B, Apaydin E, Semerci B, Altay B, Cikili N, Nazli O. Women with low libido: correlation of decreased androgen levels with female sexual dysfunction index. *Int J Impot Res* 2005 Mar-Apr;17(2):148-153.

- Davis SR. Cardiovascular and cancer safety of testosterone in women. *Curr Opin Endocrinol Diabetes Obes* 2011;18(3):198-203.

- Bolour S, Braunstein G. Testosterone therapy in women: a review. *Int J Impot Res* 2005 Sep-Oct;17(5):399-408.

- Davis SR, Braunstein GD. Efficacy and safety of testosterone in the management of hypoactive sexual desire disorder in postmenopausal women. *J Sex Med.* 2012 Apr;9(4):1134-48.

- Rosen RC, Maserejian NN, Connor MK, Krychan ML, Brown CS, Goldstein I. Characteristics of premenopausal and postmenopausal women with acquired, generalized hypoactive sexual desire disorder: the Hypoactive Sexual Desire Registry for women. *Menopause* 2012 ;19(4):396-405.

- Nastri CO, Lara LA, Ferriani RA, Rosa-E-Silva AC, Figueiredo JB, Martins WP. Hormone therapy for sexual function in perimenopausal and postmenopausal women. *Cochrane Database Syst Rev.* 2013 Jun 5;6:CD009672. doi: 10.1002/14651858.CD009672. pub2.

- Cummings SR, Ettinger B, Delmas PD, Kenemans P, Stathopoulos V, Verwij P, Mol-Arts M, Kloosterboer HJ, Mosca L, Christiansen

C, Bilesikian J, Kerzberg EM, Johnson S, Zanchetta JR, Grobbee De, Seifert W, Easell R, LIFT (Long-term Intervention on Fractures with Tibolone) Trial Investigators. The effects of tibolone in older postmenopausal women. *New Engl J Med* 2008;359:697-708.

- Bots ML, Evans GW, Riley W, McBride KH, Paskett ED, Helmond FA, Grobbee DE, for the OPAL (Osteoporosis Prevention and Arterial Effects of Tibolone) Trial Investigators. The effect of of tibolone and continuous combined conjugated equine estrogens plus medroxyprogesterone acetate on progression of carotid intima-media thickness. *Eur Heart J* 2006 Mar;27(6)746-55.

- Morais-Socorro Maria, et al. Safety and efficacy of tibolone and menopausal transition: a randomized, double-blind placebo-controlled trial. *Gynecological Endocrinology* 2012; 28(6):483-487.

- Formoso G, Perrone E, et al. Short and long term effect of tibolone in postmenopausal women. *Cochrane Database Syst Rev.* 2012 Feb 15;2:CD008536. Doi: 10.1002/14651858, CD008536.pub2.

Chapter 23: BLADDER BLUNDERS – DRY, but LEAKY

- Moegele M, Buchholz S, Seitz S, Ortmann O. Vaginal estrogen therapy in postmenopausal breast cancer patients treated with aromatase inhibitors. *Arch Gynecol Obstet* 2012;285(5):1397-1302.

- Wu J, Matthews C, Conover M, Pate V, Funk M. Lifetime risk of stress urinary incontinence and pelvic organ prolapse surgery. *Obstetrics & Gynecology* 2014;123 (6):1201-1206.

- Trutnovsky G, Rojas R et al. Urinary incontinence: the role of menopause. *Menopause* 2014;21(4):399-402.

- Cody JD, Richardson K, Moehrer B, Hextall A, Glazener CM. Estrogen therapy for urinary incontinence in postmenopausal women. *Cochrane Databas Syst Rev.*2009;(4):CD001405.

- Hendrix SL, Cochrane BB, Nygaard ID, et al. Effects of estrogen with and without progestin on urinary incontinence. *JAMA.* 2005;293(8):935-948.

- Luthje P, Brauner H, Ramos N, Ovregaard A, Glasser R et al. Estrogen supports uroepithelial defense mechanisms. *Science Translational Medicine* 2013;5(190).
- Perrotta C, Aznar M, Mejia R, Albert X, Ng CW. Estrogens for preventing recurrent urinary tract infection in postmenopausal women. *Concrane Datatbase Syst Rev.* 2008; 2:CD005131.
- Barucha AE, Zinsmeister AR, Locke GR, Seide BM, McKeon K, Schleck CD et al. Prevalence and burden of fecal incontinence: A population based study in women; *Gastroenterology* 2005; 129(1):42-49.
- Archer DF. Efficacy and tolerability of local estrogen therapy for urogenital atrophy. *Menopause* 2010;17(1):194-203.
- Suckling J, Lethaby A, Kennedy R. Local estrogen for vaginal atrophy in postmenopausal women. *Cochrance Databas Syst Rev.* 2006 Oct 18;(4)CD001500
- Al-Baghdadi O, Ewies AA. Topical estrogen therapy in the management of postmenopausal vaginal atrophy: an up-to-date overview. *Climacteric* 2009 Apr;12(2):91-105.
- Pal L, Hailpern SM, Santoro NF, Freeman R, Barad D, Kipersztok S, Barnabei VM, Wassertheil-Smoller S. Association of pelvic organ prolapse and fractures in postmenopausal women: analysis of baseline data from the Women's Health Initiative Estrogen plus Progestin trial. *Menopause* 2008 Jan-Feb;15(1):59-66.
- Pal L. Pelvic organ prolapse and relationship with skeletal integrity. *Womens Health (Lond Engl)* 2009 May;5(3):325-33.
- Berecki-Gisolf J, Spallek M, Hockey R, Dobson A. Height loss in elderly women is preceded by osteoporosis and is associated with digestive problems and urinary incontinence. *Osteoporosis Intl.* 2010;21:479-485.
- Rahn, David D, Carberry, Cassandra, Sanses, Tatiana V, Mamik, Mamta M, Ward, Renee M, Meriwether, Kate V, Olivera, Cedric K, Abed, Husam, Balk, Ethan M, and Murphy, Miles for the Society of Gynecologic Surgeons Systematic Review Group. Vaginal estrogen

for genitourinary syndrome of menopause. *Obstetrics & Gynecology* 2014 December; 124(6):1147-56.

Chapter 24: WITHERING SENSES

- Velez Edwards, DR, Gallins P, Polk M, Ayala-Haedo J, Schwartz SG, Kovach JL, Spencer K, Wang, G, Agarwal A, Postel EA, Haines JL, Pericak-Vance M, Scott W. Inverse association of female hormone replacement therapy with age-related macular degeneration and interactions with ARMS2 polymorphism. *Invest. Ophthalmol. Vis. Sci.* 2010 Apr;51(4):1873-1879.
- Freeman EE, Munoz B, Bressler SB, West SK. Hormone replacement therapy, reproductive factors, and age-related macular degeneration: the Salisbury Eye Evaluation Project. *Ophthalmic Epidemiol.* 2005 Feb;12(1):37-45.
- Feskanich D, Cho E, Schaumberg DA, Colditz GA, Hankinson SE. Menopausal and reproductive factors and risk of age-related macular degeneration. *Arch Ophthalmol* 2008 Apr;126(4):519-24.
- Eisner A, Luoh, S-W. Breast cancer medications and vision: effects of treatments for early-stage disease. *Curr Eye Res.* 2011 Oct; 36(10):867-885.
- Wang J, Yan H. Preventive effect of estrogen on cataract development. *Yan Ke Zue Bao* 2006 Mar;22(1):20-4.
- Younan C, Mitchell P, Cumming RG, Panchapakesan J, Rochtchina E, Hales AH. Hormone replacement therapy, reproductive factors, and the incidence of cataract and cataract surgery- the Blue Mountains Eye Study. *Am J Epidemiol* 2002;155:997-1006.
- Lindblad B, Hakansson N, Philipson B, Wolk A. Hormone replacement therapy in relation to risk of cataract extraction: a prospective study of women. *Opthalmology* 2010 Mar; 117(3):424-30.
- Pasquale LR, Kang JH. Female reproductive factors and primary open-angle glaucoma in the Nurse's Health Study. *Eye* 2011;25:633-641.

- Deschenes MC, Descovich D, Moreau M, et al. Postmenopausal hormone therapy increases retinal blood flow and protects the retinal nerve fiber layer. *Invest Ophthalmol Vis Sci* 2010;51:2587-2600.
- Crovetto MA, Whyte J, Rodriguez OM, Lecumberri I, Martinez C, Fernandez C, Crovetto R, Municio A, Vrotsou K. Influence of aging and menopause in the origin of the superior semicircular canal dehiscence. *Otol Neurotol.* 2012 Jun;33(4):681-4.
- Tremere, LA, Jeong JK, Pinaud R. Estradiol shapes auditory processing in the adult brain by regulating inhibitory transmission and plasticity-associated gene expression. *The Journal of Neuroscience* 2009 May;29(18): 5949-5963.
- Kilicdag EB, Yavuz H, Bagis T, Tarim E, Erkan AN, Kazanci F. Effects of estrogen therapy on hearing in postmenopausal women. *Am J Obstet Gynecolog.* 2004 Jan;190(1):77-82.
- Volpe A, Lucenti V, Forabosco A, Boselli F, Latessa AM, Pozzo P, Petraglia F, Genazzani AR. Oral discomfort and hormone replacement therapy in the postmenopause. *Maturitas* 1991; 13(1):1-5.
- Norderyd OM, Grossi SG, Machtel EE, Zambon JJ, Hausmann E, Dunford RG, Genco RJ. Periodontal status of women taking postmenopausal estrogen supplementation. *J Periodontol.* 1993 Oct;64(10):957-62.
- Harris TM. The pharmacological treatment of voice disorders. *Folia Phoniatr (Basel).* 1992:44(3-4):143-54.

Chapter 25: GUT FEELING

- Paganini-Hill A. The benefits of estrogen replacement on oral health. The Leisure World cohort. *Arch Intern Med.* 1995 Nov 27;155(21):2325-9.
- Grodstein F, Colditz GA, Stampfer MJ. Postmenopausal hormone use and tooth loss: a prospective study. *J Am Dent Assoc.* 1996 Mar;127(3):370-7.

- Triadafilopoulos G., Finlayson M, Grelllet C. Bowel dysfunction in postmenopausal women. *Womens Health* 1998;27(4): 55-66.
- Lowe DA, Baltgalvis KA, Greising SM. Mechanisms behind estrogen's beneficial effect on muscle strength in females. *Exerc Sport Sci Rev* 2010;38(2):61-67.
- Infantino M. The prevalence and pattern of gastroesophageal reflux symptoms in perimenopausal and menopausal women. *J Am Acad Nurse Pract.* 2008 May;20(5):266-72.
- Lin D, Kramer JR, Ramsey D, Alsarraj A, Verstovsek G, Rugge M, Parente P, Graham DY, El-Serag HB. Oral bisphosphonates and the risk of Barrett's esophagus: case-control analysis of US veterans. *Am J Gastroenterol.* 2013 Oct;108(10):1576-83.
- Jacobson B, Somers S, Fuchs C, et al. Body-mass indes and symptoms of gastroesophageal reflux in women. *N Engl J Med* 2006;354:2340-48.
- Allen A, Flemstrom G. Gastroduodenal mucus bicarbonate barrier: protection against acid and pepsin. *Am J Physiol Cell Physiol.* 2005;288:C1-19.
- Tuo B, Wen G, Wei J, Liu X, Wang X, Zhang Y, Wu H, Dong X, Chow JYC, Vallon V, Dong H.
- Estrogen regulation of duodenal bicarbonate secretion and sex-specific protection of human duodenum. *Gastroenterology* 2011 Sep;141(3): 854-863.
- Vessey MP, Villard-Mackintosh L, Painter R. Oral contraceptives and pregnancy in relation to peptic ulcer. *Contraception* 1992;46:349-57.
- Redchits IV, Petrov EE. The age-related characteristics of the clinical picture of duodenal ulcer in women. *Lik Sprava* 1995:149-52.
- Racine A, Bijon A, Fournier A, Mesrine S, Clavel-Chapelon F, Carbonnel F, Boutron-Ruault, MC. Menopausal hormone therapy and risk of cholecystectomy: a prospective study based on the French E3N cohort. *CMAJ* 2013 Apr;185(7):555-561.

- Liu B, Beral V, Balkwill A, Green J, Sweetland S, Reeves G; Million Women Study Collaborators. Gallbladder disease and use of transdermal versus oral hormone replacement therapy in postmenopausal women: prospective cohort study. *BMJ* 2008 Jul; 337:a386.

- Houghton LA, Lea R, Jackson N, Whorwell PJ. The menstrual cycle affects rectal sensitivity in patients with irritable bowel syndrome but not healthy volunteers. *Gut* 2002 Apr; 50(4): 471-474.

- Kane SV, Sable K, Hanauer SB. The menstrual cycle and its effect on inflammatory bowel disease and irritable bowel syndrome: a prevalence study. *Am J Gastroenterol* 1998; 93:1867-72.

- Whitehead WE, Cheskin LJ, Heller BR, et al. Evidence of exacerbation of irritable bowel syndrome during menses. *Gastroenterology* 1990;98:1485-9.

- Lewis MJV, Houghton LA, Whorwell PJ. Abdominal distension in females with irritable bowel syndrome: the effect of menopause and hormone replacement therapy. *Gut* 2001 Mar; 48(suppl1):A43-A47.

- Kane SV, Reddy D. Hormone replacement therapy after menopause is protective of disease activity in women with inflammatory bowel disease. *The American Journal of Gastroenterology* 2008 May;103: 1193-1196.

- Guerin A, Mody R, Fok B, Lasch KL, Zhou Z, Wu EZ, Zhou W, Talley NJ. Risk of developing colorectal cancer and benign colorectal neoplasm in patients with chronic constipation.

- *Ailment Pharmacol Ther.* 2014 Jul;40(1):83-92.

- Brandstedt J, Wangefjord S, Nodin B, Eberhard J, Jirstrom K, Manjer J. Associations of hormone replacement therapy and oral contraceptives with risk of colorectal cancer defined by clinico-pathological factors, beta-catenin alterations, expression of cyclin D1, p53, and microsatellite-instability. *BMC Cancer* 2014 May 25;14:371.

- Tsilidis KK, Allen NE, Key TJ, et al. Oral contraceptives, reproductive history and risk of colorectal cancer in the European Prospective Investigation into Cancer and Nutrition. *Br J Cancer* 2010 Nov 23;103(11):1755-9.
- Soderlund S, Granath F, Brostrom O, Karlen P, Lofberg R, Ekbom A, Askling J. Inflammatory bowel disease confers a lower risk of colorectal cancer to females than to males. *Gastroenterology* 2010 May;138(5): 1697-703.
- Hendifar A, Yang D, Lenz F, Lurje G, Pohl A, Lenz C, Ning Y, Zhang W, Lenz HJ. Gender disparities in metastatic colorectal cancer survival. *Clin Cancer Res* 2009 Oct;15(20): 6391-7.
- Rennert G, Rennert HS, Pinchev M, Lavie O, Gruber SB. Use of hormone replacement therapy and the risk of colorectal cancer. *J Clin Oncol.* 2009 Sep 20;27(27):4542-7.
- Barzi A, Lenz AM, Labonte M, Lenz H-J. Molecular pathways: estrogen pathway in colon cancer. *Clin Cancer Res* 2013 Nov 1;19(21):5842-8.
- Hannaford P, Elliot A. Use of exogenous hormones by women and colorectal cancer: Evidence from the Royal College of General Practitioners' Oral Contraception Study. *Contraception* 2005;71:95-98.
- Chlebowski RT, Wactawski-Wende J, Ritenbaugh C, Hubbell FA, Ascensao J, Rodabough RJ, Rosenberg CA, Taylor VM, Harris R, Chen C, Adams-Campbell LL, White E; Women's Health Initiative Investigators. Estrogen plus progestin and colorectal cancer in postmenopausal women. *N Engl J Med* 2004 Mar 4;350(10):991-1004.
- Cook NR, Lee IM, Zhang SM, Moorthy MV, Buring JE. Alternate-day, low-dose aspirin and cancer risk: long-term observational follow-up of a randomized trial. *Ann Intern Med.* 2013 Jul 16;159(2):77-85.

Chapter 26: BREAST MATTERS

- Hashemi SH, Karimi S, Mahboobi H. Lifestyle changes for prevention of breast cancer. *Electron Physician.* 2014 Jul 1; 6(3):894-905.

- Li CI Baeber EF, Tang MT, Porger PL, Daling JR, Malone KE. Reproductive factors and risk of estrogen receptor positive, triple-negative, and HER2-neu overexpressing breast cancer among women 20-44 years of age. *Breast Cancer Res Treat.* 2013 Jan; 137(2):579-87.
- Collaborative Group on Epidemiological Studies of Ovarian Cancer. Menopausal hormone use and ovarian cancer risk: individual participant meta-analysis of 52 epidemiological studies. Published on line: *The Lancet.* 12 Feb 2015. DOI: http:dx.doi.org/10.1016/S1040-6736(14)61687-1.
- Manson JE, Chlebowski RT, Stefanick ML, Aragaki AK, Rossouw JE, Prentice RL, Anderson G, Howard BV, Thomson CA, LaCroix AZ, Wactawski-Wende J, Jackson RD, Limacher M, Margolis KL, Wassertheil-Smoller S, Beresford SA, Cauley JA, Eaton CB, Gass M, Hsia J, Johnson KC, Kooperberg C, Kuller LH, Lewis CE, Liu S, Martin LW, Ockene JK, O'Sullivan MJ, Powell LH, Simon MS, Van Horn L, Vitolins MZ, Wallace RB. Menopausal hormone therapy and health outcomes during the intervention and extended poststopping phases of the Women's Health Initiative randomized trials. *JAMA.* 2013 Oct 2;310(13): 1353-68.
- Nyante SJ, Gierach GL, Dallal CM, Freedman ND, Park Y, Danforth KN, Hollenbeck AR, Brinton LA. Cigarette smoking and postmenopausal breast cancer risk in a prospective cohort. *British Journal of Cancer* 2014 Apr 29; 110: 2339-2347.
- Kawai M, Malone KE, Tang M and Li CI. Active smoking and risk of estrogen receptor-positive and triple-negative breast cancer among women ages 20 to 44 years. *Cancer.* 2014 Apr 1; 120 (7): 1026-1034.
- Flynn-Evans EE, Stevens RG, Tabandeh H, Schemhammer ES, Lockley SW. Total visual blindness is protective against breast cancer. *Cancer Causes Control.* 2009 Nov 1; 20 (9): 1753-6.
- Viswanathan AN, Schemhammer ES. Circulating melatonin and the risk of breast and endometrial cancer in women. *Cancer Lett.* 2009 Aug 18; 281 (1): 1-7.

- Grant SC, Melan MA, Latimer JJ, Witt-Enderby PA. Melatonin and breast cancer: cellular mechanisms, clinical studies and future perspectives. *Expert Rev Mol Med.* 2009 Feb 9; 11: e5.
- Kliukiene J, Tynes T, Andersen A. Risk of breast cancer among Norwegian women with visual impairment. *Br J Cancer.* 2001 Feb 2; 84(3): 397-9.
- Culver AL, Ockene IS, Balasubramanian R, Olendzki BC, Sepavich DM, Wactawski-Wende J, Manson JE, Qiao Y, Liu S, Merriam PA, Rahilly-Tierny C, Thomas F, Berger JS, Ockene JK, Curb JD, Ma Y. Statin use and risk of diabetes mellitus in postmenopausal women in the Women's Health Initiative. *Arch Intern Med.* 2012 Jan 23; 172(2):144-52.
- Goodarzi MO, Li X, Krauss RM, Rotter JI, Chen Y-DI. Relationship of sex to diabetes risk in statin trials. *Diabetes Care.* 2013 Jul; 36(7): e100-e101.
- McDougall JA, Malone KE, Daling JR, Cushing-Haugen KL, Porter PL, Li CI. Long-term statin use and risk of ductal and lobular breast cancer among women 55 to 74 years of age. *Cancer Epidemiol Biomarkers Prev.* 2013 Sep; 22(9): 1529-37.
- Desai P, Chlebowski R, Cauley JA, Manson JE, Wu C, Martin LW, Jay A, Bock C, Cote M, Petrucelli N, Rosenberg CA, Peters U, Agalliu I, Budrys N, Abdul-Hussein M, Lane D, Luo J, Park HL, Thomas F, Wactawski-Wende J, Simon MS. Prospective analysis of association between statin use and breast cancer risk in the Women's Health Initiative. *Cancer Epidemiol Biomarkers Prev.* 2013 Oct; 22(10):1868-76.
- Campbell PT, Newton CC, Patel AV, Jacobs EJ, Gapstur SM. Diabetes and cause-specific mortality in a prospective cohort of one million U.S. adults. *Diabetes Care.* 2012 Sep; 35(9): 1835-44.
- Kim Y, Je Y. Vitamin D intake, blood 25(OH)D levels, and breast cancer risk or mortality: a meta-analysis. *Br J Cancer.* 2014 Apr 8. doi: 10.1038/bjc.2014.175.

- Crew JD. Vitamin D: are we ready to supplement for breast cancer prevention and treatment. *ISRN Oncol.* 2013;2013:483687. doi: 10.1155/2013/483687. Epub 2013 Feb 26.
- Shao T, Klein P, Grossbard ML. Vitamin D and breast cancer. *Oncologist.* 2012;17(1): 36-45.
- Beaber EF, Buist DS, Barlow WE, Malone KE, Reed SD, Li CI. Recent oral contraceptive use by formulation and breast cancer risk among women 20 to 49 years of age. *Cancer Res.* 2014 Aug 1; 74(15): 4078-89.
- Charlton BM, Rich-Edwards JW, Colditz GA, Missmer SA, Rosner BA, Hankinson SE, Speizer FE, Michels KB. Oral contraceptive use and mortality after 36 years of follow-up in the Nurses' Health Study: prospective cohort study. *BMJ.* 2014 Oct 31; 349:g6356.
- Hunter DJ, Colditz GA, Hankinson SE, Malspeis S, Spiegelman D, Chen W, Stampfer MJ, Willett WE. Oral contraceptive use and breast cancer: a prospective study of young women. *Cancer Epidemiol Biomarkers Prev.* 2010 Oct; 19(10):2496-502.
- Havrilesky LJ, Moorman PG, Lowery WJ, Geirisch JM, Coeytaux RR, Urrutia RP, Dinan M, McBroom AJ, Hasselblad V, Sanders GD, Myers ER. Oral contraceptive pills as primary prevention for ovarian cancer: a systematic review and meta-analysis. *Obstet Gynecol.* 2013 Jul; 122(1):139-47.
- Francis PA, Regan MM, Fleming GF, Lang I, Ciruelos E, Bellet M, Bonnefoi HR, Climent MA, Da Prada GA, Burstein HJ, Martino S, Davidson NE, Geyer CE Jr, Walley BA, Coleman R, Kerbrat P, Buchholz S, Ingle JN, Winer EP, Rabaglio-Poretti M, Maibach R, Ruepp B, Giobbie-Hurder A, Price KN, Colleoni M, Viale G, Coates AS, Goldhirsch A, Gelber RD, Suppression of Ovarian Function Trial (SOFT) Investigators; International Breast Cancer Study Group. Adjuvant ovarian suppression in premenopausal breast cancer. *N Engl J Med.* 2015 Jan 29; 372(5):436-46.
- Barron TI, Flahavan EM, Sharp L, Bennett K, Visvanathan K. Recent prediagnostic aspirin use, lymph node involvement, and

5-year mortality in women with stage I-III breast cancer: a nation-wide population-based cohort study. *Cancer Res.* 2014 Aug 1; 74(15):4065-77.

- Bowers LW, Maximo IX, Brenner AJ, Beeram M, Hursting SD, Price RS, Tekmal RR, Jolly CA, deGraffenried LA. NSAID use reduces breast cancer recurrence in overweight and obese women: role of prostaglandin-aromatase interactions. *Cancer Res.* 2014 Aug 15; 74 (16): 4446-57.

- Harris RE, Chlebowski RT, Jackson RD, Frid DJ, Ascenseo JL, Anderson G, Loar A, Rodabough RJ, White E, McTiernan A. Breast cancer and nonsteroidal anti-inflammatory drugs: prospective results from the Women's Health Initiative. *Cancer Res.* 2003 Sep 15; 63: 6096-6101.

- Cuzick J, Thorat MA, Bosetti C, Brown PH, Burn J, Cook NR, Ford LG, Jacobs EJ, Jankowski JA, LaVecchia C, Law M, Meyskens F, Rothwell PM, Senn HJ, Umar A. Estimates of benefits and harms of prophylactic use of aspirin in the general population. *Ann Oncol.* 2015 Jan; 26 (1): 47-57.

- Luo T, Yan HM, He P, Luo Y, Yang YF, Zheng H. Aspirin use and breast cancer risk; a meta-analysis. *Breast Cancer Res Treat.* 2012 Jan; 131(2):581-7.

- Santen RJ, Song Y, Yue W, Wang JP, Heitjan DF. Effects of menopausal hormonal therapy on occult breast tumors. *J Steroid Biochem Mol Biol.* 2013 Sep; 137:150-6.

- Senten RJ, Yue W, Heitjan DF. Modeling of the growth kinetics of occult breast tumors: role in interpretation of studies of prevention and menopausal hormone therapy. *Cancer Epidemiology Biomarkers & Prevention.* 2012 July; 21(&): 1038-48.

- Santen RJ. Menopausal hormone therapy and breast cancer. *J Steroid Biochem Mol Biol.* 2014 Jul; 142:52-61.

- Collins JA, Blake JM, Crosignani PG. Breast cancer risk with post-menopausal hormonal treatment. *Hum Reprod Update.* 2005 Nov-Dec; 11(6):545-60.

- McTiernan A, Chlebowski RT, Martin C, Peck JD, Aragaki A, Pisano ED, Wang CY, Johnson KC, Manson JE, Wallace RB, Vitolins MZ, Heiss G. Conjugated Equine Estrogen influence on mammographic density in postmenopausal women in a substudy of the Women's Health Initiative Randomized Trial. *J Clin Oncol.* 2009 Dec 20; 27(36): 6135-6143.

- McTiernan A, Martin CF, Peck JD, Aragaki AK, Chlebowski RT, Pisano ED, Wang CY, Brunner RL, Johnson KC, Manson JE, Lewis CE, Kotchen JM, Hulka BS; Women's Health Initiative Mammogram Density Study Investigators. *J Natl Cancer Inst.* 2005 Sep 21; 97 (18): 1366-76.

- Stefanick ML, Anderson GL, Margolis KL, Hendrix SL, Rodabough RJ, Paskett ED, Lane DS, Hubbell FA, Assaf AR, Sarto GE, Schenken RS, Yasmeen S, Lessin L, Chlebowski RT; WHI Investigators. Effects of conjugated equine estrogens on breast cancer and mammography screening in postmenopausal women with hysterectomy. *JAMA.* 2006 Apr 2; 295(14): 1647-57.

- Chlebowski RT, Hendrix SL, Langer RD, Stefanick ML, Gass M, Lane D, Rodabough RJ, Gilligan MA, Cyr MG, Thomson CA, Khandekar J, Petrovitch H, McTiernan A; WHI Investigators. Influence of estrogen plus progestin on breast cancer and mammography in healthy postmenopausal women: the Women's Health Initiative Randomized Trial. *JAMA.* 2003 Jun 25; 289(4):3243-53.

- Anderson GL, Limacher M, Assaf AR, Bassford T, Beresford SA, Black H, Bonds D, Brunner R, Brzyski R, Caan B, Chlebowski R, Curb D, Gass M, Hays J, Heiss G, Hendrix S, Howard BV, Hsia J, Hubbell A, Jackson R, Johnson KC, Judd H, Kotchen JM, Kuller L, LaCroix AZ, Lane D, Langer RD, Lasser N, Lewis CE, Manson JE, Margolis K, Ockene J, O'Sullivan MJ, Phillips L, Prentice RL, Ritenbaugh C, Robbins J, Rossouw JE, Sarto G, Stefanick ML, Van Horn L, Wactawski-Wende J, Wallace R, Wassertheil-Smoller S; Women's Health Initiative Steering Committee. Effects of conjugated equine estrogen in postmenopausal women with hysterectomy:

the Women's Health Initiative randomized controlled trial. *JAMA.* 2004 Apr 14; 291(14):1701-12.

- LaCroix AZ, Chlebowski RT, Manson JE, Aragaki AK, Johnson KC, Martin L, Margolis KL, Stefanick ML, Brzyski R, Curb JD, Howard BV, Lewis CE, Wactawski-Wende J; WHI Investigators. Health outcomes after stopping conjugated equine estrogens among postmenopausal women with prior hysterectomy: a randomized controlled trial. *JAMA.* 2011 Apr 6; 305(13):1305-14.

- Chen WY, Manson JE, Hankinson SE, Rosner B, Holmes MD, Willett WC, Colditz GA. Unopposed estrogen therapy and the risk of invasive breast cancer. [Nurses' Health Study] *Arch Intern Med.* 2006; 166(9):1027-1032.

- Li CI, Malone KE, Porter PL, Weiss NS, Tang MT, Cushing-Haugen KL, Daling JR. Relationship between long durations and different regimens of hormone therapy and risk of breast cancer. *JAMA* 2003 Jun 25;289(24):3254-63.

- Fournier A, Berrino F, Clavel-Chapelon F. Unequal risks for breast cancer associated with different hormone replacement therapies: results from the E3N cohort study. *Breast Cancer Res Treat.* 2008 Jan; 107(1):103-11.

- Shapiro S, Farmer RD, Stevenson JC, Burger HG, Mueck AO, Gompel A. Does hormone replacement therapy (HRT) cause breast cancer? An application of causal principles to three studies. *J Fam Plann Reprod Health Care.* 2013 Apr; 39(2):80-8.

- Narod SA. Hormone replacement therapy and the risk of breast cancer. *Natl Rev Clin Oncol.* 2011 Aug 2; 8 (11):669-76.

- Collaborative Group on Hormonal Factors in Breast Cancer. Breast cancer and hormone replacement therapy: collaborative reanalysis of data from 51 epidemiological studies of 52,705 women with breast cancer and 108,411 women without breast cancer. *Lancet.* 11 Oct 1997; 350 (9084): 1047-1059.

- Rossouw JE, Anderson GL, Prentice RL, LaCroix AZ, Kooperberg C, Stefanick ML, Jackson RD, Beresford SA, Howard BV, Johnson

KC, Kotchen JM, Ockene J; Writing Group for the Women's Health Initiative Investigators. Risks and benefits of estrogen plus progestin in healthy postmenopausal women: principal results from the Women's Health Initiative randomized controlled trial. *JAMA.* 2002 Jul 17; 288(3): 321-33.

- Beral V; Million Women Study Collaborators. Breast cancer and hormone replacement therapy in the Million Women Study. *Lancet.* 2003 Aug 9; 362(9382):419-27.

- Beral V, Reeves G, Bull D, Green J; Million Women Study Collaborators. Breast cancer risk in relation to the interval between menopause and starting hormone therapy. *J Natl Cancer Inst.* 2011 Feb 16; 103(4):296-305.

- Saxena T, Lee E, Henderson KD, Clarke CA, West D, Marshall SF, Deapen D, Bernstein L, Ursin G. Menopausal hormone therapy and subsequent risk of specific invasive breast cancer subtypes in the California Teachers Study. *Cancer Epidemiol Biomarkers Prev.* 2010 Sep; 19(9):236678.

- Chlebowski RT, Manson JE, Anderson GL, Cauley JA, Aragaki AK, Stefanick ML, Lane DS, Johnson KC, Wactawski-Wende J, Chen C, Lihong ZI, Shagufta Y, Newcomb PA, Prentice RL. Estrogen plus progestin and breast cancer incidence and mortality in the Women's Health Initiative Observational Study. *J Natl Cancer Inst.* 2013; 105(8):526-535.

- Shapiro S, DeVilliers TJ, Pines A, Sturdee DW, Archer DF, Baber RJ, Pana N, Farmer RDT, Stevenson JC, Mueck AO, Burger HG, Gompel A. RE: Estrogen plus progestin and breast cancer incidence and mortality in the Women's Health Initiative Observational Study. *J Natl Cancer Inst.* 2014 Feb; 106 (2): djt372.

- Kabat GC, Kamensky V, Heo M, Bea JW, Hou L, Lane DS, Liu S, Qi L, Simon MS, Wactawski-Wende J, Rohan TE. Combined conjugated esterified estrogen plus methyltestosterone supplementation and risk of breast cancer in postmenopausal women. *Maturitas.* 2014 Sep; 79(1):70-6.

- Dimitrakakis C, Jones RA, Liu A, Bondy CA. Breast cancer incidence in postmenopausal women using testosterone in addition to usual hormone therapy. *Menopause*. 2004 Sep-Oct; 11(5): 531-5.
- Lewis-Wambi JS, Kim H, Curpan R, Grigg R, Sarker MA, Jordan VC. The selective estrogen receptor modulator bazedoxifene inhibits hormone-independent breast cancer cell growth and down-regulates estrogen receptor alpha and cyclin D1. *Mod Pharmacol*. 2011 Oct; 80(4): 610-620.
- Wardell SE, Nelson ER, Chao CA, McDonnell DP. Bazedoxifene exhibits antiestrogenic activity in animal models of tamoxifen resistant breast cancer; implications for treatment of advanced disease. *Clin Cancer Res*. 2013 May 1; 19(9): 2420-2431.

Chapter 27: BONES, BABY, BONES

- Berecki-Gisolf J, Spallek M, Hockey R, Dobson A. Height loss in elderly women is preceded by osteoporosis and is associated with digestive problems and urinary incontinence. *Osteoporosis Int* 2010;21:479-485.
- Verbalis J. and team from Georgetown University. "Chronic hyponatremia increases risk of osteoporosis and fragility fractures. " Retrospective database study presented at joint meeting of the International Congress of Endocrinology and Endocrine Society, Chicago, IL, June 2014.
- Sugimura Y. Osteoporosis associated with chronic hyponatremia. *Clin Calcium* 2013 Sep; 23(9):1293-8.
- Gray SL, LaCroix AZ, Larson J, Robbins J, Cauley JA, Manson JE, Chen Z. Proton pump inhibitor use, hip fracture and change in bone mineral density in postmenopausal women: results from the Women's Health Initiative. *Arch Intern Med*. 2010 May 10;170(9):765-71.
- Fraser LA, Leslie WD, Targownik LE, Papaioannou A, Adachi JD; CaMoS Research Group. The effect of proton pump inhibitors on

fracture risk: report from the Canadian Multicentre Osteoporosis Study (CaMoS). *Osteoporosis Int.* 2013 Apr;24(4):1161-8.

- Bruyere O, Reginster JY. Osteoporosis in patients taking selective serotonin reuptake inhibitors: a focus on fracture outcome. *Endocrine* 2015 Feb;48(1):65-8.

- Moura C, Bernatsky S, Abrahamowicz M et al. Antidepressant use and 10-year incident fracture risk: the population-based Canadian Multicentre Osteoporosis Study (CaMoS). *Osteoporosis Int.* 2014 May;25(5):1473-81.

- Ak E, Bulut SD, Bulut S, Akdag HA, Oter GB, Kaya H, Kaya OB, Sengul CB, Kisa C. Evaluation of the effect of selective serotonin reuptake inhibitors on bone mineral density: an observational cross-sectional study. *Osteoporosis Int.* 2015 Jan;26(1):273-9.

- Moura C, Bernatsky S, Abrahamowicz M, Papaioannou A, Bessette L, Adachi J, Goltzman D, Prior J, Kreiger N, Towheed T, Leslie WD, Kaiser S, Joannidis G, Pickard L, Fraser LA, Rahme E. Antidepressant use and 10-year incident fracture risk: the population-based Canadian Multicentre Osteoporosis Study (CaMoS). *Osteoporosis Int.* 2014 May;25(5):1473-81.

- Diem SJ, Blackwell TL, Stone KL, Yaffe K, Haney EM, Bliziotes MM, Ensrud KE. Use of antidepressants and rates of hip bone loss in older women: the Study of Osteoporotic Fractures, *Arch Intern Med* 2007 Jun 25; 167(12):1240-5.

- Jobbins JA, Aragaki A, Crandall C, Manson JE, Carbone L, Jackson R, Lewis CE, Johnson KC, Sarto G, Stefanick ML, Wactawski-Wende J. Women's Health Initiative clinical trials: interaction of calcium and vitamin D with hormone therapy. *Menopause: The Journal of the North American Menopause Society* 2014;24(2):116-123.

- Jackson RD, LaCroix AZ, Gass M, et al. Calcium plus vitamin D supplementation and the risk of fractures. *N Engl J Med* 2006;354:669-683.

- Li K, Kaaks R, Linseisen J, Rohrmann S. Associations of dietary calcium intake and calcium supplementation with myocardial infarction and stroke risk and overall cardiovascular mortality in the Heidelberg cohort of the European Prospective Investigation into Cancer and Nutrition stucy (EPIC-Heidelberg). *Heart* 2012;98:920-925.

- Bolland MJ, Grey A, Avenell A, Gamble GD, Reid IR. Calcium supplements with or without vitamin D and risk of cardiovascular events: reanalysis of the Women's Health Initiative limited access dataset and meta-analysis. *BMJ* 2011;342:D2040.

- Sharma A, Einstein AJ, Vallakati A, Arbab-Zadeh A, Walker MD, Mukherjee D, Homel P, Borer JS, Lichstein E. Risk of atrial fibrillation with use of oral and intravenous bisphosphonates. *Am J Cardiol.* 2014 Jun 1;113(1):1815-21.

- Diab DL, Watts NB. Use of drug holidays in women taking bisphosphonates. *Menopause: The Journal of the North American Menopause Society.* 2013;21(2):195-197.

- McCaslin FE Jr, Janes JM. The effect of strontium lactate in the treatment of osteoporosis. *Proc Staff Meetings Mayo Clinic* 1959; 34:329-334.

- Riyat M, Sharma DC. An experimental study of the effect of strontium pre-treatment on calcium release from carious and non-carious teeth. *Biol Trace Elem Res.* 2010 Mar; 133(3):251-4.

- Reginster JY, Sarlet N, Lejeune E, Leonori L. Strontium ranelate: a new treatment for postmenopausal osteoporosis with a dual mode action. *Curr Osteoporos Rep.* 2005 Mar; 3(1):30-4.

- Brixen K, Krogsgaard K, Christgau S, Weis M, Eastell R. Effect of three doses of strontium malonate on markers of bone turnover and bone mineral density: the STRONG study. *Calcif Tissue Int.* 2008;82:S217.

- Meunier PJ, Roux C, Seeman E, et al. The effects of strontium ranelate on the risk of vertebral fracture in women with postmenopausal osteoporosis. *N Engl J Med* 2004; 350:459-68.

- Reginster JY, Seeman E, De Vernejoul MC, et al. Strontium ranelate reduces the risk of nonvertebral fractures in postmenopausal women with osteoporosis: Treatment of Peripheral Osteoporosis (TROPOS) study. *J Clin Endocrinol Metab* 2005;90:2816-22.

- Reginster JY, Kaufman JM, Goemaere S, et al. Maintenance of antifracture efficacy over 10 years with strontium ranelate in postmenopausal osteoporosis. *Osteoporos Int.* 2012; 23: 1115-22.
- Cooper C, Fox KM, Borer JS. Ischaemic cardiac events and use of strontium ranelate in postmenopausal osteoporosis: a nested case-control study in CPRD. *Osteoporosis Int.* 2014 Feb;25(2):737-45.
- Reginster JY. Cardiac concerns associated with strontium ranelate. *Expert Opin Drug Saf.* 2014 SEP;13(9):1209-13.
- Ettinger B. Tibolone for prevention and treatment of postmenopausal osteoporosis. *Maturitas* 2007; 57: 35-38.
- Avisar E, Wasrbrout Z, Lin E, Agashi M. The thumb in agony- osteoarthritis of the thumb. *Harefuah* 2011 Oct;150(10):797-800.
- Stevenson JC. A woman's journey through the reproductive, transitional and postmenopausal periods of life: impact on cardiovascular and musculo-skeletal risk and the role of estrogen replacement. *Maturitas* 2011 Oct:70(2):197-205.
- Chlebowski RT, Cirillo DJ, Eaton CB, Stefanick ML, Pettinger M, Carbone L, Johnson KC, Simon MS, Woods NF, Wactawski-Wende J. Estrogen alone and joint symptoms in the Women's Health Initiative Randomized Trial. *Menopause* 2013;20(6):600-608.
- Cirillo DJ, Wallace RB, Wu L, Yood RA. Effect of hormone therapy on risk of hip and knee joint replacement in the Women's Health Initiative. *Arthritis Rheum* 2006; 54: 3294-3204.
- Tanamas SK, Wijethilake P, Wluka AE, et al. Sex hormones and structural changes in osteoarthritis: a systematic review. *Maturitas* 2011; 69: 141-156.
- Sammaritano LR. Menopause in patients with autoimmune diseases. *Autoimmun Rev.* 2012 May;11(6-7):A430-6.

- Pikwer M, Bergstrom U, Nilsson JA, Jacobsson L, Turesson C. Early menopause is an independent predictor of rheumatoid arthritis. *Ann Rheum Dis.* 2012 Mar; 71(3):378-81.
- Wilson FC, Icen M, Crowson DS, McEvoy MT, Gabriel SE, Kremers HM. Incidence and clinical predictors of psoriatic arthritis in patients with psoriasis: a population-based study. *Arthritis Rheum.* 2009 Feb 15; 61(2): 233-239.
- Nilas L, Christiansen C. Bone mass and its relationship to age and the menopause. *J Clin Endocrinol Metab* 1987 Oct;65(4):697-702.
- Richelson LS, Wahner HW, Melton LJ 3rd, Riggs BL. Relative contributions of aging and estrogen deficiency to postmenopausal bone loss. *N Engl J Med* 1984 Nov 15;311(20): 1273-5.
- Greendale GA, Sowers MF, Han W, et al. Bone mineral density loss in relation to the final menstrual period in a multiethnic cohort: results from the Study of Women's Health Across the Nation (SWAN). *J Bone Miner Res* 2012;27:111-118.
- Pal L, Hailpern SM, Santoro NF, Freeman R, Barad D, Kipersztok S, Barnabei VM, Wassertheil-Smoller S. Association of pelvic organ prolapse and fractures in postmenopausal women: analysis of baseline data from the Women's Health Initiative estrogen plus progestin trial. *Menopause* 2008 Jan-Feb;15(1):59-66.
- Sran MM. Prevalence of urinary incontinence in women with osteoporosis. *J Obstet Gynaecol Can.* 2009 May;31(5):434-9.
- Banks E, Beral V, Reeves G, Balkwill A, Barnes I, for the Million Women Study Collaborators. Fracture incidence in relation to the pattern of use of hormone therapy in postmenopausal women. *JAMA* 2004;291:2212-2220.
- Greising SM, Baltgalvis KA, Lowe DA, Warren GL. Hormone therapy and skeletal muscle strength: a meta-analysis. *J Gerontol A Biol Sci Med Sci* 2009 Oct;64(10):1071-81.
- Karim R, Dell RM, Greene DF, Mack WJ, Gallagher JC, Hodis HN. Hip fracture in postmenopausal women after cessation of hormone therapy: results from a prospective

study in a large health maintenance organization. *Menopause* 2011;18:1172-1177.

- Rossouw JE, Anderson GL, Prentice RL, LaCroix AZ, Kooperberg G, Stefanick ML, Jackson RD, Beresford SA, Howard BV, Johnson KC, Kotchen JM, Ockene J; Writing Group for the Women's Health Initiative Investigators. Risks and benefits of estrogen plus progestins in healthy postmenopausal women: principal results from the Women's Health Initiative randomized controlled trial. *JAMA* 2002 July 17;288(3):321-33.

- Bath PMW, Gra LJ. Association between hormone replacement therapy and subsequent stroke: a meta-analysis. *BMJ* 2005 Feb 12;330(7487):342

- Quigley MET, Martin PL, Burnier AM, Brooks P. Estrogen therapy arrests bone loss in elderly women. *Am J Obstet Gynecol* 1987 Jun; 156(6):1516-23.

- Prestwood KM, Kenny AM, Kleppinger A, Kulldorff M. Ultralow-dose micronized 17beta-estradiol and bone density and bone metabolism in older women: a randomized controlled trial. *JAMA* 2003 Aug 27;290(8):1042-8.

- Villareal DT, Binder EF, Williams DB, Schechtman KB, Yarasheski KE, Kohrt WM. Bone mineral density response to estrogen replacement in frail elderly women: a randomized controlled trial. *JAMA* 2001 Aug 15;286(7):815-20.

- Crandall CJ, Aragaki A, Cauley JA, Manson JE, LeBlanc E, Wallace R, Wactawski-Wende J, LaCroix A, O'Sullivan MJ, Vitolins M, Watts NB. Associations of menopausal vasomotor symptoms with fracture incidence. *J Clin Endocrinol Metab.* 2015 Feb; 100(2): 524-34.

- Naessen T, Lindmark B, Larsen HC. Better postural balance in elderly women receiving estrogens. *Am J Obstet Gynecol.* 1997 Aug; 177(2):412-6.

- Naessen T, Lindmark B, Lagerstrom C, Larsen HC, Persson I. Early postmenopausal hormone therapy improves postural balance. *Menopause.* 2007 Jan-Feb;14(1):14-19.

- Naessen T, Lindmark B, Larsen HC. Hormone therapy and postural balance in elderly women. *Menopause.* 2007 Nov-Dec; 14(6):1020-4.
- De Villiers TJ. 8th Pieter van Keep Memorial Lecture. Estrogen and bone: have we completed a full circle? *Climacteric* 2014 Dec; 17 Suppl 2:4-7.

Chapter 28: LET'S GET CARDIOVASCULAR

- Hodis HN, Mack WJ. A "winow of opportunity:" the reduction of coronary heart disease and total mortality with menopausal therapies is age- and time-dependent. *Brain Res.* 2011 Mar 16; 1379: 244-52.
- Wild RA, Carmina E, Diamanti-Kandarakis E, Dokras A, Escobar-Morreale HF, Futterweit W, Lobo R, Norman RJ, Talbott E, Dumesic DA. Assessment of cardiovascular risk and prevention of cardiovascular disease in women with polycystic ovary syndrome: a consensus statement by the Androgen Excess and Polycystic Ovary Syndrome (AE-PCOS) Society. *J Clin Endocrinol Metab.* 2010 May; 95(5):2038-49.
- Hodis HN, Mack WJ, Azen SP, Lobo RA, Shoupe D, Mahrer PR, Faxon DP, Cashin-Hemphill L, Sanmarco ME, French WJ, Shook TL, Gaarder TD, Mehra AO, Rabbani R, Sevanian A, Shil AB, Torres M, Vogelbach KH, Selzer RH: Women's Estrogen-Progestin Lipid-Lowering Hormone Atherosclerosis Regression Trial Research Group. Hormone therapy and the progression of coronary-artery atherosclerosis in postmenopausal women. *N Engl J Med.* 2003 Aug 7; 349(6):535-45.
- Van der Schouw YT, Grobbee DE. Menopausal complaints, oestrogens, and heart disease risk: an explanation for discrepant findings on the benefits of postmenopausal hormone therapy. *Eur Heart J.* 2005 July;26(14):1358-61.

- Thurston RC, Sutton-Tyrrell K, Everson-Rose SA, Hess R, Powell LH, Matthews KA. Hot flashes and carotid intima media thickness among midlife women. *Menopause* 2011 Apr; 18(4):352-8.
- Huang AJ, Sawaya GF, Vittinghoff E, Lin F, Grady D. Hot flushes, coronary heart disease, and hormone therapy in postmenopausal women. *Menopause* 2009 July-Aug; 16(4):639-43.
- Thurston RC, Sutton-Tyrell K, Everson-Rose SA, Hess R, Matthews KA. Hot flashes and subclinical cardiovascular disease: findings from the Study of Women's Health Across the Nation (SWAN) Heart Study. *Circulation* 2008 Sep 16; 118(12):1234-40.
- Karim R, Mack WJ, Lobo RA, Hwang J, Liu C, Liu C, Sevanian A, Hodis HN. Determinants of the effect of estrogen on the progression of subclinical atherosclerosis: Estrogen in Prevention of Atherosclerosis Trial. *Menopause* 2005 July-Aug;12(4): 366-73.
- Kannel WB. Metabolic risk factors for coronary heart disease in women: perspective from the Framingham Study. *Am Heart J.* 1987 Aug; 114(2):413-9.
- Salpeter SR, Walsh JM, Ormiston TM, Greyber E, Buckley NS, Salpeter EE. Meta-analysis: effect of hormone replacement therapy on components of the metabolic syndrome in postmenopausal women. *Diabetes Obes Metab.* 2006 Sep;8(5):538-54.
- Jensen LB, Vestergaard P, Hermann AP, Gram J, Eiken P, Abrahamsen B, Brot C, Kolthoff N, Sorenson OH, Beck-Nielsen H, Nielsen SP, Mosekilde L. Hormone replacement therapy dissociates fat mass and bone mass, and tends to reduce weight gain in early postmenopausal women: a randomized controlled 5-year clinical trial of the Danish Osteoporosis Prevention Study (DOPS). *J Bone Miner Res.* 2003 Feb;18(2):333-42.
- Sumino H, Ichikawa S, Yoshida A, Murakami M, Kanda T, Mizunuma H, Sakamake T, Kurabayashi M. Effects of hormone replacement therapy on weight, abdominal fat distribution, and lipid

levels in Japanese posmenopausal women. *International Journal of Obesity* 2003;27:1044-1051.

- Issa Z, Seely EW, Rahme M, Fuleihan GE-H. Effects of hormone therapy on blood pressure. *Menopause.* 2015 Apr; 22(4): 456-468.

- Margolis KL, Bonds DE, Rodabough RJ, Tinker L, Phillips LS, Allen C, Bassford T, Burke G, Torrens J, Howard BV; Women's Health Initiative Investigators. Effect of oestrogen plus progestin on the incidence of diabetes in postmenopausal women: results from the Women's Health Initiative Hormone Trial. *Diabetologia.* 2004 July; 47(7):1175-87.

- Bonds DE, Lasser N, Qi L, Brzyski R, Caan B, Heiss G, Limacher MC, Liu JH, Mason E, Oberman A, O'Sullivan MJ, Phillips LS, Prineas RJ, Tinker L. The effect of conjugated equine estrogen on diabetes incidence: the Women's Health Initiative randomized trial. *Diabetologia.* 2006 Mar; 49(3):459-68.

- de Lauzon-Guillain B, Fournier A, Fabre A, Simon N, Mesrine S, Boutron-Ruault MC, Balkau B, Clavel-Chapelon F. Menopausal hormone therapy and new-onset diabetes in the French Etude Epidemiologique de Femmes de la Mutuelle Generale de l'Education Nationale (E3N) cohort. *Diabetologia.* 2009 Oct;52(10):2092-100.

- Macedo AF, Taylor FC, Casas JP, Adler A, Prieto-Merino D, Ebrahim S. Unintended effects of statins from observational studies in the general population: systematic review and meta-analysis. *BMC Med.* 2014 Mar 22;12:51.

- Culver AL, Ockene IS, Balasubramanian R, Olendzki BC, Sepavich DM, Wactawski-Wende J, Manson JE, Qiao Y, Liu S, Merriam PA, Rahilly-Tierny C, Thomas F, Berger JS, Ockene JK, Curb JD, Ma Y. Statin use and risk of diabetes mellitus in postmenopausal women in the Women's Health Initiative. *Arch Intern Med.* 2012 Jan 23;172(2): 144-52.

- Ridker PM, Cook NR, Lee IM, Gordon D, Gaziano JM, Manson JE, Hennekens CH, Buring JE. A randomized trial of low-dose aspirin in the primary prevention of cardiovascular disease in women. *N Engl J Med.* 2005 Mar 31; 352(13): 1293-304.

- Harris RE, Chlebowski RT, Jackson RD, Frid DJ, Ascenseo JL, Anderson G, Loar A, Rodabough RJ, White E, and McTiernan A. Breast cancer and nonsteroidal anti-inflammatory drugs: prospective results from the Women's Health Initiative. *Cancer Research* 2003 Sep 15; 63; 6096-6101.
- Mendelsohn ME. Protective effects of estrogen on the cardiovascular system. *Am J Cardiol.* 2002 Jun 20;89(12A):12E-17E; discussion 17E-18E.
- The Writing Group for the PEPI Trial. Effects of estrogen or estrogen/progestin regimens on heart disease risk factors in postmenopausal women. The Postmenopausal Estrogen/Progestin Interventions (PEPI) Trial. [Erratum in *JAMA* 1995 DEC 6; 274(21): 1676] *JAMA* 1995 Jan 18; 273(3):199-208.
- Hulley S, Grady D, Bush T, Furberg C, Herrington D, Riggs B, Vittinghoff E. Randomized trial of estrogen plus progestin for secondary prevention of coronary heart disease in postmenopausal women. Heart and Estrogen/progestin Replacement Study (HERS) Research Group. *JAMA* 1998 Aug 19; 280(7);605.13.
- Grady D, Herrington D, Bittner V, Blumenthal R, Davidson M, Hlatky M, et al. Cardiovascular disease outcomes during 6.8 years of hormone therapy: Heart and Estrogen/progestin Replacement Study follow-up (HERS-II). HERS Research Group [published erratum appears in *JAMA* 2002;288:1064]. *JAMA* 2002;288:49-57.
- Manson JE. Postmenopausal hormone therapy and atherosclerotic disease. *Am Heart J.* 1994 Dec; 128(6 Pt 2):1337-43.
- Stampfer MJ, Colditz GA, Willett WC, Manson JE, Rosner B, Speizer FE, Hennekens CH. Postmenopausal estrogen therapy and cardiovascular disease. Ten-year follow-up from Nurses' Health Study. *N Engl J Med.* 1991 Sep 12; 325(11):756-62.
- Rossouw JE, Anderson GL, Prentice RL, LaCroix AZ, Kooperberg C, Stefanick ML, et al. Risks and benefits of estrogen plus

progestin in healthy postmenopausal women: principal results from the Women's Health Initiative randomized controlled trial. Writing Group for the Women's Health Initiative Investigators. *JAMA* 2002 Jul 17; 288(3):321-33.

- Manson JE, Hsia J, Johnson KC, Rossouw JE, Assaf AR, Lasser NL, et al. Estrogen plus progestin and the risk of coronary heart disease. Women's Health Initiative Investigators. *N Engl J Med* 2003;349:523-34.

- Rossouw JE, Prentice RL, Manson JE, Wu L, Barad D, Barnabei VM, et al. Postmenopausal hormone therapy and risk of cardiovascular disease by age and years since menopause [published erratum appears in *JAMA* 2008;299:1426]. *JAMA* 2007;297:1465-77.

- Manson JE, Allison MA, Rossouw JE, Carr JJ, Langer RD, Hia J, et al. Estrogen therapy and coronary-artery calcification. WHI and Women's Health Initiative Coronary Artery Calcium Study (WHI-CACS) Investigators. *N Engl J Med* 2007 Jun 21; 356(25):2591-602.

- Barrett-Connor, E, Laughlin GA. Hormone therapy and coronary artery calcification in asymptomatic postmenopausal women: the Rancho Bernardo Study. *Menopause.* 2005 Jan-Feb;12(1):40-48.

- Grodstein F, Manson JE, Stampfer MJ. Hormone therapy and coronary heart disease: the role of time since menopause and age at hormone initiation. *J Womens Health (Larchmt).* 2006 Jan-Feb;15(1):35-44

- Harman SM, Black DM, Naftolin F, Brinton EA, Budoff MJ, Cedars MI, Hopkins PN, Lobo RA, Manson JE, Merriam GR, Miller VM, Neal-Perry G, Santoro N, Taylor HS, Vittinghoff E, Yan M, Hodis HN. Arterial imaging outcomes and cardiovascular risk factors in recently menopausal women: a randomized trial. (Kronos Early Estrogen Prevention Study-KEEPS) *Ann Intern Med.* 2014 Aug 19; 161(4):249-260.

- Hodis HN, Mack WJ, Shoupe D, Azen ST, Stanczyk FZ, Hwang-Levine J, Budoff MJ, Henderson VW. Testing the Menopausal Hormone Therapy Timing Hypothesis: The Early versus Late Intervention Trial with Estradiol (ELITE). *Circulation* 2014; 130: A13283.

- Hodis HN, Mack WJ, Soupe D, Azen ST, Stanczyk FZ, Hwang-Levine J, Budoff MJ, Henderson VW. Methods and baseline cardiovascular data from the Early versus Late Intervention Trial with Estradiol (ELITE) testing the menopausal hormone timing hypothesis. *Menopause* 2015 Apr; 22(4): 391-401.

- Schierbeck LL, Rejnmark L, Tofteng CL, Stilgren L, Eiken P, Mosekilde L, Kober L, Jensen JE. Effect of hormone replacement therapy on cardiovascular events in recently postmenopausal women: randomized trial. *BMJ* 2012 Oct 9; 345:e6409.

- Tuomikoski P, Lyytinen H, Korhonen P, et al. Coronary heart disease mortality and hormone therapy before and after the Women's Health Initiative. *Obstet Gynecol.* 2014; 124(5):947-953.

- Boardman HMP, Hartley L, Eisinga A, Main C, Figuls MR, Cosp XB, Sanchez RG, Knight B. Hormone therapy for preventing cardiovascular disease in post-menopausal women. Cochrane Database of Sytematic Reviews. Published on line 10 Mar 2015. doi:10.1002/14651858.CD002229.pub4

- Henderson VW, Lobo RA. Hormone therapy and the risk of stroke: perspectives 10 years after the Women's Health Initiative trials. *Climacteric* 2012 Jun;15(3):229-34.

- Rodker PM, Cook NR, I-Min L, Gordon, D, Gaziano M, Manson JE, Hennekens CH and Buring JE. A randomized trial of low-dose aspirin in the primary prevention of cardiovascular disease in women. (Women's Health Study). *N Engl J Med* 2005 Mar 31;352:1293-1304.

- Hendrix SL, Wassartheil-Smoller S, Johnson KC, et al. Effects of conjugated equine estrogen on stroke in the Women's Health Initiative. *Circulation* 2006 May 23; 113(20):2425-34.

- Wassertheil-Smoller S, Hendrix SL, Limacher M, et al. Effect of estrogen plus progestin on stroke in postmenopausal women: the Women's Health Initiative: a randomized trial. *JAMA* 2003 May 23; 289(20):2673-84.
- Smith NL, Blondon M, Wiggins KL, Harrington LB, van Hylckama Vlieg A, Floyd JS, Hwang M, Bis JC, McKnight B, Rice KM, Lumley T, Rosendaal FR, Heckbert SR, Psaty BM. Lower risk of cardiovascular events in postmenopausal women taking oral estradiol compared with oral conjugated equine estrogens. *JAMA Intern Med.* 2014 Jan;174(1):25-31.
- Lindsay R, Gallagher JC, Kleerekoper M, Pickar JH. Effect of lower doses of conjugated equine estrogens with and without medroxyprogesterone acetate on bone in early postmenopausal women. *JAMA* 2002 May 22-29; 287(20):2668-76.
- Simon JA. What's new in hormone replacement therapy: focus on transdermal estradiol and micronized progesterone. *Climacteric* 2012 April;15(S1):3-10.
- Mueck AO. Postmenopausal hormone replacement therapy and cardiovascular disease: the value of transdermal estradiol and micronized progesterone. *Climacteric* 2012 April; 15(S1): 11-17.
- L'Hermite M. HRT optimization, using transdermal estradiol plus micronized progesterone, a safer HRT. *Climacteric* 2013 Aug;16(S1):44-53.
- Renoux C, Dell'aniello S, Garbe E, Suissa S. Transdermal and oral hormone replacement therapy and the risk of stroke: a nested case-control study. *BMJ* 2010 Jun 3; 340:c2519.
- Shufelt CL, Merz CN, Prentice RL, et al. Hormone therapy dose, formulation, route of delivery, and risk of cardiovascular events in women: findings from the Women's Health Initiative Observational Study. *Menopause.* 2014; 21(3): 260-266.
- Boardman HMP, Hartley L, Eisinga A, Main C, Roque I Figuls M, Bonfill Cosp X, Gabriel Sanchez R, Knight B. Hormone therapy for preventing cardiovascular disease in both healthy

postmenopausal women and postmenopausal women with preexisting cardiovascular disease. *Cochrane Database Syst. Rev.* 2015 March 10 [doi:10.1002/14651858. CD002229.pub4].

Chapter 29: A WOMAN'S BRAIN – the FINAL FRONTIER

- Rasgon NL, Geist CL, Kenna HA, Wroolie TE, Williams KE, Silverman DH. Prospective randomized trial to assess effects of continuing hormone therapy on cerebral function in postmenopausal women at risk for dementia. *PLoS One.* 2014 Mar 12; (9)3: e89095.
- Pike CJ, Carroll JC, Rosario ER, Barron AM. Protective actions of sex steroid hormones in Alzheimer's disease. *Front Neuroendocrinol.* 2009 Jul; 30(2):239-58.
- Craig MC, Murphy DG. Estrogen: effects on normal brain function and neuropsychiatric disorders. *Climacteric.* 2007 Oct 10 Suppl 2: 97-104.
- Naessen T, Lindmark B, Lagerstrom C, Larsen HC, Persson I. Early postmenopausal hormone therapy improves postural balance. *Menopause.* 2007 Jan-Feb; 14(1): 14-9.
- Naessen T, Lindmark B, Larsen HC. Hormone therapy and postural balance in elderly women. *Menopause.* 2007 Nov-Dec; 14(6):1020-4.
- Nathan L, Chaudhur G. Estrogens and atherosclerosis. *Annual Review of Pharmacology and Toxicology.* 1997 Apr; 37: 477-515.
- Erickson KI, Colcombe SJ, Raz N, Korol DL, Scalf P, Webb A, Cohen NJ, McAuley E, Kramer AF. Selective sparing of brain tissue in postmenopausal women receiving hormone replacement therapy. *Neurobiol Aging.* 2005 Aug-Sep; 26(8): 1205-13.
- Alonso de Lecinana M, Egido JA. Estrogens as neuroprotectants against ischemic stroke. *Cerebrovasc Dis.* 2006; 21 Suppl 2: 48-53. Epub 2006 May 2.
- Markou A, Duka T, Prelevic GM. Estrogens and brain function. *Hormones (Athens).* 2005 Jan-Mar; 4(1):9-17.

- Bove R, Secor E, Chibnik LB, Barnes LL, Schneider JA, Bennett DA, De Jager PL. Age at surgical menopause influences cognitive decline and Alzheimer pathology in older women. *Neurology.* 2014 Jan 21; 82(3):222-9.

- Crivello F, Tzourio-Mazoyer N, Tzourio C, Mazoyer B. Longitudinal assessment of global and regional rate of grey matter atrophy in 1, 172 healthy older adults: modulation by sex and age. *PLoS One.* 2014 Dec 3; 9(12): e114478.

- Abbassi-Ghanavati M, Greer LG, Cunningham FG. Pregnancy and laboratory studies: a reference table of clinicians. *Obstet Gynecol.* 2009 Dec; 114(6): 1326-31.

- Sichel DA, Cohen LS, Robertson LM, Ruttenberg A, Rosenbaum JF. Prophylactic estrogen in recurrent postpartum affective disorder. *Biol Psychiatry.* 1995 Dec 15; 38(12):814-8.

- Ahokas A, Kaukoranta J, Wahlbeck K, Aito M. Estrogen deficiency in severe postpartum depression: successful treatment with sublingual physiologic 17beta-estradiol: a preliminary study. *J Clin Psychiatry.* 2001 May; 62(5):332-6.

- Kumar C, McIvor RJ, Davies T, Brown N, Papadopoulos A, Wieck A, Checkley SA, Campbell IC, Marks MN. Estrogen administration does not reduce the rate of recurrence of affective psychosis after childbirth. *J Clin Psychiatry.* 2003 Feb; 64(2): 112-8.

- Sit D, Rothschild AJ, Wisner KL. A review of postpartum psychosis. *J Womens Health (Larchmt).* 2006 May; 15(4): 352-368.

- Ahokas A, Aito M, Rimon R. Positive treatment effect of estradiol in postpartum psychosis: a pilot study. *J Clin Psychiatry.* 2000 Mar; 61(3): 166-9.

- Rocca WA, Bower JH, Maraganore DM, Ahlskog JE, Grossardt BR, de Andrade M, Melton LJ 3rd. Increased risk of parkinsonism in women who underwent oophorectomy before menopause. *Neurology.* 2008 Jan 15; 70(3): 200-9.

- Goveas JS, Hogan PE, Kotchen JM, Smoller JW, Denburg NL, Manson JE, Tummala A, Mysiw WJ, Ockene JK, Woods NF,

Espeland MA, Wassartheil-Smoller S. Depressive symptoms, antidepressant use, and future cognitive health in postmenopausal women: the Women's Health Initiative Memory Study. *Int Psychogeriatr.* 2012 Aug; 24(8): 1252-64.

- Goveas JS, Espeland MA, Hogan PE, Tindle HA, Shih RA, Kotchen JM, Robinson JG, Barnes DE, Resnick SM. Depressive symptoms and longitudinal changes in cognition: Women's Health Initiative Study of Cognitive Aging. (WHISCA). *J Geriatr Psychiatry Neurol.* 2014 Feb 28; 27(2): 94-102.

- Smoller JW, Allison M, Cochrane BB, Curb JD, Perlis RH, Robinson JG, Rosal MC, Wenger
NK, Wassertheil-Smoller S. Antidepressant use and risk of incident cardiovascular morbidity and mortality among postmenopausal women in the Women's Health Initiative Study. (WHI). *Arch Intern Med.* 2009 Dec; 169(22): 2128-2139.

- Richards JB, Papaioannou A, Adachi JD, Joseph L, Whitson HE, Prior JC, Goltzman D, Canadian Osteoporosis Study Research Group. Effect of selective serotonin reuptake inhibitors on the risk of fracture. *Arch Intern Med.* 2007 Jan 22; 167(2): 188-94.

- Dieleman ZG, van der Cammen TJ, Hofman A, Pols HA, Stricker BH. Selective serotonin reuptake inhibiting antidepressants are associated with an increased risk of nonvertebral fractures. *J Clin Psychopharmacol.* 2008 Aug; 28(4): 411-7.

- Kawas C, Resnick S, Morrison A, Brookmeyer R, Corrada M, Zonderman A, Bacal C, Lingle DD, Metter E. A prospective study of estrogen replacement therapy and the risk of developing Alzheimer's disease: the Baltimore Longitudinal Study of Aging. (BLSA). *Neurology.* 1997 Jun; 48(6): 1517-21.

- Shao H, Breitner JCS, Whitmer RA, Wang J, Hayden K, Wengreen H, Corcoran C, Tschanz J, Norton M, Munger R, Welsh-Bohmer K, Zandi PP; Cache County Memory Study County Investigators. Hormone therapy and Alzheimer disease dementia. *Neurology.* 2012 Oct 30; 79(18): 1846-1852.

- Zandi PP, Carlson MC, Plassman BL, Welsh-Bohmer KA, Mayer LS, Steffens DC, Breitner JC; Cache County Memory Study Investigators. Hormone replacement therapy and incidence of Alzheimer disease in older women: the Cache County Study. *JAMA.* 2002 Nov 6; 288(17): 2123-9.
- Paganini-Hill A, Henderson VW. Estrogen deficiency and risk of Alzheimer's disease in women. (Leisure World Cohort). *American Journal of Epidemiology.* 1994; 140: 256-61.
- Shumaker SA, Legault C, Rapp SR, Thal L, Wallace RB, Ockene JK, Hendrix SL, Jones BN 3rd , Assaf AR, Jackson RD, Kotchen JM, Wassertheil-Smoller S, Wactawski-Wende J; WHIMS Investigators. Estrogen plus progestin and the incidence of dementia and mild cognitive impairment in postmenopausal women: the Women's Health Initiative Memory Study: a randomized controlled trial. (WHIMS). *JAMA.* 2003 May 28; 289(20): 2651-62.
- Resnick SM, Espeland MA, Jaramillo SA, Hirsch C, Stefanick ML, Murray AM, Ockene J, Davatzikos C. Postmenopausal hormone therapy and regional brain volumes: the WHIMS-MRI Study. *Neurology.* 2009 Jan 13; 72(2): 135-42.
- Colker LH, Hogan PE, Bryan NR< Kuller LH, Margolis KL, Bettermann K, Wallace RB, Lao Z, Freeman R, Stefanick ML, Shumaker SA. Postmenopausal hormone therapy and subclinical cerebrovascular disease: the WHIMS-MRI Study. *Neurology.* 2009 Jan 13; 72(2): 125-34.
- Erickson KI, Colcombe SJ, Raz N, Korol DL, Scalf P, Webb A, Cohen NJ, McAuley E, Kramer AF. Selective sparing of brain tissue in postmenopausal women receiving hormone replacement therapy. *Neurobiol Aging.* 2005 Aug-Sep; 26(8): 1205-13.
- Ghidone R, Boccardi M, Benussi L, Testa C, Villa A, Pievani M, Gigola L, Sabattoli F, Barbiero L, Frisoni GB, Binetti G. Effects of estrogens on cognition and brain morphology: involvement of the cerebellum. *Maturitas.* 2006 Jun 20; 54(3): 222-8.

- Lord C, Buss C, Lupien SJ Pruessner JC. Hippocampal volumes are larger in postmenopausal women using estrogen therapy compared to past users, never users and men: a possible window of opportunity effect. *Neurobiol Aging.* 2008 Jan; 29(1): 95-101.
- Espeland MA, Shumaker SA, Leng I, Manson JE, Brown CM, LeBlanc ES, Vaughan L, Robinson J, Rapp SR, Goveas JS, Wactawski-Wende J, Stefanick ML, Li W, Resnick SM; WHIMSY Study Group. Long-term effects on cognitive function of postmenopausal hormone therapy prescribed to women aged 50 to 55 years. *JAMA Intern Med.* 2013 Aug 12; 173(15): 1429-36.
- Asthana S, Gleason CE, Wharton W, et al. The Kronos Early Estrogen Prevention Study (KEEPS): results of the cognitive and affective study. In: *Abstracts of the North American Society 23rd Annual Meeting;* October 3-6, 2012; Orlando, FL.
- Hodis HN, Mack WJ, Shoupe D, Azen SP, Stanczyk FZ, Hwang-Levine J, Budoff MJ, Henderson VW. Testing the menopause hormone therapy timing hypothesis: the Early versus Late Intervention Trial with Estradiol (ELITE). *Circulation.* 2014 Nov; 130: A13283.
- Zandi PP, Anthony JC, Hayden KM, Mehta K, Mayer L, Breitner JC; Cache County -Study Investigators. Reduced incidence of AD with NSAID but not H2 receptor antagonists: the Cache County Study. *Neurology.* 2002 Sep 24; 59(6): 880-6.

Chapter 30: BLOOD CLOTS

- Rossouw JE, Anderson GL, Prentice RL, et al; Writing Group for the Women's Health Initiative Investigators. Risks and benefits of estrogen plus progestin in healthy postmenopausal women: principal results from the Women's Health Initiative randomized controlled trial. *JAMA.* 2002 July 17; 288: 321-33.
- Anderson GL, Limacher M, Assaf AR, et al; Women's Health Initiative Steering Committee. Effects of conjugated equine estrogen in postmenopausal women with hysterectomy: the Women's

Health Initiative randomized controlled trial. *JAMA*. 2004 Apr 14; 291(14): 1701-12.

- Cushman M, Kuller LH, Prentice R, Rodabough RJ, Psaty BM, Stafford RS, Sidney S, Rosendaal FR; Women's Health Initiative Investigators. Estrogen plus progestin and risk of venous thrombosis. *JAMA*. 2004 Oct 6; 292(13): 1573-80.

- Curb JD, Prentice RL, Bray PF, Langer RD, Van Horn L, Barnabei VM, Block MJ, Cyr MG, Gass M, Lepine L, Rodabough RJ, Sidney S, Uwaifo GI, Rosendaal FR. Venous thrombosis and conjugated equine estrogen in women without a uterus. *Arch Intern Med*. 2006 Apr 10; 166(7): 772-80.

- Prentice RL, Manson JE, Langer RD, Anderson GL, Pettinger M, Jackson RD, Johnson KC, Kuller LH, Lane DS, Wactawski-Wende J, Brzyski R, Allison M, Ockene J, Sarto G, Rossouw JE. Benefits and risks of postmenopausal hormone therapy when it is initiated soon after menopause. *Am J Epidemiol*. 2009 Jul 1; 170(1): 12-23.

- Di Minno MN, Tufano A, Ageno W, Prandoni P, Di Minno G. Identifying high-risk individuals for cardiovascular disease: similarities between venous and arterial thrombosis in perspective. A 2011 update. *Intern Emerg Med*. 2012 Feb; 7(1): 9-13.

- Canonico M, Oger E, Plu-Bureau G, Conard J, Meyer G, Levesque H, Trillot N, Barrellier M-T, Wahl D, Emmerich J, Scarabin P-Y; Estrogen and Thromboembolism Risk (ESTHER) Study Group. Hormone therapy and venous thromboembolism among postmenopausal women: Impact of route of estrogen administration and progestogens: the ESTHER study. *Circulation*. 2007 Feb 20; 115(7): 840-5.

- Canonico M, Plu-Bureau Genevieve, Lowe GD, Scarabin P-Y. Hormone replacement therapy and risk of venous thromboembolism in postmenopausal women: systematic review and meta-analysis. *BMJ*. 2008 May 31; 336(7655): 1227-31.

- Peragallo Urrutia R, Coeytaux RR, McBroom AJ, Gierisch JM, Havrilesky LJ, Moorman PG, Lowery WJ, Dinan M, Hasselblad

V, Sanders GD, Myers ER. Risk of acute thromboembolic events with oral contraceptive use: a systematic review and meta-analysis. *Obstet Gynecol* 2013 Aug;122(2 Pt 1):308-9.

- Galson, Steven K. Prevention of deep vein thrombosis and pulmonary embolism. *Public Health Rep.* 2008 July-Aug;123(4):420-21.

- Deitelzweig SB, Johnson BH, Lin J, Schulman KL. Prevalence of clinical venous thromboembolism in the USA: current trends and future projections. *Am J Hematol.* 2011 Feb;86(2):217-20

- Freeman AL, Pendleton RC, Rondina MT. Prevention of venous thromboembolism in obesity. *Expert Rev Cardiovas Ther.* 2010 Dec;8(12):1711-21.

- Laliberte F, Dea K, Duh MS, Kahler K, Rolli M, Lefebvre P. Does the route of administration for estrogen hormone therapy impact the risk of venous thromboembolism? Estradiol transdermal system versus oral estrogen-only hormone therapy. *Menopause.* 2011 Oct; 18(10):1052-9.

- American College of Obstetricians and Gynecologists (ACOG). ACOG committee opinion no. 556: Postmenopausal estrogen therapy: route of administration and risk of venous thromboembolism. *Obstet Gynecol.* 2013 Apr; 121(4): 887-90.

- Canonico M. Hormone therapy and hemostasis among postmenopausal women: a review. *Menopause.* 2014 Jul; 21(7): 753-62.

- Pulmonary Embolism Prevention (PEP) Trial Collaborative Group. Prevention of pulmonary embolism and deep vein thrombosis with low dose aspirin: Pulmonary
Embolism Prevent (PEP) trial. *Lancet.* 2000 Apr 15; 355(9212): 1295-302.

- Li L, Zhang P, Tian JH, Yang K. Statins for primary prevention of venous thromboembolism. *Cochrane Database Syst Rev.* 2014 Dec 18; 12: CD008203.

- Herrington DM, Vittinghoff E, Lin F, Fong J, Harris F, Hunninghake D, Bittner V, Schrott HG, Blumenthal RS, Levy R; HERS Study Group. Statin therapy, cardiovascular events, and total mortality in the Heart and Estrogen/Progestin Replacement Study (HERS). *Circulation.* 2002 Jun 25; 105(25): 2962-7.

- Berglind IA, Andersen M, Citarella A, Linder M, Sundstrom A, Kieler H. Hormone therapy and risk of cardiovascular outcomes and mortality in women treated with statins. *Menopause.* 2015 Apr; 22(4): 369-76.

- Hodis H, Mack W. Hormone therapy and risk of all-cause mortality in women treated with statins. *Menopause.* 2015 Apr; 22(4): 363-364.

Chapter 31: MENOPAUSE HORMONE THERAPY – TYPE, TIME, and TIMING

- The Writing Group for the PEPI Trial. Effects of estrogen or estrogen/progestin regimens on heart disease risk factors in postmenopausal women. The Postmenopausal Estrogen/Progestin Interventions (PEPI) Trial. *JAMA* 1995 Jan 18;273(3):199-208. (Erratum in *JAMA* 1995 Dec 6;274(21):1676)

- Grodstein F, Manson JE, Colditz GA, Willett WC, Speizer FE, Stampfer MJ. A prospective, observational study of postmenopausal hormone therapy and primary prevention of cardiovascular disease. *Ann Intern Med* 2000 Dec 19;133(12):933-41.

- Hulley S, Grady D, Bush T, Furberg C, Herrington D, Riggs B, Vittinghoff E. Randomized trial of estrogen plus progestin for secondary prevention of coronary heart disease in postmenopausal women. Heart and Estrogen/progestin Replacement Study (HERS) Research Group. *JAMA* 1998 Aug 19;280(7):605-13.

- Grady D, Herrington D, Bittner V Blumenthal R, Davidson M, Hlatky M, Hsia J, Hulley S, Herd A, Khan S, Newby LK, Waters D, Vittinghoff E, Wenger N; HERS Research Group. Cardiovascular disease outcomes during 6.8 years of hormone therapy: Heart and Estrogen/progestin Replacement Study follow-up (HERS II). *JAMA* 2002 Jul 3; 288(1):49-57.

- Grodstein F, Manson JE, Stampfer MJ. Postmenopausal hormone use and secondary prevention of coronary events in the nurses' health study; a prospective, observational study. *Ann Intern Med.* 2001 July 3; 135(1):1-8.

- Rossouw JE, Anderson GL, Prentice RL, LaCroix AZ, Kooperberg C, Stefanick ML, Jackson RD, Beresford SA, Howard BV, Johnson KC, Kotchen JM, Ockene J; Writing Group for the Women's Health Initiative Investigators. Risks and benefits of estrogen plus progestin in health postmenopausal women: principal results from the Women's Health Initiative randomized controlled trial. *JAMA* 2002 Jul 17; 288(3): 321-33.

- Anderson GL, Limacher M, Assaf AR, Bassford T, Beresford SA, Black H, Bonds D, Brunner R, Brzyski R, Caan B, Chlebowski R, Curb D, Gass M, Hays J, Heiss G, Hendrix S, Howard BV, Hsia J, Hubbell A, Jackson R, Johnson KC, Judd H, Kotchen JM, Kuller L, LaCroix AZ, Lane D, Langer RD, Lasser N, Lewis CE, Manson JE, Margolis K, Ockene J, O'Sullivan MJ, Phillips L, Prentice RL, Ritenbaugh C, Robbins J, Rossouw JE, Sarto G, Stefanick ML, Van Horn L, Wactawski-Wende J, Wallace R, Wassertheil-Smoller S; Women's Health Initiative Steering Committee. Effects of conjugated equine estrogen in postmenopausal women with hysterectomy: the Women's Health Initiative randomized controlled trial. *JAMA* 2004 Apr 14;291(14):1701-12.

- Rossouw JE, Prentice RL, Manson JE, Wu L, Barad D, Barnabei VM, Ko M, LaCroix AZ, Margolis KL, Stefanick ML. Postmenopausal hormone therapy and risk of cardiovascular disease by age and years since menopause. *JAMA* 2007 Apr 4; 297(13);1465-77.

- Manson JE, Allison ME, Rossouw JE, Carr JJ, Langer RD, Hsia J, Kuller LH, Cochrane BB, Hunt JR, Ludlam SE, Pettinger MB, Gass M, Margolis KL, Nathan L, Ockene JK, Prentice RL, Robbins J, Stefanick ML; WHI and WHI-CACS Investigators. Estrogen therapy and coronary-artery calcification. *N Engl J Med.* 2007 Jun 21; 356(25):2591-602.

- Hsia J, Langer RD, Manson JE, Kuller L, Johnson KC, Hendrix SL, Pettinger M, Heckbert SR, Greep N, Crawford S, Eaton CB, Kostis JB, Caralis P, Prentice R; Women's Health Initiative Investigators. Conjugated equine estrogens and coronary heart disease: the Women's Health Initiative. *Arch Intern Med.* 2006 Feb 13; 166(3):357-65.
- Stevenson JC, Hodis HN, Pickar JH, Lobo RA. Coronary heart disease and menopause management: the swinging pendulum of HRT. *Atherosclerosis* 2009 Dec;207(2):336-40.
- Manson JE, Chlebowski RT, Stefanick ML, Aragaki AK, Rossouw JE, Prentice RL, Anderson G, Howard BV, Thomson CA, LaCroix AZ, Wactawski-Wende J, Jackson RD, Limacher M, Margolis KL, Wassertheil-Smoller S, Beresford SA, Cauley JA, Eaton CB, Gass M, Hsia J, Johnson KC, Kooperberg C, Kuller LH, Lewis CE, Liu S, Martin LW, Ockene JK, O'Sullivan MJ, Powell LH, Simon MS, Van Horn L, Vitolins MZ, Wallace RB. Menopausal hormone therapy and health outcomes during the intervention and extended poststopping phases of the Women's Health Initiative randomized trials. *JAMA* 2013 Oct 2; 310 (13) 1353-68.
- Schierbeck LL, Rejnmark L, Tofteng CL, Stilgren L, Eiken P, Mosekilde L, Kober L, Jensen JEB. Effect of hormone replacement therapy on cardiovascular events in recently postmenopausal women: randomized trial. (DOPS) *BMJ* 2012; 345:e6490.
- Hodis HN, Mack WJ, Shoupe D, Azen SP, Stanczyk FZ, Hwang-Levine J, Budoff MJ, Henderson VW. Testing the Menopausal Hormone Therapy Timing Hypothesis: The Early versus Late Intervention Trial with Estradiol (ELITE). *Circulation* 2014 Nov; 130: A13283.
- Harman SM, Black DM, Naftolin F, Brinton EA, Budoff MJ, Cedars MI, Hopkins PN, Lobo RA, Manson JE, Merriam GR, Miller VM, Neal-Perry G, Santoro N, Taylor HS, Vittinghoff E, Yan M, Hodis HN. Arterial imaging outcomes and cardiovascular risk factors in

recently menopausal women: a randomized trial. (KEEPS). *Ann Intern Med.* 2014; 161(4):249-260.

- Hodis HN, Mack WJ, Soupe D, Azen ST, Stanczyk FZ, Hwang-Levine J, Budoff MJ, Henderson VW. Methods and baseline cardiovascular data from the Early versus Late Intervention Trial with Estradiol testing the menopausal hormone timing hypothesis. *Menopause* 2015 Apr; 22(4): 391-401.

- Haring B, Leng X, Robinson J, Johnson KC, Jackson RD, Beyth R, Wactawski-Wende J, von Ballmoos MW, Goveas JS, Kuller LH, Wassertheil-Smoller S. Cardiovascular disease and cognitive decline in postmenopausal women: results from the Women's Health Initiative Memory Study. (WHIMS) *J Am Heart Assoc.* 2013 Dec 18; 2(6):e000369.

- Maki PM, Henderson VW. Hormone therapy, dementia, and cognition: the Women's Health Initiative 10 years on. *Climacteric.* 2012 Jun; 15(3):256-62.

- Espeland MA, Shumaker SA. Leng I, Manson JE, Brown CM, LeBlanc ES, Vaughan L, Robinson J, Rapp SR, Goveas JS, Wactawski-Wende J, Stefanick ML, Li W, Resnick SM; Women's Health Initiative Memory Study of Younger Women (WHIMSY) Study Group.
Long-term effects on cognitive function of postmenopausal hormone therapy prescribed to women aged 50 to 55 years. *JAMA Intern Med.* 2013 Aug 12; 173(15):1429-36.

- Zandi PP, Carlson MC, Plassman BL, Welsh-Bohmer KA, Mayer LS, Steffens DC, Breitner JC, Cache County Memory Study Investigators. Hormone replacement therapy and incidence of Azlheimer disease in older women: the Cache County Study. *JAMA.* 2002 Nov 6; 288 (17): 2123-9.

- Rapp SR, Espeland MA, Shumaker SA, Henderson VW, Brunner RL, Manson JE, Gass ML, Stefanick ML, Lane DS, Hays J, Johnson KC, Coker LH, Dailey M, Bowen D; WHIMS Investigators. Effect of estrogen and progestin on global cognitive function in postmenopausal women: the Women's Health Initiative Memory Study (WHIMS): a randomized controlled trial. *JAMA.* 2003 May 28; 289(20):2663-72.

-   Shumaker SA, Legault C, Rapp SR, Thal L, Wallace RB, Ockene JK, Hendrix SL, Jones BN 3rd, Assaf AR, Jackson RD, Kotchen JM, Wassartheil-Smoller S, Wactawski-Wende J: WHIMS Investigators. Estrogen plus progestin and the incidence of dementia and mild cognitive impairment in postmenopausal women: the Women's Health Initiative Memory Study (WHIMS): a randomized controlled trial. *JAMA.* 2003 May 28; 289(20); 2651-62.

-   Shumaker SA, Legault C, Kuller L, Rapp SR, Tal L, Lane DS, Fillit H, Stefanick ML, Hendrix SL, Lewis CE, Masaki K, Coker LH; WHIMS Investigators. Conjugated equine estrogens and incidence of probable dementia and mild cognitive impairment in postmenopausal women: Women's Health Initiative Memory Study (WHIMS). *JAMA.* 2004 Jun 23;291(24): 2947-58.

-   Espeland MA, Rapp SR, Shumaker SA, Brunner R, Manson JE, Sherwin BB, Hsia J, Margolis KL, Hogan PE, Wallace R, Dailey M, Freeman R, Hays J; WHIMS Investigators. Conjugated equine estrogens and global cognitive function in postmenopausal women: Women's Health Initiative Memory Study (WHIMS). *JAMA.* 2004 Jun 23;291 (24): 2959-68.

-   Million Women Study Collaborators. Patterns of use of hormone replacement therapy in one million women in Britain, 1996-2000. *BJOG* 2002 Dec; 109(12):1319-30.

-   Hodis HN, Mack WJ. Hormone replacement therapy and the association with coronary heart disease and overall mortality: clinical application of the timing hypothesis. *J Steroid Biochem Mol Biol.* 2014 July; 142:68-75.

-   Goveas JS, Espeland MA, Hogan PE, Tindle HA, Shih RA, Kotchen JM, Robinson JG, Barnes DE, Resnick SM. Depressive symptoms and longitudinal changes in cognition: Women's Health Initiative

Study of Cognitive Aging (WHISCA). *J Geriatr Psychiatry Neurol.* 2014 Feb 28; 27(2):94-102.

- Shao H, Breitner JC, Whitmer RA, Wang J, Hayden K, Wengreen H, Corcoran C, Tschanz J, Norton M, Munger R, Welsh-Bohmer K, Zandi PP; Cache County Investigators. Hormone Therapy and Alzheimer disease dementia: new findings from the Cache County Study. *Neurology.* 2012 Oct 30; 79(18):1846-52.

- Whitmer RA, Quesenberry CP, Zhou J, Yaffe K. Timing of hormone therapy and dementia: the critical window theory revisited. *Ann Neurol.* 2011 Jan;69(1):163-9.

- Rapp SR, Espeland MA, Manson JE, Resnick SM, Bryan NR, Smoller S, Coker LH, Phillips LS, Stefanick ML, Sarto GE; Women's Health Initiative Memory Study (WHIMS). Educational attainment, MRI changes, and cognitive function in older postmenopausal women from the Women's Health Initiative Memory Study. *Int J Psychiatry Med.* 2013; 46(2):121-43.

- O'Brien J, Jackson JW, Grodstein F, Blacker D, Weuve J. Postmenopausal hormone therapy is not associated with risk of all-cause dementia and Alzheimer's disease. *Epidemiol Rev.* 2014;36(1):83-103.

- Chen WY, Manson JE, Hankinson SE, Rosner B, Holmes MD, Willett WC, Colditz GA. Unopposed estrogen therapy and the risk of invasive breast cancer. [Nurses' Health Study] *Arch Intern Med.* 2006; 166(9): 1027-1032.

- Welton AJ, Vickers MR, Kim J, Ford D, Lawton BA, MacLennan AH, Meredith SK, Martin J, Meade TW; WISDOM study team. Health related quality of life after combined hormone replacement therapy: randomized controlled trial. *BMJ.* 2008 Aug 21; 337: a1190.

- Shufelt CL, Merz CN, Prentice RL, Pettinger MB, Rossouw JE, Aroda VR, Kaunitz AM, Lakshminarayan K, Martin LW, Phillips LS, Manson JE. Hormone therapy dose, formulation, route of delivery, and risk of cardiovascular events in women: findings from the

Women's Health Initiative Observational Study. *Menopause.* 2014 Mar; 21(3):260-6.

- Hendrix SL, Wassartheil-Smoller S, Johnson KC, Howard BV, Kooperberg C, Rossouw JE, Trevisan M, Aragaki A, Baird AE, Bray PF, Buring JE, Criqui MH, Herrington D, Lynch JK, Rapp SR, Torner J; WHI Investigators. Effects of conjugated equine estrogen on stroke in the Women's Health Initiative. *Circulation.* 2006 May 23; 113(20):2425-34.

- Smith NL, Blondon M, Wiggins KL, Harrington LB, van Hylckama Vlieg A, Floyd JS, Hwang M, Bis JC, McKnight B, Rice KM, Lumley T, Rosendaal FR, Heckbert SR, Psaty BM. Lower risk of cardiovascular events in postmenopausal women taking oral estradiol compared with oral conjugated equine estrogens. *JAMA Intern Med.* 2014 Jan; 174(1):25-31.

- Novensa L, Selent J, Pastor M, Sandberg K, Heras M, Dantas AP. Equine estrogens impair nitric oxide production and endothelial nitric oxide synthase transcription in human endothelial cells compared with the natural 17beta-estradiol. *Hypertension.* 2010 Sep; 56(3):405-11.

- Cordina-Duverger E, Truong T, Anger A, Sanchez M, Arveux P, Kerbrat P, Guenel P. Risk of breast cancer by type of menopausal hormone therapy: a case-control study among postmenopausal women in France. *PLoS One.* 2013 Nov 1; 8(11):e78016.

- Fournier A, Berrino F, Riboli E, Avenel V, Clavel-Chapelon F. Breast cancer risk in relation to different types of hormone replacement therapy in the E3N-EPIC cohort. *Int J Cancer.* 2005 Apr 10; 114(3):448-54.

- Fournier A, Berrino F, Clavel-Chapelon F. Unequal risks for breast cancer associated with different hormone replacement tharpies: results from the E3N cohort study. *Breast Cancer Res Treat.* 2008 Jan; 107(1): 103-111.

- Rosano GM, Webb CM, Chierchia S, Morgani GL, Gabraele M, Sarrel PM, de Ziegler D, Collins P. Natural progesterone, but not medroxyprogesterone acetate, enhances the beneficial effect of estrogen on exercise-induced myocardial ischemia in postmenopausal women. *Am Coll Cardiol.* 2000 Dec; 36(7):2154-9.

- Ryan N, Rosner A. Quality of life and costs associated with micronized progesterone and medroxyprogesterone acetate in hormone replacement for non-hysterectomized, postmenopausal women. *Clin Ther.* 2001;23:1099-1115.

- Montplaisir J, Lorrain J, Denesle R, Petit D. Sleep in menopause: differential effects of two forms of hormone replacement therapy. *Menopause.* 2001;8:10-16.

- Goodman MP. Are all estrogens created equal? A review of oral vs. transdermal therapy. *J Womens Health (Larchmt).* 2012 Feb;21(2):161-9.

- Sanada M, Tsuda M, Kodama I, Sakashita T, Nakagawa H, Ohama K. Substitution of transdermal estradiol during oral estrogen-progestin therapy in postmenopausal women: effects on hypertriglyceridemia. *Menopause.* 2004 May-Jun;11(3):331-6.

- Racine A, Bijon A, Fournier A, Mesrine S, Clavel-Chapelon F, Carbonnel F, Boutron-Ruault MC. Menopausal hormone therapy and risk of cholecystectomy: a prospective study based on the French E3N cohort. *CMAJ.* 2013 Apr 16; 185(7):555-61.

- Canonico M, Oger E, Plu-Bureau G, Conard J, Meyer G, Levesque H, Trillot N, Barrellier MT, Wahl D, Emmerich J, Scarabin PY. Estrogen and Thromboembolism Risk (ESTHER) Study Group. *Circulation.* 2007 Feb 20; 115(7):840-5.

- Renoux C, Dell-aniello S, Garbe E, Suissa S. Transdermal and oral hormone replacement therapy and the risk of stroke: a nested case-control study. *BMJ* 2010 Jun 3;340:c2519.

- Speroff L. Transdermal hormone therapy and the risk of stroke and venous thrombosis. *Climacteric.* 2010 Oct; 13(5):429-32.

- LaCroix AZ, Chlebowski RT, Manson JE, Aragaki AK, Johnson KC, Martin L, Margolis KL, Stefanick ML, Brzyski R, Curb JD, Howard BV, Lewis CE, Wactawski-Wende J; WHI Investigators.

Conjugated equine oestrogen and breat cancer incidence and mortality in postmenopausal women with hysterectomy: extended follow-up of the Women's Health Initiative radomized placebo-controlled trial. *JAMA.* 2011 Apr 6; 305(13):1305-14.

- Chlebowski RT, Anderson GL, Gass M, Lane DS, Aragaki AK, Kuller LH, Manson JE, Stefanick ML, Ockene J, Sarto GE, Johnson KC, Wactawski-Wende J, Ravdin PM, Schenken R, Hendrix SL, Rajkovic A, Rohan TE, Yasmeen S, Prentice RL; WHI Investigators. Estrogen plus progestin and breast cancer incidence and mortality in postmenopausal women. *JAMA.* 2010 Oct 20;304(15):1684-92.

- Chlebowski RT, Manson JE, Anderson GL, Cauley JA, Aragaki AK, Stefanick ML, Lane DS, Johnson KC, Wactawski-Wende J, Chen C, Qi L, Yasmeen S, Newcomb PA, Prentice RL. Estrogen plus progestin and breast cancer incidence and mortality in the Women's Health Initiative Observational Study. *J Natl Cancer Inst.* 2013 Apr 17; 105(8):526-35.

- Shapiro S, DeVilliers TJ, Pines A, Sturdee DW, Archer DF, Baber RJ, Panay N, Farmer RDT, Stevenson JC, Mueck AO, Burger HG, Gompel A. RE: Estrogen plus progestin and breast cancer incidence and mortality in the Women's Health Initiative Observational Study. *J Natl Cancer Inst* 2014; 106 (2): djt372.

- Newcomy PA, Egan KM, Trentham-Dietz A, Titus-Ernstoff L, Baron JA, Hampton JM, Stampfer MJ and Willett WC. Prediagnostic use of hormone therapy and mortality after breast cancer. *Cancer Epidemiol Biomarkers Prev* 2008 Apr 17; 864

- Sweetland S, Beral V, Balkwill A, Liu B, Benson VS, Canonico M, Green J, Reeves GK; Million Women Study Collaborators. Venous thromboembolism risk in relation to use of different types of postmenopausal hormone therapy in a large prospective study. *J Thromb Haemost.* 2012 Nov; 19(11):2277-86.

- Doherty JA, Cushing-Haugen KL, Saltzman BS, Voight LF, Hill DA, Beresford SA, Chen C, Weiss NS. Long-term use of postmenopausal estrogen and progestin hormone therapies and the risk of endometrial cancer. *Am J Obstet Gynecol* 2007 Aug; 197(2):139.e1-7.

- Somboonporn W, Panna S, Temtanakitpaisan T, Kaewrudee S, Soontrapa S. Effects of the levonorgestrel-releasing intrauterine system plus estrogen therapy in perimenopausal and postmenopausal women: systematic review and meta-analysis. *Menopause.* 2011 Oct; 18(10): 1060-6.

- Parker WH, Broder MS, Chang E, Feskanich D, Farquhar C, Liu Z, Shoupe D, Berek JS, Hankinson S, Manson JE. Ovarian conservation at the time of hysterectomy and long-term health outcomes in the Nurse's Health Study. *Obstet Gynecol.* 2009 May; 113(5): 1027-37.

- Rivera CM, Grossardt BR, Rhodes DJ, Brown RD Jr, Rober VL, Melton LJ 3rd, Rocca WA.
Increased cardiovascular mortality after early bilateral oophorectomy. *Menopause.* 2009
Jan-Feb; 16(1): 15-23.

- Rivera CM, Grossardt BR, Rhodes DJ, Rocca WA. Increased mortality for neurological and mental diseases following early bilateral oophorectomy. *Neuroepidemiology.* 2009; 33(1): 32-40.

- Rocca WA, Bower JH, Maraganore DM, Ahlskog JE, Grossardt BR, de Andrade M, Melton LJ 3rd. Increased risk of parkinsonism in women who underwent oophorectomy before menopause. *Neurology.* 2008 Jan 15; 70(3):200-9.

- Lobo RA, Davis SR, De Villiers TJ, Gompel A, Henderwon VW, Hodis HN, Lumsden MA, Mack WJ, Shapiro S, Baber RJ. Prevention of diseases after menopause. *Climacteric.* 2014 Oct; 17(5): 540-56.

- Gurney EP, Nachtigall MJ, Nachtigall LE, Naftolin F. The Women's Health Initiative trial and related studies: 10 years later: a clinician's view. *J Steroid Biochem Mol Biol.* 2014 Jul; 142: 4-11.

- L'Hermite M. Hormone replacement therapy (HRT) optimization, using transdermal estradiol plus micronized progesterone, a safer HRT. *Climacteric.* 2013 Aug; 16(S1): 44-53.
- Simon JA. What's new in hormone replacement therapy: focus on transdermal estradiol and micronized progesterone. *Climacteric.* 2012 Apr; 15(S1): 3-10.
- Mueck AO. Postmenopausal hormone replacement therapy and cardiovascular disease: the value of transdermal estradiol and micronized progesterone. *Climacteric.* 2012 Apr; 15(S1): 11-17.
- Sarrel PM, Njike VY, Vinante V, Katz DL. The mortality toll of estrogen avoidance: an analysis of excess deaths among hysterectomized women aged 50 to 59 years. *Am J Public Health.* 2013 Sep; 103(9): 1583-8.
- Boardman HMP, Hartley L, Eisinga A, Main C, Roque I Figuls M, Bonfill Cosp X, Gabriel Sanchez R, Knight B. Hormone therapy for preventing cardiovascular disease in both healthy postmenopausal women and postmenopausal women with preexisting cardiovascular disease. *Cochrane Database Syst. Rev.* 2015 March 10 [doi:10.1002/14651858. CD002229.pub4].

Chapter 32: GERIPAUSE COCKTAIL

- Hodis HN, Mack WJ. Postmenopausal hormone therapy in clinical perspective. *Menopause* 2007; 14:944-957.
- Rossouw JE, Anderson GL, Prentice RL, et al. Risks and benefits of estrogen plus progestin in healthy postmenopausal women: principal results from the Women's Health Initiative randomized control trial. *JAMA* 2002;288:321-333.
- Coker LH, Espeland MA, Rapp SR, Legault C, Resnick SM, Hogan P, Gaussoin S, Dailey M, Shumaker SA. Postmenopausal hormone therapy and cognitive outcomes: the Women's Health Initiative Memory Study (WHIMS). *J Steroid Biochem Mol Biol* 2010 Feb 28;118(4-5):304-10.

- Resnick SM, Coker LH, Maki PM, Rapp SR, Espeland MA, Shumaker SA. The Women's Health Initiative Study of Cognitive Aging (WHISCA): a randomized clinical trial of the effects of hormone therapy on age-associated decline. *Clin Trials* 2004; 1(5):440-50.
- Canonico M, Oger E, Plu-Bureau G; Estrogen and Thromboembolism Risk (ESTHER) Study Group. Hormone therapy and venous thromboembolism among postmenopausal women: impact of the route of estrogen administration and progestogens: the ESTHER study. *Circulation* 2007;115:840-845.
- LeCroix AZ, Chlebowski RT, Manson JE, Aragaki AK, Johnson KC, Martin L, Margolis KL, Stefanick ML, Brzyski R, Curb JD, Howard BV, Lewis CE, Wactawski-Wende J; WHI Investigators. Health outcomes after stopping conjugated equine estrogens among postmenopausal women with prior hysterectomy: a randomized controlled trial. *JAMA* 2011 Apr 6;305(13):1305-14.
- Fournier A, Berrino F, Clavel-Chapelon F. Unequal risks for breast cancer associated with different hormone replacement therapies: results from the E3N cohort study. *Breast Cancer Res Treat* 2008 Jan;107(1):103-111.
- Mosca L, Benjamin EJ, Berra K, et al. Effectiveness-based guidelines for the prevention of cardiovascular disease in women – 2011 update: a guideline from the American Heart Association. *J Am Coll Cardiol* 2011;57:1404-1423.
- Marcucci R, Cioni G, Giusti B, Fatini C, Rossi L, Pazzi M, Abbate R. Gender and anti-thrombotic therapy: from biology to clinical implications. *J Cardiovasc Transl Res* 2014 Feb;7(1):72-81.
- Speroff L. Transdermal hormone therapy and the risk of stroke and venous thrombosis. *Climacteric* 2010 Oct;13(5):429-32.
- Mueck AO. Postmenopausal hormone replacement therapy and cardiovascular disease: the value of transdermal estradiol and micronized progesterone. *Climacteric* 2012 Apr;15 Suppl 1:11-7.

- Henderson VW, Logo RA. Hormone therapy and the risk of stroke: perspectives 10 years after the Women's Health Initiative trials. *Climacteric* 2012 Jun;15(3):229-34.
- L'Hermite M. HRT optimization, using transdermal estradiol plus micronized progesterone, a safer HRT. *Climacteric* 2013 Aug;16 Suppl 1:44-53.
- Shufelt CL, Merz CN, Prentice RL, Pettinger MB, Rossouw JE, Aroda VR, Kaunitz AM, Lakshminarayan K, Martin LW, Phillips LS, Manson JE. Hormone therapy dose, formulation, route of delivery, and risk of cardiovascular events in women: findings from the Women's Health Initiative Observational Study. *Menopause* 2014 Mar;21(3):260-6.
- Noyes AM, Thompson PD. A systematic review of the time course of atherosclerotic plaque regression. *Atherosclerosis* 2014 May;234(1):75-84.
- Espeland MA, Applegate W, Furgerg CD, Lefkowitz D, Rice L, Hunninghake D, the ACAPS Investigators. Estrogen replacement therapy and progression of intimal-medial thickness in the carotid arteries of postmenopausal women. *Am J Epidemiol* 1995;142:1011.
- Akkad A, Hartshorne T, Bell PRF, Al-Azzawi F. Carotid plaque regression on oestrogen replacement: a pilot study. *Eur J Vasc Endovasc Surg* 1996;11:347.
- Clarkson TB. Estrogen effects on arteries vary with stage of reproductive life and extent of subclinical atherosclerosis progression. *Menopause* 2007 May-Jun; 14 (3 Pt 1):373-84.
- Berglind IA, Andersen M, Citarella A, Linder M, Sundstrom A, Kieler H. Hormone therapy and risk of cardiovascular outcomes and mortality in women treated with statins. *Menopause.* 2015 Apr; 22(4): 369-376.
- Buhling KJ, von Studnitz FS, Jantke A, Eulenberg C, Mueck AO. Use of hormone therapy by female gynecologists and female partners of male gynecologists in Germany 8 years after the Women's

Health Initiative study: results of a survey. *Menopause* 2012; 19: 1088-1091.

- Pederson AT, Iversen OE, Lukkegaard E, et al. Impact of recent studies on attitudes and use of hormone therapy among Scandinavian gynecologists. *Acta Obstet Gynecol Scand 2007;86:*1490-1495.
- Biglia N, Ujcic E, Kubatzki F, et al. Personal use of hormone therapy by postmenopausal women doctors and male doctors' wives in Italy after the publication of WHI trial. *Maturitas* 2006;54:181-192.

Chapter 33: TANTALIZING TELOMERES

- Sikora E, Bielak-Zmijewska A, Mosieniak G. Cellular senescence in aging, age-related disease and longevity. *Curr Vasc Pharmacol.* 2014;12(5):698-706.
- Boccardi V, Paolisso G. Telomerase activation: a potential key modulator for human healthspan and longevity. *Ageing Res Rev* 2014 May;15:1-5.
- Fyhrquist F, Saijonmae O. Telomere length and cardiovascular aging. *Ann Med.* 2012 Jun;44 Suppl 1:S138-42.
- Leung CW, Laraia BA, Needham BL, Rehkopf DH, Adler NE, Lin J, Blackburn EH, Epel ES. Soda and cell aging: associations between sugar-sweetened beverage consumption and leukocyte telomere length in healthy adults from the national health and nutrition examination surveys. *Am J Public Health* 2014 Dec;104(2):2425-31.
- Crous-Bou M, Fung TT, Prescott J, Julin B, Du M, Sun Q, Rexrode KM, Hu FB, De Vivo I. Mediterranean diet and telomere length in Nurses' Health Study: population-based cohort study. *BMJ* 2014 Dec 2;349:g6674.
- Du M, Prescott J, Kraft P, Han J, Giovannucci E, Hankinson SE, De Vivo I. Physical activity, sedentary behavior, and leukocyte telomere length in women. *Am J Epidemiol* 2012 Mar 1;175(5):414-22.

- Epel ES, Blackburn EH, Lin J, Dhabhar FS, Adler NE, Morrow JD, Cawthon RM. Accelerated telomere shortening in response to life stress. *Proc Natl Acad Sci.* 2004;101:17312-17315.
- Vina J, Borras C, Gambini J, Sastre J, Pallardo FV. Why females live longer than males: control of longevity by sex hormones. *Sci Aging Knowledge Environ.* 2005 Jun 8;23 pe17.
- Borras C, Gambini J, Vina J. Mitochondrial oxidant generation is involved in determining why females live longer than males. *Front Biosci* 2007 Jan 1;12:1008-13.
- Kalpouzos G, Rizzuto D, Keller L, Fastborn J, Santoni G, Angleman S, Graff C, Backman L, Fratiglioni L. Telomerase Gene (hTERT) and Survival: Results from two Swedish Cohorts of Older Adults. *J Gerontol A Biol Sci Med Sci* 2014 Nov 30;pii: glu222.
- Cha Y, Kwon SJ, Seol W, Park KS. Estrogen receptor-alpha mediates the effects of estradiol on telomerase activity in human mesenchymal stem cells. *Mol Cells* 2008 Nov 30;26(5):454-8.
- Lee DC, IM JA, Kim JH, Lee HR, Shim JY. Effect of Long-Term Hormone Therapy on Telomere Length in Postmenopausal Women. *Yonsei Medical Journal* 2005 Aug 31; 46(4): 471-479.
- Lin J, Kroenke CH, Epel E, Kenna HA, Wolkowitz OM, Blackburn E, Rasgon NL. Greater endogenous estrogen exposure is associated with longer telomeres in postmenopausal women at risk for cognitive decline. *Brain Res.* 2011 Mar 16;1379:224-31.